Save the Babies

The Henry E. Sigerist Series in the History of Medicine

Sponsored by The American Association for the History
of Medicine
and The Johns Hopkins University Press

The Development of American Physiology:
Scientific Medicine in the Nineteenth Century, by W. Bruce Fye

Save the Babies: American Public Health Reform and the Prevention of Infant Mortality,
1850–1929, by Richard A. Meckel

Politics and Public Health in Revolutionary Russia, 1890–1918, by John F. Hutchinson

Save the Babies

American Public Health Reform and the Prevention of Infant Mortality 1850–1929

Richard A. Meckel

THE JOHNS HOPKINS UNIVERSITY PRESS
Baltimore and London

Brought to publication with the generous assistance of a grant from the American
Association for the History of Medicine

The Johns Hopkins University Press
701 West 40th Street, Baltimore, Maryland 21211
The Johns Hopkins Press Ltd., London

The paper used in this publication meets
the minimum requirements of American National Standard
for Information Sciences—Permanence of Paper
for Printed Library Materials, ANSI Z39.48–1984.

Library of Congress Cataloging-in-Publication Data

Meckel, Richard A., 1948–
Save the babies : American public health reform and
the prevention of infant mortality, 1850–1929 / Richard
M. Meckel.
    p.   cm.—(The Henry E. Sigerist series in the
history of medicine)
Bibliography: p.
Includes index.
ISBN 0-8018-3879-7 (alk. paper)
1. Infants—Death—United States—Prevention—
History.   2. Infant health services—United States—
History.   3. Maternal health services—United States—
History.   I. Title.   II. Series.
RJ102.M43 1990
362.1′9892′01097309034—dc20   89-15389   CIP

To Joseph G. Meckel

Contents

Tables

Acknowledgments

The research and writing of this book, as with most, was primarily a solitary endeavor. However, it was not done entirely alone, and I would like to use this opportunity to thank those who assisted me along the way.

My research could not have been done without the kind help of the staffs of the Rockefeller and Science Libraries at Brown University, the Francis A. Countway Library of Medicine, the New York Academy of Medicine Library, the Boston Public Library, and the New York Public Library. Nor could my revisions have been done without the helpful comments of those who read all or part of the manuscript. Among these were Mari Jo Buhle, James Cassedy, Howard Chudacoff, Judith Walzer Leavitt, James Patterson, Morris Vogel, and Maris Vinovskis. I would also like to thank Henry Y. K. Tom and the editorial staff at the Johns Hopkins University Press for the unfailing courtesy and professionalism they displayed in dealing with me and the manuscript.

Most of all, however, I would like to thank my family. I owe an incalculable debt to my wife, Mary Paula Hunter, for her close reading, critical comments, and unflagging faith in me. I also owe an incalculable debt to my daughter, Katherine and son, Peter, whose births and infancies during the preparation of this book reminded me daily just how great was the personal and social tragedy I was writing about. Finally, I would like to thank my father, Joseph G. Meckel, to whom this book is dedicated. In bequeathing me his passion for reading and learning, he gave me a most precious legacy.

Introduction

Of all the health revolutions that have taken place in the United States since 1850, the reduction of infant mortality is arguably the most dramatic and far-reaching. Because of the incompleteness and unreliability of surviving vital records, we will probably never know precisely the rate of infant death a century ago. But an informed estimate would be that somewhere between 15 and 20 percent of all American infants born in the second half of the nineteenth century died before they could celebrate their first birthdays.[1] It also seems probable that in some large cities and industrial towns, as well as in certain areas of the South, the rates were considerably higher, ranging upward to 30 percent.[2] In sharp contrast, only 1 percent of all American infants born today die under the age of one.[3]

What do these percentages mean in actual deaths? A few simple comparisons provide some illustration. From July 1, 1987, to June 30, 1988, 38,300 of the 3,855,000 infants born in the United States died. If the infant mortality rate had been 15 percent rather than 1.0 percent, well over half a million would have died. More specifically, in 1985, of the 81,780 infants born in Massachusetts, 743 died in their first year. One hundred years earlier, in 1885, less than 60 percent as many babies were born but more than ten times as many died. Similarly, in 1985, New York City, with one of the nation's highest urban infant mortality rates, was the scene of 1,670 infant deaths. Yet if the infant mortality rate in 1985 had been what it was in the city one hundred years earlier, 28,266 infants would have died.[4] In sheer numbers, then, and in the concentration of those numbers in a single year of the life cycle, no other modern reduction of mortality—not that accomplished among older children and adults by the virtual eradication of tuberculosis, nor that effected by the diminution of venereal disease, nor even that which followed the serologic control of epidemic infectious diseases—comes near comparing with the reduction of infant mortality.[5]

Behind this profound health revolution lay several causal developments. Prior to the 1930s, declining fertility and better nutrition and housing, accompanying a rising standard of living, played important roles in reducing infant mortality. So too did the environmental improvements, particularly in urban areas, brought about by state and municipal construction of water supply and sewage systems and the implementation of effective refuse removal. Also crucial was the work of public health officials and their allies in social work and medicine in controlling milk-borne diseases and in educating the public in the basics of preventive infant and maternal hygiene.[6] After 1930, further declines in fertility and family size along with economic, environmental, nutritional, and educational improvements continued to drive infant mortality rates downward. But unlike in the earlier period, they were substantially assisted by increases in the quality and availability of medical care.[7] Indeed, in the last half century, medical advances have played a critical role in reducing infant mortality. The perfection of effective fluid and electrolyte therapy, the development of pediatric hematology, the discovery and use of antibiotics to control infectious and parasitic diseases and, most recently, the design and implementation of surgical, therapeutic, and intensive care techniques to correct congenital deformities and to counter the risks faced by low birthweight or premature babies: all have significantly lessened the risk of death faced by the nation's infants.[8]

Compared to that accomplished by many other nations, however, America's success in saving her infants pales somewhat. Although having one of the world's highest standards of living and possessing one of the most technologically advanced health care systems, the United States continues to have one of the highest infant mortality rates among developed nations. Indeed, twenty-one countries currently have lower infant mortality rates.[9] Moreover, although only 1 percent of all babies born nationwide die in infancy, the rate is considerably higher in certain inner cities and among specific racial minorities. In 1986, for instance, infant mortality in central Harlem was over two-and-a-half times the national rate. And nationwide, black infants continue to die almost twice as often as do white babies.[10] Especially since the late 1950s, the comparative excess of U.S. infant mortality rates, as well as the strikingly higher rates among poor blacks, have generated considerable debate among American health professionals, social welfare advocates, and government policy makers over the efficacy of the way that the United States combats mortality among its youngest citizens.

While the evidence is anything but clear and the issues complex and not easily disentangled, the debate revolves around certain questions initially raised 130 years ago when infant mortality was first defined as a significant public health problem demanding remedial action. These questions involve the relative importance of poverty, race, and personal behavior in determining rates of infant mortality and the ways in which government can and

should intervene to reduce those rates.[11] Critics of current American policy
and programs argue that the United States has failed to reduce infant mortality adequately and evenly because, unlike those countries with lower
rates, it has not seen fit to adopt comprehensive national health and maternal support systems. In particular, critics charge that the United States has
chosen to fight infant mortality in the comparatively narrow way it has
chosen to fight most health problems: by channeling the majority of appropriated public funds into medical education, health facility construction,
and the development of advanced medical technologies, and by urging the
public to avail themselves of quality medical care and advice. Such an
approach, it is argued, while representing a critical component of any strategy to reduce infant mortality, is both incomplete and costly. Organized
around the provision of expensive medical care to correct problems once
they occur, it gives short shrift to comparatively inexpensive preventive
programs designed to assist women to carry, bear, and raise healthy infants.
Indeed, historically, maternal assistance programs have been not only relatively meager in the United States but also politically vulnerable. Much of
the most heated debate on American infant mortality during the last decade,
for instance, has revolved around federal cuts in what many infant welfare
advocates regard as already inadequate "bare-bones health, nutrition,
childcare and family support programs."[12]

Critics also maintain that aside from being both costly and less effective
than a comprehensive one, the U.S. approach to combating infant mortality
is made problematic by unequal access to health care. Observing that access
to health care is essentially tied to access to health insurance, they contend
that American infant mortality is comparatively high in part because the
United States does not have universal health insurance. Rather, it has a
three-tiered system: employer- or individual-provided private insurance for
those who are well off or have good jobs; government-provided insurance
(Medicaid) for those in poverty who qualify; and no or inadequate insurance for millions of others. Even if medical care could alone combat infant
mortality, critics thus assert, many Americans would not have access to it.

Defenders of American infant and maternal health policy, while conceding that some problems and inequities exist, have generally argued that the
observed higher rate of infant mortality in the United States is not the
consequence of existing medical and social services being inadequate, but
rather the result of unique sociocultural conditions combined with dysfunc-
tional behavior among high-risk groups (currently, teenage pregnancy and
drug addiction among those minorities with high infant mortality rates).
Additionally, they have suggested that such groups, whether through ignorance or obduracy, fail to take full advantage of existing medical and social
services. Indeed, because infant mortality in the United States is highest
among minorities, and particularly among black Americans, both defenders

and critics of the U.S. policy frequently discuss infant mortality, not as a generalized American problem, but as one specific to minorities and especially to blacks.[13]

I do not intend the following study as a definitive evaluation of the specific arguments of either side of this on-going debate, although it will be manifestly clear where my sympathies lie. Though related, my intent is somewhat different. First, I hope to lend the debate a historical dimension, specifically by providing an analysis of that period in public health and social welfare history—roughly from 1850 to 1929—when Americans first engaged in an intensive discourse on infant mortality and, in so doing, not only raised many of the questions debated today, but also outlined an approach to infant and maternal welfare that is still apparent in contemporary policies and programs. Most of the attention thus far paid to the history of maternal and infant health policies in the United States has focused on the last half-century, and particularly on the period since the 1960s when the discovery that the United States was lagging ever farther behind other developed nations in combating infant death prompted a renewed effort to save America's babies.[14] And, in many respects, that focus is justified. For current policies and programs owe much of their specific shape and organization to developments in social welfare, medical care delivery, and health insurance that have occurred since then.[15]

Yet, if current maternal and infant health programs are the specific products of the New Deal and following eras, their essential approach to the problem of infant mortality is the product of a discourse on infant mortality that took place in the late nineteenth and early twentieth centuries. Indeed, the maternity and infancy provisions of the 1935 Social Security Act— which along with their various amendments continue to provide the legislative basis for American infant and maternal health programs—owe much of their shape and orientation to a formula for combating infant mortality developed during the first decades of the century. So, too, the orientation of medical care designed to prevent infant deaths, as well as many of the problems and inequities attending the delivery of that care, have their roots in turn-of-the-century developments in the organization of American medicine and health care. Finally, most of the fundamental issues being debated today in regard to infant mortality—its relationship to poverty, race, and ethnicity, the extent to which it is a behavioral as well as a socioeconomic problem, the scope of government responsibility to combat it, and the breadth or comprehensiveness of required corrective measures—were all initially raised when Americans first confronted infant mortality as a social problem in the late nineteenth and early twentieth centuries. It is my hope, then, that an analysis of the initial American discourse on infant mortality may shed some light on the fundamental issues, questions, and sociomedical arrangements that continue to inform American debate on infant welfare.

Second, and more importantly, I intend this study to illumine a central but still largely unexamined part of the late nineteenth- and early twentieth-century public health movement, both because it is a historically significant phenomenon in and of itself and because it offers insight into several questions of interest to historians of reform, and particulary of public health reform.[16] Infant mortality was central to the development of American public health policy for a number of reasons. Perhaps most important, it came to be regarded as a particulary sensitive index of community health and well-being and of the effectiveness of existing public health measures. It also came to be seen and employed as an emotionally and politically powerful issue strategically useful in securing government funding for related health and social assistance measures. Consequently, it preoccupied late nineteenth- and early twentieth-century public health reformers in a way that many other forms of mortality did not.

Concern over infant mortality developed almost contemporaneously with the appearance of sanitary reform as the first phase of the essentially urban public health movement that emerged in America in the second half of the nineteenth century. Mapping out variances in mortality in order to determine the relative impact of environmental conditions on health and to prompt government action to counter morbific influences, sanitarians soon turned to the infant death rate as a more sensitive and politically useful measure than the crude death rate. In so doing, they revealed and publicized the extent of infant mortality (especially in cities), helped transform a demographic condition into a social problem, and made its reduction a measure of the degree to which their sanitary programs were succeeding.

Discovered and defined in the mid-nineteenth century as a problem in need of amelioration, infant mortality prompted a reform effort to reduce it that stretched over approximately eight decades and evolved through three overlapping and cumulative, but recognizably discrete, conceptual and strategic stages. In the first stage, lasting roughly from 1850 through 1880, the conception of the problem embraced and the remedial strategy adopted emphasized general environmental reform. Convinced that infants died in such great numbers because of hereditary debility and direct exposure to morbific influences, public health reformers sought to reduce infant mortality by improving general health through sanitizing the environment. The second stage, beginning around 1880 and stretching through the second decade of the century, witnessed a narrowing of reform focus, from the conditions in which infants lived to the condition of that which they were fed. Prompted by frustration over their inability to reduce infant mortality through general environmental reform, made aware from collected vital statistics that the greatest proportion of infant deaths were from digestive and nutritional disorders, and influenced by developments within both pediatrics and the emerging science of bacteriology, public health reformers

reconceptualized infant mortality and refocused their attention on improving the quality and purity of the urban milk supply and on making clean and
wholesome milk available to those infants at highest risk. The third stage,
beginning near the end of the first decade of this century and lasting until the
end of the third, witnessed yet another reconceptualization of infant mortality and the adoption of another strategy to combat it. Increasingly questioning the efficacy of narrowly focusing on milk reform and prompted by
new sociomedical research and by a concurrent reorientation in public
health and social welfare work, infant health reformers defined infant mortality as a problem of motherhood and turned their attention to improving
mothers' abilities to carry, bear, and rear healthy infants. By far generating
the most publicity and reform activity, this final stage in the campaign to
reduce infant mortality witnessed a number of critical developments within
public health, social welfare, and medicine that continue to impact on
American infant and maternal health policy.

Linking all three stages was an informing conviction that was itself historically constructed: that infant mortality was by far highest among the poor,
and particularly among the urban immigrant poor. As a consequence, at
issue in the late nineteenth- and early twentieth-century discourse on infant
mortality was the causal relationship between poverty, ethnicity, and infant
death. Infant welfare was thus structured by a number of related and fundamental questions. To what extent was infant mortality the consequence of
the privations and environmental conditions of poverty; and to what extent
was it the result of ignorance, obdurance, and unhygienic behavior among
the poor? Were all impoverished infants equally at risk; or was risk scaled
according to the customs and physiological characteristics of various racial
and ethnic groups?[17] Would infant mortality most effectively be reduced
through programs of social assistance and environmental reform; or would it
respond best to parental education? Did the reduction of infant mortality
require the eradication of all the physical conditions attending poverty; or
could the influence of those conditions be offset by narrow and specific
health measures?

Americans were not the only ones debating these questions. Nor were the
answers they arrived at solely their own. Like a number of other reform
movements of the time, the infant welfare movement was international.
Both reformers and reform ideas readily criss-crossed national boundaries.
So, too, did medical and statistical findings. American infant welfare activists borrowed heavily from the ideas and data published by their counterparts in other countries and shared with them a number of basic assumptions
concerning the nature and causes of infant mortality. Yet the American
discourse on infant mortality was different in a number of critical structural
and ideological respects. From the beginning, both the propositions put forth
and the participants involved ranged along a narrower political spectrum

than they did in the other developed nations pursuing infant welfare. More-over, the American discourse took place largely outside the arena of institu-tional political power and was more decentralized and never as truly nation-al as elsewhere. It also tended to focus on narrower solutions, and to promote the adoption of a comparatively narrower approach to assisting mothers.[18] And finally, it gave as much or more attention to race and eth-nicity as it did to socioeconomic class.

Chapter One examines the construction of the conviction that infant mortality was a problem of the urban poor, and particularly the urban immigrant poor. Focusing on the first stage of the campaign to improve infant survival, it explores how and why infant mortality was discovered and defined as a social problem, and places that discovery and definition within the context of an emerging urban sanitary reform movement. It also looks at the impact that English sanitary reform and the publishing of vital statistics had on the way that Americans came to conceptualize and ap-proach infant mortality. Chapter Two examines the development of pedi-atrics as a medical specialty in America and explores the ways in which developments in the science of nutrition, as well as the professional needs and orientation of the new specialists, helped shift attention from the en-vironment to infant care and feeding. Chapter Three looks at urban milk reform, exploring the political, institutional, and scientific obstacles that such reform faced and speculating on its effectiveness. It also examines the various strategies proposed, describing the development of infant milk sta-tions and the debate that surrounded pasteurization and certified milk. Chapter Four details the reconceptualization of infant mortality as a prob-lem of motherhood and the international emergence of voluntary associa-tions dedicated to publicizing the problem of infant mortality, researching its causes, and promoting its reduction. In particular, it focuses on the founding and work of the American Association for Study and Prevention of Infant Mortality.

Chapter Five examines the maternal reform campaign that occupied a central position in the nation's effort to combat infant mortality during the second decade of the century. Chapter Six illumines the discovery of neona-tal mortality and the broadening of infant welfare to include prenatal care and instruction for pregnant women. Chapter Seven explores the renewed interest in poverty as a factor in infant mortality following publication of the U.S. Children's Bureau's studies on the causes and rates of infant death in specific American communities. It also examines the debate over and rejection of maternity insurance, arguing that it represented a critical junc-ture in the development of American infant welfare policy. The eighth and last chapter looks at the rise and fall of the Sheppard-Towner Act, the seminal but relatively conservative federal welfare measure establishing the formula that American maternal and infant health programs have essentially followed ever since. The epilogue traces the development of American infant and maternal health policy from the repeal of Sheppard-Towner to the present. An overview, its primary intent is to explore the legacy left by the late nineteenth- and early twentieth-century reform movement. It is meant, and should be read, as a provocative postscript rather than a detailed analysis.

Like all public health reform campaigns or even general reform movements, that which was aimed at reducing infant mortality confronts the scholar who would recount and analyze its genesis and evolution with a number of difficult methodological questions. The first and perhaps most problematic of these is how to conceptualize and talk about the campaign or movement as a singular, recognizable, and distinct form of collective activity without artificially homogenizing it or separating it from the contexts in which it appeared and developed. This is essentially a definitional problem and a particularly challenging one, since the scholarly literature on reform and reform movements, though voluminous, is anything but conceptually uniform and consistent.[19] As the author of a recent overview of American reform observed: "The first thing that one notices in approaching the subject of reform is that everyone uses the term differently."[20]

I have chosen to conceptualize, describe, and analyze the American infant welfare movement as a discourse. Some clarification is necessary here, however, because discourse may be the most overused and vague term in the current scholarly lexicon. By discourse, I mean something straightforward and specific: a public discussion that is neither independent of nor strictly determined by the sociocultural and political setting in which it takes place, and that is primarily among but not limited to a definable community of activists who agree that a certain condition represents a problem, share a general conception of its nature, are committed to its remedy, and are actively engaged, through research, argument, experimentation, and the implementation of policies and programs in defining its general and particular causes and in promoting and instituting general and specific courses of remedial action.[21] While less theoretically complex than some of the philosophical and linguistic definitions of discourse currently employed in social and cultural history, this definition nevertheless shares with them an emphasis on the determinacy of structure.[22] Indeed, if there is a central theoretical assumption guiding this study, it is that the direction that the American discourse on infant mortality took and the programs and policies it produced were profoundly shaped by the way it was structured—conceptually, rhetorically, and in terms of who participated.

I have chosen to approach the infant welfare movement as a discourse for essentially two reasons. First, the movement was considerably less uniform than it appears in historical retrospect. It can best be described as a coalition of individuals and groups who agreed on general principles but held somewhat competing ideas and agendas. The way that infant mortality was variously defined and the remedies advocated were as much a product of competition between those ideas and agendas as they were of consensual thinking. Second, while focused on a specific problem, the infant welfare discourse was suspended in a web of general reform discussion and was never only about saving babies. The shape and direction that infant welfare took thus owed much to the general reform context in which it took place. Because it developed within the context of a larger discourse on the effects of urbanization, industrialization, and immigration, infant welfare was a reform movement initially centered in the urban areas and industrial towns of the Northeast and the near Midwest. It was not, indeed, until late in the second decade of the twentieth century that mortality among rural infants began to attract any significant attention.

A second and related problem centers on the limitations that should be imposed on the scope of the discourse and the size of the community of participants. My concern here is with the American infant welfare movement and, therefore, my primary focus is on the discourse that took place in the United States among interested public health officials, physicians, and charity and social welfare workers. Yet because of the international character of the overall movement, it would be both irresponsible and historically inaccurate to treat the American discourse as if it took place isolated from what was being said and done on the other side of the Atlantic. My study is thus international and comparative, at least in the limited sense that it endeavors to illustrate what American infant welfare activists borrowed and rejected from their European counterparts and the ways in which the courses of action they chose to follow differed. Indeed, if there is a second theoretical assumption around which this study is organized, it is that the development of American infant welfare policy cannot be fully appreciated unless it is examined within an international context.

A third problem involves the amount of attention that should be devoted to determining actual rates and trends of morbidity and mortality, to detailing actual environmental conditions, and to illuminating the responses of those groups and individuals targeted by reformers. How one chooses to deal with this problem is largely determined both by the goals pursued and by the evidence available. My primary concern in this study is with reformers and what motivated them to conceptualize and approach infant mortality in the ways that they did. While I do attempt to define what actual rates and trends of infant mortality probably were, I devote greater effort to illustrating what they were perceived to be and why. I therefore pay close attention to what statistics were available and when they became available, to how much credibility they were given, and to how they were interpreted.[23] Similarly, while I describe the conditions in which infants at risk lived and discuss the responses of their parents to the advice and programs offered by infant welfare reformers, doing so is not my main objective.[24]

How to treat medical theory, reasearch, and knowledge and how to conceptualize their roles in reform constitute a fourth major methodological problem. The relationship between medicine and public health reform is problematic, to say the least. It has been and continues to be the subject of heated debate, especially between those who see medical theory, research, and knowledge as socially constructed and those who argue that as science they are comparatively insulated from social context.[25] I have attempted to chart a middle course between the competing positions in that debate by examining both the scientific and social construction of medical theory, research, and knowledge on infant pathologies. Essentially, I view them as the products of a scientific discourse that had its own cumulative history and formal logic and was governed by certain rules of analysis and evidence; yet was necessarily shaped by the social, political and cultural context and by the needs, aspirations, material interests and ideologies of those who took part in the discourse. I also approach medicine with an acute appreciation that more than many forms of science it is fundamentally an applied science, and is especially so when incorporated into public health reform. I pay close attention, then, to the ways in which medical theory, research, and knowledge on infant mortality were translated into advocated and implemented policies and programs. In short, I attempt to follow the sound advice offered by William Farr, the English sanitarian and vital statistician who was a major participant in the early part of infant welfare reform. Writing 150 years ago on the history of British medicine and its influence on public health, Farr assured his readers that he intended to give ample attention to the internal development of medical theory. But he also advised that "the state of Medical Science is only one of the elements of the inquiry; for the problem is—given a certain quantity of science, how has that science been brought into contact with the people, by what class of persons, by what institutions, and with what effect."[26]

1

Cities as Infant Abattoirs:
Anglo-American Sanitary Reform
and the
Discovery of Urban Infant Mortality

On July 19, 1876, the *New York Times* sadly editorialized: "There is no more depressing feature about our American cities than the annual slaughter of little children of which they are the scene."[1] The editorial was in direct response to a health department bulletin reporting that each day during the preceding week more than a hundred infants under the age of one year had died in the city. But it was not the first time the *Times* had felt compelled to comment on infant mortality. For almost two decades, it had been lamenting that each summer, with unfailing regularity, an already high urban infant death rate climbed to catastrophic levels. Indeed, by 1876 it had become almost impossible for any observer of the urban scene not to conclude that whatever else American cities happened to be, they were for infants, and especially for the infants of the immigrant poor, giant abattoirs in which a large proportion of all those born were destined to be slaughtered before they could celebrate their first birthday.

The conclusion that cities were inimical to the preservation of infant life, indeed inimical to the preservation of life at any age, was certainly not one that was reached for the first time in the latter half of the nineteenth century. Thomas Malthus had ranked great cities, along with war, famine, and epidemics, as one of the major checks on population. Thomas Jefferson had called them pestilential. And Benjamin Rush, America's preeminent Revolutionary era physican, had considered them one of the great killers of the new nation's infants and young children. Yet the conclusion took on a new importance and something of a new meaning in the decades straddling 1850, when the United States, along with England and a number of other Western nations, began to confront the profound social, cultural, and economic changes that were both cause and consequence of a vast and unprecedented migration from country to city.

Although nineteenth-century urbanization in the United States came

11

later and to a lesser extent than in England, its scale and pace were nonetheless striking. In 1800, out of a population of 5,308,000, less than 4 percent of
all Americans lived in communities with 2,500 or more people; by 1860
almost 20 percent did. Concurrently, the number of such communities vastly increased. Whereas in 1800 there were only 33, by 1860 there were 392.
Individual cities also grew at a startling pace. Among the established eastern
cities, New York began the period with 60,489 inhabitants and ended it with
813,669. Boston saw its population increase from 24,937 in 1800 to 177,840
in 1860; and Philadelphia from 69,403 to 565,529 during the same time.
Along the shifting frontier, growth was even more dramatic. Chicago had
fewer than 5,000 residents in 1840, but 109,260 twenty years later. And in
the same two decades, St. Louis grew from a bustling but modest trading
center of 14,470 people to a major metropolis with a population of 160,773.[2]

The dramatic growth of the nation's cities during the first half of the
century immensely complicated their internal management. The rate at
which rural migrants and foreign immigrants poured into urban areas far
outstripped any increases in housing, water supplies, and sanitary facilities
and made grossly inadequate the traditional methods employed by urban
authorities to maintain social order and administer to the needs of residents.
Also, the tendency of many of the newcomers to crowd into the city core,
where they could be close to day-labor opportunities, combined with the
willingness of landlords to capitalize on that tendency, operated to create a
type of densely packed urban slum previously unseen in the United States.[3]
The abject poverty and squalor prevailing in these slums, the threat to the
social order they seemed to pose, and the increasingly obvious need for new
methods to control and administer the vastly changed urban environment
launched a national discourse on urbanization that occupied public consciousness through the early decades of the twentieth century.[4] Not the least
important part of that discourse was debate over the consequences of urban
growth on the health of city residents. Wide-ranging and tied into a similar
discourse taking place in England, that debate gave rise to sanitary reform,
the first phase of a public health movement that remained essentially urban
in focus until the early part of the twentieth century. Indeed, because
sanitary reform and the public health movement in general developed out of
a discourse on urban growth, it tended to be less a national movement than
one spearheaded by and finding its greatest activity in the large urban
centers of the Northeast and near Midwest.[5]

Like many other urban reform movements that took shape in the middle of
the nineteenth century, sanitary reform was in large part motivated by a
perception that existing methods of regulating the urban environment and
administering to the needs of city residents had become profoundly inadequate in the face of dramatic population growth. Through the early part of
the century, what public health activity was pursued by American cities

was largely ameliorative and reactive rather than preventive. Neither en-demic disease nor the sanitary condition of the urban environment seemed to elicit much concern, although some effort was made to control the most noxious environmental nuisances. When authorities did take action, it was to contain epidemics through quarantine and sequestration and to relieve the indigent sick.[6] As in other areas of municipal management, antebellum city officials seemed to regard a laissez-faire approach to protecting the public health as quite sufficient.

By the 1840s, however, as American cities, already swollen by early native in-migration, struggled to accommodate a massive influx of foreign immigrants, a few physicians and health reformers began questioning whether a laissez-faire policy was indeed sufficient to safeguard the health of urban residents. Concerned over the spiraling cost of relieving those new-comers who became sick or impoverished, shocked by the filth and squalor in which many of the immigrants lived, and fearful that slum neighborhoods might serve as breeding grounds for epidemic diseases such as cholera, they exhumed what mortality records existed and used them as a basis for in-creasingly pessimistic judgments about the consequences of urban growth.

One of the first to do so was Lemuel Shattuck, a Boston book publisher who established himself during the 1840s and 1850s as one of America's most sophisticated social statisticians, or "statists," as they were then known.[7] In 1841 Shattuck published an essay in the *American Journal of Medical Sci-ences* in which he took issue with the still popular belief that American cities were relatively healthy places. Developing a theme he expanded upon in later publications, he argued that quite the contrary was true, that life expectancy had begun to spiral downward as urban growth spiraled up-ward. Using a variety of records, but chiefly relying on bills of mortality—death records collected by sextons—Shattuck demonstrated that while the longevity of Bostonians had steadily increased from the eighteenth through the early nineteenth centuries, the trend had dramatically reversed itself between 1811 and 1820, when in-migration from rural areas had fueled a process of rapid population growth which had further accelerated during the 1830s as large numbers of foreign immigrants began arriving in the city.[8]

At the same time that Shattuck was surveying the health of Bostonians, John Griscom was doing the same for New Yorkers.[9] In 1842, while serving a one-year term as city inspector, he conducted a sanitary survey of New York and sent a written report of his findings to the mayor. The mayor, how-ever, shuttled the report to a city council committee, which returned it to its author, declaring it inappropriate for its consideration. Undeterred, Griscom presented it in 1844 as a talk before the American Institute and the following year published it under the title *The Sanitary Condition of the Laboring Class of New York*. As Shattuck had done, Griscom hammered away at one point: that mortality was rising consonant with urban growth and that this was cause for great individual and civic concern.[10]

Shattuck and Griscom were in the vanguard of a small group of American sociomedical investigators who, in the decades straddling midcentury, actively participated in and promoted the collection and analysis of vital statistics, thereby laying the groundwork on which public health reform was built. In so doing, they found great inspiration and example from the comparative health surveys issuing from the sanitary reform movement in England. Although the principles of sanitary reform found earliest expression on the continent, the English sanitary reform movement had the most significant impact on Americans. In part this was because, throughout much of the nineteenth century, the American popular and medical presses excerpted heavily from their English counterparts, and in part it was because the social, political, and economic developments that generated sanitary reform in the United States more closely approximated the English experience than the continental one. As was the case here, English sanitary reform developed within the context of a national discourse over the most effective means by which to measure, rationalize, and ameliorate the consequences of the social and economic changes that were fueling urbanization and creating a large and highly visible population of urban poor. Moreover, England and the United States not only shared a common Liberal political tradition but also had welfare systems originating in the Elizabethan Poor Law Statutes. Thus, the English discourse on how government and society should respond to meet the social and relief crisis posed by urbanization had particular relevance for Americans.

In discussing what appeared to them an increasing and dangerous amount of urban social dislocation, early Victorian reformers articulated a wide variety of opinions as to causation and amelioration. Social conservatives and romantic moralists tended to interpret such dislocation as the consequence of moral degeneration inspired by the "civilized" temptations that city life offered to migrants from rural and necessarily simpler locales. Anti-industrialists and economic radicals, on the other hand, tended to blame emerging industrial capitalism, and particularly the factory system, for dehumanizing workers and lowering wages, thereby creating poverty, ill health, and other social miseries.[11]

Sanitarian ideas developed as something of a synthetic compromise between these two interpretations. While accepting the moralist contention that social progress could not proceed without moral progress, sanitarians turned the moralist causal equation around and, in so doing, constructed a rationale for government intervention. Conceding that education and moral suasion were necessary if the new urban underclass were to escape the social miseries besetting it, they argued that both were useless so long as the conditions in which that class lived were rife with physically degenerative influences.[12] They thus came to advocate a public health reform strategy that focused attention on urbanization rather than industrialization as the cause of social ills, yet located that causation in environmental filth rather than moral degeneration due to "civilized" urban temptations. In short, they offered an interpretation of poverty and ill health that was environmental and hygienic rather than moral or economic. Convinced that filth caused disease and that disease promoted poverty and vice, they argued that social ills and the cost of relieving them could most effectively be reduced by sanitizing the urban domain through facilitating sewage and garbage removal, cleansing city streets, providing clean water supplies, and improving ventilation in both individual domiciles and the areas they occupied.

Beginning in the 1830s with the publication of sanitary surveys by private individuals and associations, sanitary reform in England had developed by midcentury into a statistically sophisticated and politically effective movement. A national registration system was in place and a General Register Office (GRO) had been created, which, beginning in 1839, began issuing detailed annual reports compiled and written by William Farr. In 1842 the Poor Law Commission released its monumental *Report on the Sanitary Conditions of the Labouring Population of Great Britain*. Written chiefly by Edwin Chadwick, the report had an immense influence on promoting sanitary reform on both sides of the Atlantic. And in 1848, Parliament created a National Board of Health.[13]

Although anything but monolithic, the English sanitary reform movement did revolve around a few basic beliefs. One of these was that there existed an empirically identifiable relationship between the place and circumstances in which an individual lived and the health he or she enjoyed. As a consequence, especially during the initial stage of the movement, sanitary reformers sought to map out numerically a spatial and social geography of death and disease. As they did so, they increasingly illustrated that this geography had rural-urban and intraurban dimensions. In the first five reports of the General Register Office, Farr established the convention of comparing mortality rates of urban and rural districts, as well as those of various districts within individual cities. Those comparisons showed that mortality was generally two times higher in the city than in the country and as much as three times higher in urban districts occupied by the poor. In the Poor Law Commission report, Chadwick did the same, and likewise contended that much of the observed differences between country and city could be accounted for by high mortality rates among the urban poor.[14]

Sanitarians also believed that population density and environmental insanitation were largely responsible for urban areas being less healthy than rural areas. Contending that disease, "excited" by decaying organic matter, found its most frequent victims where population density vitiated the air and prevented poisonous miasmata from dissipating, sanitarians identified atmospheric impurity as the chief determinant of the observed mortality differentials. Indeed, so convinced were sanitarians of the link between foul air and morbidity that a few of them adopted a medically reductionist position equating every noxious odor with a threat to health. Chadwick, for instance, was fond of baldly pronouncing, "All smell is disease."[15]

Most sanitarians, however, were considerably less reductionist and doctrinaire than Chadwick and sought to reconcile sanitary doctrine with existing medical theory. Among American and English sanitarians, the most widely accepted and influential reconciliation was that conceived by Farr. Taking as a starting point the suggestion of the great German chemist Justus von Liebig, that disease processes were similar to the chemical action that occurred during fermentation and putrefaction, Farr devised an etiological theory that he labeled "zymotic," after the Greek word for fermentation. Somewhat simplified, that theory held that analogous physiological and environmental chemical processes were responsible for the origin and spread of infectious disease. When a person was sick, Farr explained, fermentation within the tissues and organs produced, as a byproduct, poisonous miasmata that were expelled into the atmosphere. Breathed in by other individuals, such miasmata introduced poisons into the bloodstream, which in turn produced sickness. Farr also contended that disease-causing miasmata were produced when animal and vegetable matter underwent putrefaction and fermentation. In his view, disease could occur both when previous disease was present and when it was not, so long as in the latter case filthy conditions prevailed. Farr thus allowed for the influence of contagion while propagating an essentially environmentalist etiology. Moreover, while claiming that the miasmata produced by physiological and environmental fermentation were present in all areas, Farr contended that they worked their greatest evil in cities and especially in the crowded urban areas occupied by the poor. In such locales, he declared, miasmata were not only produced in greater abundance because of the population density and filth prevailing but were also prevented from dissipating by the close quarters in which people lived.[16]

A third basic sanitarian belief, and the one on which advocacy of government intervention was based, was that many of the unsanitary conditions that made cities unhealthy and that produced excessive morbidity and mortality among the urban poor were beyond the abilities of private individuals to rectify. Sanitarians thus argued that if the rising tide of sickness and death in the city was to be stemmed, government would have to intervene and sanitize the environment. Indeed, while not discounting the importance of personal reform, sanitarians asserted that personal moral and social progress were impossible in an environment where filth and sickness prevailed.

Widely reported in the American popular and medical press, English sanitary surveys and theory, along with the statistics published by the General Register Office, served to fuel concern about urban health.[17] While

most social commentators believed that American cities were not nearly as ·
bad as their English counterparts, they increasingly voiced the suspicion
that urban growth was producing a widening gap between the life expectancy of city and rural inhabitants. In 1849 that suspicion was given strong
confirmation when, at its second annual meeting, the American Medical
Association (AMA) issued a report showing that mortality rates in the
nation's ten largest cities were strikingly higher than they were anywhere
else in the country.[18]

As it had in England, the publication of statistics showing that higher
mortality rates characterized the urban setting generated considerable discourse among antebellum American social commentators, physicians, and
urban reformers. The American discourse, however, was different from its
English counterpart in a number of important respects. For one thing, it took
place in something of a political and institutional vacuum. In England those
involved in the discourse on public health wielded considerable political
influence and were soon able to institutionalize their reform ideas within
increasingly powerful and centralized government regulatory agencies. In
antebellum America, however, sanitarians were largely outside the political
framework.[19] Neither Shattuck nor Griscom ever held a government appointment after the issuance of their sanitary reports. And although their
recommendations were modest, neither report had any real immediate effect
on the way that states and municipalities dealt with the public health.
Indeed, it was not until the 1860s and 1870s that states and municipalities
began to form permanent boards of health, thereby giving American sanitary reform an institutional base. Moreover, as was true well into the twentieth century, the American discourse and whatever action it promoted was
fractured by the lack of any national coordination. Unlike in England, where
the first National Board of Health, then the Privy Council, and finally the
Local Government Board provided a certain degree of unity, direction, and
impetus to the sanitary reform discourse and to the development of public
health programs at the local level, in the United States, public health reform
was primarily a state and municipal matter.

The American discourse was also considerably less comprehensive in
scope than its English counterpart. Almost entirely absent was the radical
economic interpretation that was prominent in England, especially after the
ideas of Germany's "medical democrats" began filtering in around midcentury.[20] One probable reason for the relative narrowness of the American
discourse was that the factory system, which significantly shaped the agenda of the English discourse, was as yet in an embryonic stage in the United
States and did not excite the concern it did on the other side of the Atlantic.
Furthermore, the early phase of American sanitary reform may have been
much more deeply steeped in evangelical Protestantism, moral philosophy,
and Romantic self-perfectionism than was the case in England.[21] But, cer-

tainly, a critical reason was that many of the new urban poor in the United States were foreign immigrants, whose rate of morbidity and mortality could be ascribed to habits and customs imported from less-developed societies. During the cholera epidemics of 1832 and 1849, immigrants had suffered heavy losses, and native-born Americans were quick to blame their way of life. The New York Board of Health, for instance, reported in 1832 that "the low Irish suffered the most, being exceedingly dirty in their habits, much addicted to intemperance and crowded together into the worst portions of the city."[22] Similarly, Shattuck emphasized that much of Boston's mortality increase was among "unacclimated foreigners," who showed their ignorance of native customs of industriousness and cleanliness by crowding together and living in filth.[23] Indeed, it was not until after the Civil War that American sanitarians began seriously considering what had long been an accepted tenet of English sanitary reform: that many of the morbific conditions attending urban poverty were beyond the poor's individual abilities to rectify.

If, initially at least, American sanitarians tended to place primary emphasis on behavior and customs and to disagree with their English counterparts as to the ability of the urban poor to control the unsanitary conditions in which they lived, they expressed no disagreement with the conviction that those conditions were responsible for increasing urban mortality or that they were worsening with continued urban growth. While they might blame the immigrant poor for the filthy and overcrowded conditions of their neighborhoods, they had no doubt that such conditions caused excessive morbidity and mortality. Moreover, they early and readily accepted another English sanitarian conviction: that a disproportionate amount of that excessive morbidity and mortality was taking place among infants and young children.

The conviction that it was those just beginning life who suffered most the effects of the insanitation accompanying urban growth developed gradually but steadily as sanitarians statistically documented their belief that urban living was deleterious to health and survival. Both Chadwick and Farr noted the seemingly disproportionate mortality suffered by the urban young. So too did other early English sanitary investigators. An 1839–43 study of York, for instance, concluded that 42 percent of all the deaths during that period were among children less than five years.[24] In the United States, as early as 1841, the editors of the *New York Journal of Medicine and Surgery*, pointing to statistics recently released by the city inspector, observed that mortality among those under five seemed to have risen from 32 percent in 1810 to 50 percent in 1840, and connected that rise to urban growth. Shattuck made the same point, as did Griscom, who observed that the social and environmental changes accompanying urbanization seemed to be taking their greatest toll among the young.[25]

By the 1850s the observations of the early sanitary investigators had been sufficiently substantiated so that sociomedical investigators and medical journals were beginning to express some alarm over what was perceived as a tragically high and rising mortality rate among the urban young. An 1856 editorial in the *Boston Medical and Surgical Journal*, citing statistics released by Farr of the GRO and by the Massachusetts Secretary of the Commonwealth, ominously called attention to the current "frightful" waste of urban infant life and warned that rising mortality among the young could be interpreted as a "telling fact against the morbid growth of cities."[26] Also in 1856, the American Medical Association commissioned a special report on urban infant mortality to be delivered the following year, at its tenth annual meeting. Written principally by D. Meredith Reese, a New York physician, the report was statistically unsophisticated and somewhat contradictory in its conclusions and recommendations. But on one point it was clear and emphatic: "In our large cities a fearful ratio of infant mortality is to be found."[27] From the beginning, then, infant mortality was conceptualized as essentially an urban problem. Indeed, while infants throughout the nation were dying at what we would today consider shockingly high rates, it was only the death rate of urban infants that initially elicited significant concern among public health reformers. Hence, like nineteenth-century public health reform in general, that part of it which was aimed at the prevention of infant mortality was an urban reform activity centered in the large cities of the Northeast and near Midwest.

Along with the conviction that urban areas were inhospitable to the young, midcentury sanitary surveys and the collection of vital statistics also inspired something of a change in opinion as to which of the young were most likely to die. Like the statistics collected on general mortality, those on mortality among the young seemed to offer compelling evidence that the infants and children of the urban poor suffered disproportionately from premature death. In 1840 Alexander Finlaison showed that, among artisans, laborers, and servants in Bath, the ratio of child death to all deaths was one out of two, while among the gentry and professional classes it was one out of eleven. Not long after, Southwood Smith did the same for London, concluding that "of the children born in the best part of town, one-fifth die before they attain the fifth year; of the children born in the worst, one-half die before they attain the fifth year."[28] On this side of the Atlantic, Shattuck suggested that mortality was particularly high among those newly arrived immigrant children whose families crowded into Boston's Broad Street section. And John Griscom, in his 1845 sanitary survey, expressed the conviction that those New York children who occupied the city's growing slum areas faced a particularly difficult battle for survival.[29] Yet, especially in the United States, the idea that the infants and children of the urban poor were death's most frequent victims was not one that gained immediate and universal acceptance. For it contradicted certain Romantic assumptions that continued to undergird much popular and medical thinking on health, and especially on the health of the young.

From the mid-eighteenth century, when Anglo-American medicine first began to show real interest in infant and child health, one of the most cherished beliefs concerning mortality among the young was that early indulgence undermined constitutional development and thus promoted premature death. Evolving out of a nascent medical nihilism that found early expression in Locke's theories on the necessity of early hardening and shaped by the connection that Romantics made between health and the simple life of the poor, it was popularized by the English physician William Cadogan, in his pioneering and immensely influential 1748 pediatric manual *An Essay upon the Nursing and Management of Children.* "In the lower class of mankind," Cadogan wrote,

> especially in the country, disease and mortality are not so frequent either among adults or their children. Health and prosperity are the portion of the poor, I mean the laborious; the want of superfluity confines them more within the limits of nature; hence they enjoy blessings they feel not, and are ignorant of their cause. The mother who only has a few rags to cover her child loosely, and little more than her own breast to feed it, sees it healthy and strong and very able to shift for itself; while the puny insect, the heir and hope of the rich family, lies languishing under a load of finery that overpowers its limbs, abhorring and rejecting the dainties he is crammed with, 'till he dies victim of the mistaken tenderness of his fond mother.[30]

Nor was Cadogan alone in his belief. That it was mistaken indulgence of the better-off classes which accounted for the majority of preventable deaths among the young was a theme repeatedly articulated by William Buchan, Hugh Smith, Michael Underwood, and other eighteenth-century English pediatric writers. So too was it a belief of those early nineteenth-century American physicians, like William Dewees, who produced this country's first pediatric texts.[31] Indeed, the idea that it was the pampered offspring of the wealthy who suffered the highest infant and child mortality rates continued to hold powerful sway through the entire first half of the nineteenth century and found considerable sympathy among antebellum American Romantic health reformers. For one of the most commonly expressed opinions of such reformers was that increasing wealth and luxury were undermining the national robustness that had traditionally followed from a simple and vigorous way of life.[32]

By the 1850s, however, an increasing number of physicians and health officials, armed with the data being collected by newly established state and municipal registry systems and aware of the findings of the English sanitarians, were beginning to dismiss with barely disguised disdain contentions that early indulgence contributed most heavily to high mortality among the young. Such, at least, was the response of Nicolas Appolino, Boston's long-time vital registrar, to an 1855 medical journal essay by William A. Alcott.[33] A physician and author of some of antebellum America's most widely read popular health manuals, Alcott quoted with approval an editorial that had appeared the previous year in the *Baltimore Patriot* suggesting that "a close examination of the subject, we doubt not, would show that it is chiefly among those who are surrounded with all the comforts, and in many instances, with the luxuries, which riches command, that the infantile diseases find their most unresisting victims."[34] On the validity of this suggestion, Appolino wasted few words. Noting that of the 971 infants who had died in Boston the previous year, 641 were of foreign parentage and occupied the poorer sections of the city, he concluded "that however true the foregoing remarks may be for other portions of the country, they are certainly not true for Boston, as the death of the above 641 children, under one year of age (who will not be considered as having been surrounded with 'the luxuries which riches command') will testify."[35]

Appolino's comment was one of many that were beginning to appear at the time in medical journals, state and municipal reports, and newspaper editorials expressing the conviction that infant and child mortality was most pronounced among the poor and immigrant classes occupying urban slums. In 1857, for instance, the health physician of Buffalo observed in his annual report that city statistics showed that the children of the well-to-do had twice the chance of surviving the first five years of life as had children of the poor. Not long afterward, the *New York Times* made a similar observation, editorializing that it was becoming increasingly obvious that mortality among the young was most common to those urban inhabitants suffering the "trying ills attendant upon dependence and poverty."[36] Similarly, in its 1857 special report, the AMA, while conceding that mortality among the young was suffered by all classes, emphasized that it was highest "among the suffering poor in our large cities." Indeed, it suggested that such mortality "has reached an extent of magnitude which demands inquiry into its causes."[37]

Statistics illustrating that it was among the young of the urban poor and especially among those of the immigrant poor that death took its heaviest toll did not, admittedly, entirely banish from popular and medical thinking the notion that increased wealth, civilized living, and overindulgence were important causes of infant and child mortality. Throughout the second half of the century, there were those who continued to insist that improved living conditions, along with unprecedented pampering, were producing successive generations of children, each less likely than the previous one to be endowed with the constitutional vigor requisite for survival. Most of those involved in public health, though, discounting such arguments as nonsense, increasingly accepted a connection between poverty and infant mortality and sought to explore and explain that connection.

Guiding that exploration continued to be the fundamental metaphor informing much nineteenth-century medical thought and therapy. Although in both theory and practice American medicine was in a constant state of change throughout the century, for all but the very last decades it remained organized around what Charles Rosenberg has described as a "deeply assumed metaphor—a particular way of looking at the body and exploring both health and disease."[38] According to Rosenberg, "the body was seen, metaphorically, as a system of dynamic interactions with its environment. Health or disease resulted from a cumulative interaction between constitutional endowment and environmental circumstances."[39] The healthy body was thus understood to be one that was able to retain a systemic equilibrium by successfully adjusting to and resisting both internal and external excitements. Conversely, the unhealthy body was one that, for any number of reasons, had weakened powers of resistance and adjustment. This informing metaphor gave nineteenth-century medicine a considerable degree of unity, despite divisive battles between regulars and irregulars, empiricists and rationalists, and localists and systematists. For instance, the growing reaction against heroic medicine and the development of more naturalistic therapies and theories during the middle third of the century did not essentially challenge this essential metaphor; it only placed greater emphasis on the body's ability to adjust without external help and therefore put a premium on maintaining the body's natural powers. Similarly, the decline of contagionism and its replacment with zymotic and other miasmatic theories of disease causation also did not challenge the metaphor. Whether the product of human contact or exposure to filth-generated miasmata, infection still called forth powers of resistance and adjustment.

Mid-nineteenth-century health reformers thus conceptualized infant and child mortality as a problem demanding the identification of those factors that made the young of the urban poor significantly less able to adjust to and resist internal excitements like teething and external excitements like disease, heat, cold, and improper feeding and foodstuffs.[40] Because the ability to resist and adjust was constitutional and since, especially in the young, constitution was as much endowed as developed, heredity was seen as crucial. Sickly parents begat sickly children, who, it was believed, were either predisposed to the diseases their parents suffered or were so consitutionally enervated as to suffer disproportionately from the traumas of teething or the excitements of morbific influences. The high rate of mortality suffered by the urban infant poor was thus conceived of as being at once a function and a reflection of the generally high morbidity and mortality suffered by the adult urban poor. It followed, then, that if infant mortality was to be reduced, the health of all urban slum residents had to be improved.

Yet not all sickly parents had infants die and not all infants who died were the offspring of sickly parents. Heredity was a factor, but not the only one. Increasingly seen as more critical were the possible postnatal influences that could affect an infant's or child's ability to resist or adjust to potentially mortal excitements. Conceptualizing that ability as the body's "vital powers," physicians and health reformers during the third quarter of the century understood such powers to be finite and exhaustible. The infant or child (or adult, for that matter) could be left incapable of adjusting to or resisting exposure to the next exciting influence.

Medical opinion held that two types of influence—both of which were connected to the infant's and child's physical and nurturant environment— contributed to this life-threatening depletion of vital powers. The first was the degree of exposure to those excitements that activated the powers of adjustment and resistance and therefore necessarily depleted them. While conceding that certain excitements like teething were universal and un- avoidable, physicians and health reformers generally agreed that others, like exposure to disease agents, excessive heat and cold, and improper food, were not. Hence, they proceeded on the assumption that if infants and children of the poor died in greater number than those of the better-off classes, it was in part because the care they received (particularly in regard to feeding and protection from heat and cold) and the physical environment they inhabited exposed them to a greater number of excitements that depleted their vital powers. In short, parental ignorance of proper care and feeding and the high concentration in urban slums of disease-causing agents were seen as combin- ing to make the earliest period of life for the poor one of constant danger. Similarly, the second and related cause of constitutional impairment and vital-power depletion was also seen as devolving from the physical and nurturant environment. Malnourishment plus constant exposure to the enervating influence of vitiated air inevitably transformed even the strong- est of the young into weaklings incapable of adjusting to or resisting morbific influences. Therefore, want of sufficient or proper food and confinement to airless tenement houses and districts were considered necessarily to enfeeble the young of the poor and predispose them to excessive mortality.

In the third quarter of the century, then, as public health officials and concerned physicians attempted to explain the high rate of mortality suf- fered by the urban young and to devise strategies for combating it, they did so within a conceptual framework that viewed health as an interactive phenomenon dependent on constitutional vitality influenced by heredity, nurture, and the character of the physical environment. As a consequence, they approached the problem as one demanding both environmental sanita- tion and parental education in the management of their young. They re- garded the latter as necessary to improve the quality of nurture. They saw the former as necessary both to improve parental health and to remove those morbific influences that not only exposed the young to excessive excitements but also, by impairing their constitutional vitality, profoundly diminished their ability to adjust to and resist those excitements.

Blaming excessive mortality among the young on parental, and especially maternal, ignorance and improper care, was certainly not new. That mothers, left to their own devices and instincts, too often mismanaged their offspring had been the dominant theme of the eighteenth- and early nineteenth-century Anglo-American pediatric writers who sought to "medicalize" infant and child care and bring it under the governance of "men of sense."[41] William Buchan, for instance, began his *Domestic Medicine* (1769), a work that went through nineteen editions and was widely read on both sides of the Atlantic, by noting "the following melancholy fact, that almost half the human species perish in infancy by neglect or improper management." He then went on to complain, "it is indeed to be regretted that more care is not bestowed in teaching the proper management of the young to those nature has designed as mothers."[42] Similarly, William Dewees opened his pioneering American pediatric text with the solemn observation that the large number of infants and children who each year were either consigned to an early grave or a life of invalidism stood as mute testimony of the need to improve infant and child management.[43] Moreover, in the initial part of the twentieth century, improving the way mothers cared for their young became the favored strategy for dealing with infant mortality.

Yet in the years after midcentury, educational reform increasingly took a back seat to environmental reform. Health reformers did not abandon their long-time conviction that mismanagement contributed to excessive mortality among the young. Indeed, developments during this period in pediatric theory, especially in regard to feeding, laid the foundation for the early twentieth-century emphasis on maternal education. Additionally, beginning in the late 1860s, a few medical societies and municipal boards of health began publishing and disseminating among the urban poor flyers containing advice on infant management. But despite this underlying and ongoing concern with reforming infant and child care, the main thrust of infant health reform activity to combat mortality among the young during this period was aimed at improving the physical environment in which the offspring of the urban poor were forced to live.

In part this environmental emphasis was the consequence of a pragmatic decision made by health reformers. Although convinced of the necessity of changing customs of care and management, they concluded that such change would take several generations, whereas environmental reform might be effected immediately.[44] To a greater extent, however, it reflected the increasing conviction of American sanitarians that education would only be effective if it followed upon the material improvement of the living conditions of those at whom it was aimed. As one Boston health official observed in an 1864 examination of the excessive mortality suffered by the city's immigrant infant poor who lived in squalid tenements,

Is there a remedy for this shocking state of things? And if so, what is it? It seems but there is one answer to this question. Not in education, which some appear to consider the great panacea for all the "ills the flesh is heir to"; not in instructing, merely, those who are the greatest sufferers, by demonstrating to them that disease and death follow a persistent disregard of the laws of health; for such attempts will result as similar attempts have always resulted, in perfect indifference and apathy. The answer is in rigid oversight and control of the erection of dwellings.[45]

Also encouraging public health officials and concerned physicians to emphasize environmental reform over educational reform was the growing conviction of many physicians that infants and children were particularly sensitive to the atmospheric impurity that pervaded slum districts and registered its densest concentration in airless tenements. That the young, along with those at other ages, were harmed by breathing impure air had, of course, been an accepted principle among sanitarians from the beginning. As early as 1845, Shattuck, while listing parental mismanagement and increasing luxury as reasons for Boston's rising infant and child death rate, had declared that the most important reasons were filth and overcrowding, both of which he declared "render the air very impure, and expose the lives of infants who are compelled to breathe it, to disease and death."[46] Similarly, Reese in his 1857 AMA report observed that "multitudes of infants" born each year in urban slums "perish in a few weeks, or months for lack of pure air; and instead of marveling at the extent of the increase of fatality among such, we might wonder that any survive."[47] Two years later, those meeting at the Third National Quarantine and Sanitary Convention agreed that "the fearful aggregate of infant mortality in New York . . . is at once the fruit and the proof of the contaminated air they breathe, in the wretched habitations of the poor, where confined and ill-ventilated apartments render healthy respiration impossible."[48]

By the 1860s, however, sanitarians were taking the logic behind these observations one step farther and arguing that while impure air was harmful to everyone, it was especially so to those at the beginning of life. After describing how the impure and vitiated air common to crowded and dirty living quarters worked its evil on all ages, one of the physicians involved in the 1864 Citizens' Association sanitary survey of New York graphically observed,

But it is on the tender and susceptible frames of infants that the effects of these influences are most speedily and strikingly manifested. Like the fabled vampires, marasmus and its kindred diseases here hover above the pillow of childhood, sipping from the dewey springs of life till life itself is gone. On the walls of these tombs DEATH hastens to inscribe the names of more than half of those whose hapless fate it is to be born within their dismal precincts.[49]

Indeed, some physicians, such as Jerome Walker, who authored a series on infant and child care for the *Sanitarian* during the early 1870s, contended that so sensitive were the young to atmospheric impurity that an unsanitary environment that might produce only slight indisposition among adults could be deadly to their offspring.[50]

Behind the argument that infants and children were particularly suscepti- ble to morbific environmental influences was the growing belief among physicians in the natural feebleness of the young. Where pediatric theorists in the eighteenth century had argued that children "are born with more health and strength than is imagined" and are therefore "able to bear great hardships," those in the middle and latter part of the nineteenth century came to equate strength and the ability to resist and adjust to health impair- ing influences with growth and maturity, and thus came to view the young as particularly fragile.[51] As one postbellum physician observed in an essay exploring the causes of infant mortality, "the infant at birth, and for a long time after, is weak, feeble, immature, imperfectly developed, unable to bear successfully the vicissitudes of climate, resist morbific influences, and main- tain a hold on life against adverse conditions."[52] Thus, if atmospheric im- purity diminished the body's ability to resist and adjust to disease and other excitements and therefore increased the incidence of morbidity and mor- tality, infants and children would necessarily be the greatest sufferers.

The belief that the young, because of their natural frailty, were most susceptible to morbific influences not only provided medical justification for emphasizing environmental reform as means of reducing infant and child mortality but also inspired the adoption of the level of that mortality as a prime index of local sanitation and the effectiveness of sanitary efforts. From the time of the first comparative sanitary surveys, health statisticians had recognized that promoting sanitary reform required those environmental influences that destroyed physical well-being be identified, their effects be proven, and the amount of excessive and thus preventable sickness be deter- mined. The ideal statistic to do this would have been morbidity rates, but the data needed to calculate these were exceptionally difficult to collect and remained largely unavailable until well into the twentieth century. As a consequence, those involved in sanitary reform were forced to turn to other indices of excessive and preventable morbidity. After initially experiment- ing with the mean length of life, they finally settled on the crude death rate (the ratio of all deaths to all those living). Contending that the crude death rate reflected the extent of sickness obtaining in various localities, sanitarians maintained that a comparison of such rates in healthy and unhealthy places could serve as an index to the degree of morbidity tied to local environmental influences and therefore preventable.[53] Crude death rates were therefore the investigative building blocks on which sanitary reform was constructed. William Farr claimed that they were as fundamental to sanitary investigation as the concept of value was to economic analysis. And John Griscom called them "the hygienic barometer, whose figures on a scale denote the state of physical health."[54]

Despite the importance of the crude death rate to sanitary reform, many sanitary investigators were never entirely satisfied with it and complained of its sensitivity to distortion by such population characteristics as age composition, migration rate, and occupational profile.[55] By the 1860s, that dissatisfaction had reached a point where health statisticians on both sides of the Atlantic were beginning to turn to age-specific death rates as more accurate indices of community health. In particular, they began employing the "infantile death rate," by which they generally meant some measure of the death rate of children under five years of age. As early as 1860, Edwin Chadwick, retired from public life but still an imposing figure in English sanitary reform, urged the members of the National Association for the Promotion of Social Science to stop relying solely on crude death rates and to begin using the infantile death rate. It was, he argued, "the best single test of the sanitary condition of a place or population, as that test is least affected by occupation, immigration, migration, and as children are most affected by aerial impurity."[56] Five years later Chadwick's recommendation was given substantial weight when Farr, in the twenty-fifth GRO report, illustrated that up to 80 percent of the difference in mortality between healthy and unhealthy districts could be accounted for by the excessive deaths of those under five years. Thus, he declared, no measure of the consequences of local morbific influences even approached the descriptive value of comparative death rates of infants and children.[57]

Not long afterward, American public health reformers were advancing the same argument. In a special report for the Massachusetts State Board of Health, Edward Jarvis cited both Farr's report and current medical theory on the natural frailty of the young to support his own contention that the rate of mortality suffered by infants and children under five years was a particularly accurate index of local health conditions.[58] Other American health statisticians did the same, and by the end of the 1870s their arguments had created something of a consensus within the public health community. As Walter D. F. Day, registrar of vital statistics for New York City, observed in his 1879 annual report: "It is generally conceded that the most sensitive test of the sanitary condition of a community is to be found in the percentage which mortality among children under five years of age bears to total mortality, at all ages, for a given period."[59]

Ironically, in adopting mortality among the young as a prime index of local sanitary conditions, public health reformers did not, initially at least, acquire a descriptive statistic significantly more accurate than the crude death rate. For what they commonly employed was not the comparatively accurate ratio of child deaths to children living, but rather the ratio of deaths recorded for those under five to all recorded deaths. This was a statistic that had been around at least since the late seventeenth century, and like the crude death rate is affected by the age composition of the population being examined.[60] If, for instance, a certain population contains a large number of children and possesses a comparatively high fertility rate, then its ratio of child deaths to all deaths will be higher than a more age-diversified and low fertility population, even if the age-specific death rates among both populations' children are the same.

One probable effect of employing the ratio of child deaths to all deaths was that American sanitarians developed a somewhat exaggerated sense of just how high mortality was among the young in urban immigrant enclaves, since such enclaves tended to be disproportionately populated with children and with adults of childbearing age whose fertility was significantly greater than that of their native counterparts.[61] Indeed, although mortality among and children of the urban immigrant poor was undoubtedly higher than that among native urbanites, it certainly was not 300–400 percent higher, as was commonly believed.[62] This can be seen in Table 1, calculated from data on death by country of parental origin collected by Massachusetts between 1866 and 1875. The actual difference between the two extreme groups—

Table 1

Infant Mortality by Nativity of Parents, Suffolk County, Massachusetts, 1866–1875[a]

Year	IMR[b] Native Parents	IMR[b] One Parent Foreign Born	IMR[b] Both Parents Foreign Born[c]
1866	181.2	188.5	198.7
1867	178.5	185.3	193.3
1868	192.2	201.6	208.4
1869	180.3	184.8	192.4
1870	196.6	204.8	212.4
1871	185.6	184.3	191.4
1872[d]	220.0	235.2	246.7
1873[d]	201.5	216.1	224.8
1874	181.6	188.7	199.9
1875	187.8	209.8	220.4

Source: Secretary of the Commonwealth of Massachusetts, *Annual Reports* (1866–1875)
[a]Exclusive of stillbirths.
[b]IMR computed as: all infant deaths in one year/all infant births in same year × 1000
[c]Includes births and deaths designated as of unknown parentage. See text note 63 for full explanation.
[d]The high rates of mortality for 1872 and 1873 were probably in large part due to the smallpox epidemic that ravished the eastern United States during those years.

infants with both parents native and those with both parents foreign—is surprisingly small.[63]

Sanitarian use of the infant and child death to all deaths ratio also seems to have inflated their estimates of the proportion of children who were dying in childhood. Although public health officials and concerned physicians must have been aware that the ratio of infant and child deaths to all deaths is not the same as the proportion of children who do not survive early childhood, one finds little evidence of such awareness in their prose. From late in the seventeenth century, when the statistic was first used to illustrate mortality among the young, through the latter half of the nineteenth century, the tendency was to equate the two.[64] If infant and child deaths constituted, say, 50 percent of total deaths recorded for a community, it was common practice to describe that as indicating that 50 percent of that community's young died in infancy and early childhood.

Finally, use of the ratio probably inflated the rate at which infant and child mortality was understood to be rising in mid-nineteenth-century American cities. In the 1860s, when the ratio became a popular index of community sanitation, a number of state and municipal registrars dredged up old mortality records and calculated tables purportedly illustrating the trend of infant and child mortality from earlier in the century to the present. Those tables showed that such mortality had dramatically risen, especially after the 1840s when immigrants began flooding into the major East Coast cities. (See Table 2.)

Given that some recent demographic studies have shown that mortality did indeed rise in correlation with immigration, some of the observed increase undoubtedly was real.[65] But a significant amount was probably due to improvements in death registration, since the greatest proportion of such improvement tended to be in the enumeration of infant and child deaths. Most nineteenth-century sanitarians, however, did not have the benefit of

Table 2

Percentage of All Deaths Accounted for by Infant and Child Deaths, Boston, 1820–1829, 1840–1865

Year	Total Deaths[a]	Deaths < 1 year[a]	%[b]	Deaths < 5 years[a]	%[b]
1820–24	5,560	336	6.0	1,282	23.0
1825–29	5,783	674	11.7	1,702	29.4
1840–44	9,846	1,209	12.3	3,680	37.4
1845–49	18,022	2,481	13.8	6,813	37.8
1850–54	19,983	4,720	23.6	9,296	46.5
1855–59	19,869	4,785	24.0	9,254	46.6
1861–65[c]	22,436	4,027	17.9	9,793	43.6

Source: Boston City Registrar. Annual Report (1865), pp. 46–47.
[a]Exclusive of stillbirths.
[b]Percentages have been recalculated to correct original compiler's mathematical errors.
[c]No registration report was published for 1860.

our hindsight and were not particularly inclined to question the accuracy of the ratio. For not only did it confirm their conviction that the environmental filth prevalent in urban immigrant slums was causing a wholesale slaughter among the young, it also gave their calls for reform considerable weight and emotional force. This last was of some significance, since it was not simply medical and statistical theory that prompted American sanitarians to adopt the level of infant and child mortality as a prime index of local sanitation. Strategic considerations also played a role. Having achieved an institutional base, yet faced with continued opposition from municipal politicians, tax-payers, and local economic interests—and well aware that even those sym-pathetic to the measures they advocated held conflicting attitudes toward the poor—sanitary reformers came to rely on infant and child mortality rates, at least in part, because of their emotional appeal and political useful-ness.

Through the middle third of the century, as the industrializing West increasingly came to embrace a definition of children as essentially innocent and undeservedly suffering the ills of adult society, reformers of all stripes began to use children to evoke sympathy for their calls for reform. Charles Dickens raised this technique to a high art form, creating a literary subgenre to call attention to the social problems besetting Victorian England. Sim-ilarly, in killing off Little Eva, Harriet Beecher Stowe played upon American sympathies toward children to further the cause of abolition. The decades after midcentury also witnessed a steady increase in societal concern over the fate of poor, destitute, and abandoned urban children. Indeed, by the 1870s a multifaceted child welfare movement was beginning to take shape, a movement predicated on the assumption that children were a unique class of citizens who deserved a special protective relationship with the state.[66]

One of the early ways in which this developing societal commitment to safeguarding the young manifested itself was in an international effort, beginning in the 1860s, to protect infants from abandonment, infanticide, and callous neglect. In France, that effort centered on reforming the wet-nurse industry and inspired the 1866 creation of the Societé Protectrice de l'Enfance and the 1874 passage of the Rousell Law, extending government protection to infants and nurslings. In England, it developed out of a dis-course on the consequences of what was perceived as a rising rate of il-legitimacy and infanticide and produced the Better Protection of Infant Life Act of 1872.[67] In the United States, it also was inspired by concern over what happened to illegitimate infants, especially following the widely pub-licized 1868 grand jury investigation of one Madame Parselle (Catherine D. Putnam). A New York City "baby farmer," Parselle had several of her charges die under suspicious circumstances. Like other so-called baby farm-ers, she ran a private lying-in hospital that took in mostly unwed mothers and for a fee promised to dispose of their infants once they were born. Critics charged that persons like Parselle more often than not kept this promise by murdering the infants, and thus urged that foundling hospitals be established to prevent commercial infanticide.[68] As the grand jury report in the Parselle case concluded: "Experience has proven that illicit intercourse between the sexes cannot sensibly be checked by legislation. If you place difficulties in the way of disposing of illegitimate children, you do not prevent illegitimacy; you only foster murder. Give us well-conducted foundling hospitals and you break up the trade of women like 'Madame Parselle' forever."[69]

In response, a number of states, municipalities, and private philanthropies established foundling hospitals and infant asylums in the 1860s and 1870s, both to prevent infanticide and to provide a place for abandoned infants who, up to this time, had generally been consigned to almshouses, where they were given over to the care of female inmates.[70] The creation of such institutions, however, proved to be less than an unqualified blessing for America's illegitimate and abandoned infants, since the mortality suffered by babies sent there was staggering. One careful analysis of the 231 "true" foundlings committed to New York's Randall's Island Infant Asylum between 1868 and 1871 found that 17 were claimed by their mothers, 19 were adopted, and 195 died.[71] Yet postbellum infant asylums and foundling hospitals did have at least an indirect beneficial effect on infant life. They provided American physicians with their first real clinical opportunity to examine and treat infant maladies and thus fostered interest in infant health and served as a training ground for the generation of medical professionals who would subsequently establish pediatrics as a medical specialty. More immediately, the shockingly high death rate their inmates suffered helped publicize the general problem of infant mortality and served to fuel public and medical interest in its prevention.

Justified by medical theory that defined the young as more susceptible than others to environmental influences, in quest of a statistic more environmentally sensitive than crude death rates, and well aware that citing mortality levels among the young would generate more public and official support for their programs than would illustrating the more generalized consequences of urban insanitation, postbellum public health officials made the death rate of those in the first few years of life an increasingly important part of the reports they published and the statistics they released to the press.[72] By the mid-1870s, most of the municipal and state boards of health so far established had come to include in their annual reports special sections dealing with "infantile mortality," and had begun supplying newspapers, especially during the summer, with weekly counts of infant and child deaths.

Three major consequences followed from public health's new focus on infant mortality. First, mortality among the urban young was given unprecedented publicity and was thereby transformed from a social condition to a social problem that increasingly occupied public consciousness. Although three decades passed before public concern over saving urban babies blossomed into a truly major reform movement, the seed had now been planted. Second, in adopting mortality among the young as an index of local sanitation, public health officials also came to consider the extent of its reduction a prime measure of how effective they were in implementing and carrying out their programs. As Jerome Walker observed before the American Public Health Association in 1890: "It has repeatedly been said that the public administration of sanitary measures in any city or town can be judged as to its efficiency by the rate of infant mortality in the city or town in question, and that a decrease in the mortality of infants means more efficient health authorities than hitherto."[73] Finally, and perhaps most importantly, the centrality that mortality among the young asssumed in postbellum public health reform inspired the collection of ever more detailed statistics on that mortality and thus generated among public health officials an increasingly sophisticated understanding of its timing and causes and a conviction that both could be manipulated. Specifically, public health officials came to regard as unnecessary that deaths among those under one vastly outnumbered deaths in the rest of childhood. The result was a shift in focus from the mortality of all children under five to the mortality of those under one, and a consequent narrowing of the definition of infantile mortality to the death rate of those in the first year of life.

Although demographers from John Graunt through Adolphe Quetelet had observed that more newborns died than older infants and more infants than children, prior to the last third of the century their observations had not inspired public health reformers to take any great pains to distinguish between mortality among infants and mortality among children, or to consider the former as disproportionately high and therefore capable of greater reduction.[74] Behind this disinclination to make sharper age distinctions were several reasons. One was a centuries-old belief that natural law dictated that a certain proportion of each age group die. That newborns died more frequently than older infants and infants more frequently than children was thus not generally regarded as a phenomenon subject to human manipulation. The early sanitarians never seriously questioned the validity of this belief. Indeed, their reformist activity was predicated on the assumption that mortality among the urban young was subject to reduction only because it was higher than the law demanded. Shattuck, for instance, never doubted that more infants than children were supposed to die and explained that, although the degree of sanitation obtaining in a particular place would affect levels of mortality, it would not change proportions. Enumerating the principles on which sanitary reform was based, he declared "that a uniform law of mortality exists, which destroys more persons at one age than at another, in all other circumstances exactly similar; and that this law is modified in its operation in a healthy and an unhealthy locality, only by its being less stringently regarded in the one than in the other."[75] It followed, then, that sanitizing the environment might reduce the number of infants who died each year, but it would not affect the law of mortality that demanded a greater number of infants perish than children.

The idea that some type of universal law demanded a certain number or percentage of infant deaths continued to hold some weight through the second half of the century and was resurrected in variant form by turn-of-the-century eugenicists. But by the 1870s, an increasing number of physicians and public health reformers were arguing that the long-observed differentials in mortality at the various ages had less to do with universal law than with the particular susceptibility of certain ages, specifically infants, to morbific influences. Job Lewis Smith, for instance, suggested that more infants than children died, not because of some immutable law, but because the vital powers of resistance and adjustment were at their lowest ebb in infancy and increased with age. If infants could be protected from morbific influences, he argued, their chances of survival could be greatly increased.[76] Other postbellum physicians and public health reformers went even farther than Smith. Henry Hartshorne frequently expressed the opinion that mortality among infants born with a healthy constitution and under favorable circumstances should be no higher than it was among any other age group.[77] Michigan's H. B. Baker agreed with Hartshorne, and argued that not only was infant mortality a more sensitive index than child mortality of local environmental conditions, it was also a more serious and pressing problem, since its astronomic levels were fully capable of being reduced by public health measures. "I have no hesitation," he declared, "subscribing to the belief that much of the infant mortality could be prevented by thorough and enlightened action by local boards of health in cities and towns."[78]

A long tradition of imprecision in conceptualizing and describing age distinctions also contributed to the lack of specificity with which infant mortality was defined and approached prior to the last third of the nineteenth century. As both Joseph Kett and Howard Chudacoff have illustrated, through the first half of the nineteenth century conceptual and linguistic age distinctions were rather fluid and vague. The term *infant*, for example, was as frequently used to refer to a child under five as it was to a baby under one.[79] Among the first generations of American public health reformers, this general fluidity and nebulousness of age distinctions manifested itself in a tendency to use infant and child mortality as interchangeable terms and to lump together the deaths of all those under the age of five. Moreover, any attempt on their part, prior to the Civil War, to be more age-specific was often complicated by a lack of requisite vital data. Most notably, birth records, required to compute infant mortality rates (the ratio of deaths under one year to births for a given period) were ridiculously incomplete. In

1843, for instance, Boston reported to the Massachusetts Secretary of the Commonwealth only nineteen births among its population of 93,383.[80]

In the postbellum period, however, age distinctions began to take on sharper conceptual and linguistic dimensions. Concurrently, public health officials began to pay closer attention to the different mortality levels of each age of childhood and in particular began computing infant mortality as a separate and meaningful statistic. Admittedly, in doing the latter they continued to be plagued by incomplete birth records. But by the 1870s, at least a few states had improved their birth registration to the point where such computation, if not entirely accurate, was at least no longer impossible. Indeed, by the late 1870s the infant mortality rate was fast replacing the ratio of child deaths to all deaths as the most respected measure of local sanitation. And as it did so, infant mortality came to be increasingly differentiated from the mortality of young children and acknowledged as one of the most pressing problems facing urban public health reformers.

Also contributing to the differentiation of infant mortality as a discrete public health problem were the increasingly detailed nosological data being collected by state and municipal registry departments. Although data on cause of death by age had long been collected, before the Civil War their accuracy left much to be desired. Not only were age distinctions imprecise, but the causes of death listed were often vague and meaningless. Deaths among infants and children were frequently attributed to such general conditions as teething and weaning or were lumped together under the headings "childhood maladies" and "infant diseases." Moreover, in the many cases where death was from acute diarrhea, the cause of death was often attributed to the convulsions that frequently attend the final phase of that disorder. However, following the adoption in the late 1850s of a standardized nosology developed by William Farr, the classification of death by cause began to improve.[81] Much imprecision still existed and would persist through the early twentieth century; but by the 1860s vital statisticians and public health reformers were rapidly gaining the ability to construct a relatively detailed picture of when during the year the various age groups died and from what causes.

Among other things, this more detailed picture showed that while older children died throughout the year from a wide variety of diseases, a large proportion of infant deaths came during the summer and were caused by diarrheal diseases.[82] Aside from providing justification for differentiating infant mortality from child mortality, revelation of this "summer diarrheal plague" among infants had three related consequences. First, since diarrheal diseases were commonly attributed to filth and atmospheric impurity, it supported public health reformers' increasing tendency to view infant mortality as one of the most serious preventable health problems resulting from the squalid conditions in which the urban poor lived. Second, the realization that infant mortality increased dramatically during the summer months lent the problem an epidemic quality that ensured it high public and official visibility. As each summer approached, public health officials and urban newspapers began warning the public of the "annual epidemic slaughter of innocent babes" that was about to commence, and continued to call attention to that slaughter until cool weather brought respite.[83] Third, although infants also died in large numbers from respiratory and congenital problems, the numerical predominance of diarrheal deaths, their association with those environmental conditions sanitary reform was aimed at, and the epidemic quality of their seasonal concentration tended to focus public health attention almost solely on them. Indeed, although public health reformers and concerned physicians were well aware that infant mortality had no single pathological cause, it was not until the twentieth century that they began approaching its reduction as if it required more than simply the prevention of gastrointestinal disorders.

The differentiation of infant mortality as a problem separate from child mortality, the increasing publicity it received, and its definition as a serious consequence of the insanitation attending urban poverty did not, however, initially motivate American public health authorities to design and implement special measures to save the lives of urban babies. Quite the contrary; for while it was believed that infants might be subject to different diseases than older children and adults, it was not believed that the general conditions producing those diseases and affecting the ability to resist and adjust to them were any different for infants than for the general populace. As William Clendenin observed before the American Public Health Association in 1873: "There are not general causes, existing and affecting persons of one age, that do not exist at every other period of life."[84] In other words, that infants died in such great numbers proved only that they suffered more from those morbific influences that affected health at all ages. Postbellum public health authorities therefore channeled their mounting concern with infant mortality into an already existing program of general environmental reform designed to improve the health of the entire urban populace.

Aside from collecting vital statistics and establishing politically independent boards of health that would oversee such environmental reform, this program consisted of essentially two parts. The first involved improving the urban service and physical infrastructure: specifically, cleansing and paving streets, establishing functioning garbage removal services, and constructing sewerage and water supply systems. The second involved upgrading the immediate living environment of urbanites, particularly the urban poor, by improving the sanitary conditions of their neighborhoods and dwellings. Convinced that health was impossible in the filthy and airless tenements occupied by the poor, public health authorities and their urban reform allies sought to get legislation passed effectively regulating what sort of housing could be built and occupied.

Although both parts of this program were given equal attention, public health reformers were considerably more successful in effecting the first than the second. Improving the service and physical infrastructure of cities bene-fited all residents and had the support of both home-owning taxpayers and the political bosses and the powerful business interests who together con-trolled what was and was not done in postbellum American cities. Like many other urban development projects, the construction of sanitary public works not only improved the urban environment but also provided a lucra-tive source of legitimate profit and illegitimate payoffs, kickbacks, and graft.[85] Tenement house reform, however, benefited no one but the urban poor. And even that benefit was questionable. The few regulations that succeeded in being passed and implemented worked to decrease the number of living spaces without providing new ones. What political power the urban immigrant community had was therefore generally not marshaled behind tenement reform.[86] Moreover, home-owning urbanites, of whom there were more in the United States than elsewhere, were at best ambiva-lent about tenement reform. While increasingly convinced that tenements and the slums they constituted were breeding grounds for disease and social pathology, they were considerably less than enthusiastic about using tax dollars to effect their improvement. At the same time, urban landlords, supported by court decisions upholding the privilege traditionally granted to property in the United States, actively and effectively opposed the imple-mentation of any rules or regulations that would curtail their entrepre-neurial freedom and their right to do what they wished with their property. Indeed, while a number of municipal and state laws regulating housing were passed during the postbellum era, they were either emasculated by taxpayer and landlord opposition or were prevented from being enforced by the refusal of state legislatures and city councils to appropriate adequate fund-ing.[87] Hence, while sanitarians and urban reformers in England, France and to a lesser extent Germany, were initiating and carrying out programs of housing reform, their counterparts in the United States were by and large frustrated in attempting to do the same.[88]

Also complicating tenement house reform was the ongoing uncertainty among reformers themselves as to the extent to which filthy tenement condi-tions resulted from the ignorance and obdurance of the poor and the extent to which they were the consequence of factors beyond the control of the poor. While most postbellum sanitarians subscribed to the principle that improving physical conditions was a prerequisite for effective educational reform, they remained convinced that no lasting improvement would come about unless the poor radically altered entrenched patterns of unhygienic behavior. Moreover, this conviction received considerable reinforcement in the late 1860s as a number of "model tenements," which had earlier been constructed amidst great reform fanfare, degenerated into appalling slum housing. Thus, the same Boston health official who in 1864 had argued that education was not the answer was capable six years later of making the obverse argument. Again examining infant mortality, he this time blamed its excess on the failure of poor parents to learn and follow basic rules of hygiene which would ensure that the domestic environment in which their infants lived and died was not so deadly. "To build spacious, well arranged tenement houses in salubrious localities," he wrote, "will not alone afford relief; for none but the instructed and the intelligent, comparatively, can secure them. Hence, it follows, that until education itself demands change, no reform in the present uncompromising condition of things can be hoped for."[89] Other public health officials agreed, noting that infants were especially vulnerable to poor domestic hygiene. As one inspector for the Brooklyn Board of Health explained in 1876: "Tenement house laws and health ordinances have their place, and should be enforced, but these only reach the border-land as it were, of the difficulty. Within the apartments where family life goes on is where the laws of health are really broken." He therefore argued that if such apartments were to be transformed from the "hetacombs of dead babies" they now were, public health officials would have to come to grips with "how to correct the modes of living among the ignorant poor."[90]

American public health reformers entered the last quarter of the nineteenth century increasingly convinced that infant mortality was a pressing urban health problem, yet stymied in their attempts to reduce it, both by external opposition and by their own uncertainty as to whether it would respond more to sanitary engineering and regulation or to parental education. Throughout the 1870s, they complained bitterly that taxpayers, landlords, and corrupt municipal officials blocked every effort they made to lower the infant death rate by improving the housing conditions of the poor. They also repeatedly lamented what they believed to be the poor's persistent apathy to improving their own condition and to observing even the most basic rules of hygiene and sanitation. In the last decades of the century, then, American public health reform was faced with what seemed an intractable dilemma. If excessive infant mortality had its causal roots in environmental conditions that persisted because of both the self-interested opposition of landlords and taxpayers to tenement reform and the ignorant and obdurate behavior of the poor, how could it be reduced without fundamentally reordering urban sociopolitical configurations and effecting massive behavioral change?

Admittedly, this was not a dilemma entirely new to public health reform. But as the last quarter of the century got under way it loomed increasingly large. For in defining infant mortality as the best index of community sanitation, public health had also defined it as the best measure of how effective sanitary authorities were. Failure to reduce it cast a pall over all other accomplishments. It was, therefore, particularly galling for public health officials to realize at the end of the 1870s that, while mortality among adults and older children had begun to drop, infant mortality remained as high as ever and in a some places seemed to be rising.[91] True, a few public health officials interpreted the perceived stability of infant mortality as proof that their efforts were having at least some effect. In 1879 the vital registrar of New York City found it "gratifying, if not entirely satisfactory" that infant mortality had not risen significantly since the creation of the Board of Health fifteen years earlier.[92] But to a greater degree the perceived stability of the infant mortality rate generated a mounting sense of frustration among public health officials. Articulating that frustration, Boston's Appolino asked in 1880 "whether there is ever to be a lessening of this 'slaughter of the innocents,'" and complained that "the same aspect is presented with unfailing regularity year after year; and while there is no dearth of advisors, nor those who profess to put their finger on the plague-spot, there does not appear anyone disposed to name a remedy."[93]

As the last quarter of the nineteenth century began, American public health officials thus came to regard the levels of infant mortality prevailing in their cities with concern heightened by a sense of impotency. Having distinguished the mortality of those under one year from that of older children and having made the reduction of the former a measure of the effectiveness of their sanitary programs, they found it particularly frustrating that infant mortality remained as high as ever. As a consequence, they began to take a few hesitant steps toward treating infant mortality as a health problem that demanded special and separate measures. One of the first such steps was taken by the New York City Health Department in 1876 when it used a special $5,000 appropriation to employ fifty doctors during the month of August to visit tenements districts and provide whatever treatment they could to sick infants.[94] At the same time, the New York Children's Aid Society set up "Summer Relief Bureaus" to provide free medical exams and hired its own summer corps of physicians.[95] Within a few years, other private agencies were doing the same. Newspapers also soon became involved. By 1880, the *New York Times*, the *Tribune*, and the *Evening World* were all hiring their own summer corps of physicians and sponsoring fresh air excursions out of the city for infants and their mothers.[96]

Treating sick infants, however, was a stopgap measure, ameliorative rather than preventive, designed to deal with consequences rather than the causes. Although they encouraged and funded such efforts, few public health officials deluded themselves into believing that relieving sick infants would ever be an adequate substitute for preventive measures. They therefore continued to concentrate on sanitary reform. But inspired by developments within pediatric medicine and motivated by their inability effectively to improve urban infants' immediate environment, they adopted an alterna- tive strategy that promised to make such improvement less critical to the saving of infant lives. In the last decades of the nineteenth century, Ameri- can public health reform shifted the thrust of its efforts to reduce infant mortality from improving the sanitary conditions in which infants lived and died to improving the sanitary condition of their nourishment. In short, the sanitary reform of commercial milk supplies came to replace tenement house reform as the primary public health strategy for combating the excessive mortality suffered by the nation's urban infants.

2

Improper Aliment:
American Pediatrics
and
Infant Feeding

Writing on digestive disorders and di-
arrheal diseases in John Keating's *Cyclopaedia of the Diseases of Children*,
the eminent American pediatrician, L. Emmett Holt, duly noted that they
accounted for the vast majority of infant mortality and found their most
frequent victims among the offspring of the urban poor. Yet Holt was quick
to caution, "still we cannot say that they are essentially diseases of the city
or of poverty." Rather, he asserted, they were diseases of faulty nutrition.
While poverty and confinement in close and ill-ventilated rooms could be
regarded as predisposing infants to digestive disorders, it was the nature of
what they were fed that actually produced diarrhea.[1] Published in 1890,
Holt's comments adumbrate a view of infant morbidity that gained wide
acceptance in the last decades of the nineteenth century and had a major
impact on the way that concerned physicians and public health officials
conceptualized infant mortality and pursued its reduction.

Concern that improper food and feeding consigned many infants to premature death was certainly not new. But not until the end of the nineteenth
century did a number of developments, both within and without medicine,
crystallize that concern and provide the impetus for concerted reform activity aimed at improving what infants were fed. In the United States, one
such development was the maturation of death registration in a few key
municipalities and states. Admittedly, death registration was still far from
complete and remained so through the first third of the twentieth century.
But by the 1870s, the data collected and published by those states and
municipalities with functioning vital registration systems were providing
public health officials and interested physicians with a numerical basis on
which to build an increasingly sophisticated understanding of the timing
and causes of infant mortality.

For the most part, the registration records confirmed what had already
been learned from the voluminous reports and careful statistics published by

England's General Register Office. But they also revealed that there were certain aspects of American infant mortality that appeared unique. In the United States, a disproportionately large number of urban infants seemed to die from gastrointestinal disorders, or as they were commonly called, diarrheal diseases and diseases of the digestive organs. In an 1873 comparative analysis of infant mortality around the world, Edward Jarvis, then president of the American Statistical Association, illuminated this apparently singular curse of American infants, demonstrating that while diarrheal diseases caused fully one-fourth of all American infant deaths, they caused less than one-ninth of such deaths in Great Britain.[2] Other physicians and health reformers made the same observation. That American infants, and particularly those who lived in the nation's cities, succumbed in shockingly large numbers to gastrointestinal disorders was a theme repeatedly hammered home by Abraham Jacobi, the German emigré who in the last quarter of the century reigned as the dean of American pediatrics. Asked to deliver the anniversary address before the 1882 annual meeting of the Medical Society of New York, Jacobi chose as his topic infant feeding and the prevention of infant death. While conceding that infants died from a wide variety of causes, he insisted that none was more significant than diseases of the digestive organs. Indeed, he noted that mortality records indicated that such diseases accounted for 40–50 percent of the infant deaths that took place each year in New York City.[3]

Whether or not it was valid—and there is good reason to suspect that it was not—the evidence showing that American infants were more prone than infants elsewhere to die from gastrointestinal disorders was widely accepted in the late nineteenth century, in part because it confirmed a long-held belief.[4] Since early in the colonial era, both popular opinion and medical theory had held that there was something about the American climate, and perhaps about the American diet and way of life, that was particularly conducive to bowel complaints.[5] Moreover, since at least the latter half of the eighteenth century, American physicians had held as an article of faith that an especially virulent gastroenteric disorder, particularly prevalent among town and city infants during the hot summer months, was especially rife on the American continent. Variously called the "summer complaint" or the "disease of the season," it was finally named *cholera infantum* by Benjamin Rush in 1777 when he published the first systematic account of the disease. Connecting it to the heated atmosphere of cities during the summer, he argued that it was more common in America than elsewhere.[6]

Cholera infantum was only one of the various digestive disorders that plagued American infants in the past. Yet it occupied a central place in American medical theory on the diseases of infancy through the early twentieth century—and with good reason. Each summer it killed tens of thousands of infants, cutting a particularly deadly swath among the urban poor.

Moreover, as described by Rush and subsequent medical writers, cholera infantum was not only deadly but frightening to behold. With the onset of the disease, an infant would develop diarrhea that persisted for eight to twelve days. Then it would begin vomiting and though wracked with thirst, would be unable to retain any liquid. Almost overnight, the infant's body would become emaciated, its belly distended, and its eyes deeply sunk within their sockets. Its skin would lose its resilience and turn ashen and cold. Continuing to vomit and purge, the infant would cry without cessation until it sank into a coma, after which it soon died.[7]

Although medical researchers never isolated the precise causes of the annual epidemics of cholera infantum, it seems likely that the disease was bacterial or viral in origin and was probably intensified by malnutrition. One or more strains of E. coli bacteria have been suggested as a possible cause, as have bacteria from the Salmonella and Shigella genera. But it is equally probable that the epidemics were caused by a virus, perhaps one of the rotaviruses visualized in the 1970s. Whatever the precise cause—and a number may have acted synergistically—infection probably resulted from ingestion of infected matter and was transmitted by unclean hands, linen, or bottles, or through contaminated milk, water, and food. Moreover, from the descriptions of the clinical features of the disease, it seems apparent that death resulted from acute electrolytic disturbance and circulatory failure brought on by severe dehydration.[8] However, not until the very end of the nineteenth century did physicians begin to understand the relationship between bacterial infection and infant diarrhea, and not until much later did they begin to comprehend the role of viruses. It was also not until the third and fourth decades of the twentieth century that they sufficiently understood the disease process to develop and employ effective fluid and electrolyte therapy.[9] Consequently, although medical discussion of the causes and treatment of infant digestive disorders grew steadily more sophisticated during the last decades of the nineteenth and first decades of the twentieth centuries, it remained marked by considerable and often erroneous speculation.

That speculation principally revolved around how to interpret the relative influences of environment, infant physiology, and infant feeding. From the late eighteenth through the early nineteenth centuries, American physicians, operating within a context of medical theory that remained essentially humoral and thus concerned with general conditions and humors, tended to regard acute infant diarrhea as the consequence of acidic imbalance brought on by a combination of intense summer heat, dentition, and improper or excessive feeding. In his 1825 Treatise on the Physical and Medical Management of Children, William Potts Dewees suggested that atmospheric heat, teething, and overfeeding were all capable of producing in infants excessive bile, which disturbed the bowels and caused them to spasm in an effort to evacuate the poison. He therefore recommended that the bowels be completely emptied through the use of emetics and cathartics and then tranquilized with coffee, calomel, laudanum, and, in extreme cases, by bleeding.[10]

Dewees' approach to cholera infantum and other serious gastrointestinal disorders in infants was only a slight modification of that earlier advanced by Rush and informed the way that many rank and file physicians conceptualized and treated severe infant vomiting and purging through much of the century. By the mid-1840s, however, opinion as to the nature and causes of acute infant gastroenteritis was beginning to change, at least among those physicians who constituted the well-educated elite of American medicine. As the influence of speculative humoral medicine receded in the face of newly developed localistic disease theories and as an environmental etiology increasingly made its presence felt in medicine, a number of American medical theorists came to view infant digestive disorders less as a result of acidic imbalance brought on by heat, overfeeding, and dentition and more as the consequence of digestive dysfunction caused by exposure to the stagnant, heated, and impure air, which was concomitant to urban living during the summer months.

By the 1840s, as the idea that impure air was deleterious to health was beginning to have an impact on general American medical thought, it also began to influence pediatric thought. While American pediatric theorists had long granted impure air a role in the causation of infant diarrhea, it was only around midcentury that changing etiological theory—culminating in William Farr's classification of cholera infantum as a zymotic disease— encouraged them to make that role a central one. Among the earliest to do so was David Francis Condie, whose 1844 *Practical Treatise on the Diseases of Children* reigned for a quarter of a century as the most respected American pediatric text until it was superseded in 1869 by Job Lewis Smith's *Treatise on the Diseases of Infancy and Childhood*.[11] Condie agreed with earlier theorists that heat was undoubtedly a factor in causing the epidemics of summer diarrhea that carried away so many urban infants. But he argued that heat alone could not account for those epidemics since they were largely absent from rural areas where temperatures were equally high. He also conceded that dentition and overfeeding could excite the alimentary canal and contribute to gastrointestinal disorders. But he contended that in most cases their influence was secondary to that which impure and stagnant air had on the digestive organs. He felt this was especially true in regard to cholera infantum. "By many writers," he observed, "dentition and errors of diet are enumerated among the causes of cholera infantum. They are unquestionably to be viewed in many cases as predisposing, and in others as exciting—but we have, in no instance, known of an attack of genuine cholera infantum to occur, without exposure to the influence of a heated, stagnant, and more or less impure atmosphere; and this alone, in the great majority of cases, would appear to be the sole cause of the attack."[12]

In seeking to prove the importance of environment in producing the summer epidemics of infant gastroenteritis, Condie necessarily downplayed the influence that pediatric writers had traditionally credited to parental mismanagement of infant feeding. Other midcentury theorists did the same. Not all American physicians, however, were happy with the emphasis being placed on environmental factors. Observing in an 1858 editorial that the "popular explanation of high infant mortality in cities and towns is a close and vitiated atmosphere," the *Boston Medical and Surgical Journal* protested that "too much importance has been given to the state of the air."[13] Suggesting that improper feeding was at least equally important, it complained that environmental explanations of infant mortality minimized the critical role that physicians should play in the management and treatment of the young. By their own admission, however, the editors were somewhat out of step with the times; at least a decade would pass before infant feeding was again granted equal causal importance with foul air.

In 1869, when Job Lewis Smith published his textbook on infant and child diseases, he showed the influence that prevailing theories of environmental etiology had on his thinking by listing impure air as one of the chief causes of infant mortality in the nation's cities.[14] Indeed, throughout his career, Smith maintained that the excessive rate of mortality suffered by urban infants was closely related to the foul and vitiated air they were forced to breathe. Asked in 1879 by the trustees of the Thomas Wilson Sanitarium to address the problem of urban infant mortality from summer digestive disorders, Smith declared that anyone familiar with the problem was aware that "each summer furnished abundant direct observations showing that foul air sustains a causative relation to infantile diarrhea."[15] Yet he was also quick to emphasize that "another important cause of summer diarrhea is diet," and noted that especially "in the families of the poor, the food given as a substitute for mother's milk is very apt to disagree with the feeble digestive powers of the infant."[16]

In adding improper feeding to exposure to foul air and arguing that "the causes of intestinal inflammation in infancy as it prevails in the cities during the summer, are mainly twofold, atmospheric and dietetic," Smith's text helped restore diet to the central place it had occupied in pediatric thinking since the second half of the eighteenth century when William Cadogan, William Buchan, and the other early English pediatric writers had brought the diseases of infants and children into the arena of Anglo-American medicine.[17] Yet it also signaled something of a departure from earlier pediatric thinking on the relation of feeding to infant digestive disorders. Although Smith and other postbellum American pediatric theorists tended to agree with their predecessors that breast milk was the best food for infants, they increasingly devoted less energy to urging mothers to nurse and more to developing safe artificial alternatives. Moreover, in focusing their attention on such alternatives, they paid less attention to the bilious qualities of foods and more to their nutritional value and digestibility.

As was true with so much in nineteenth-century American medicine, a great deal of the impetus for this new way of looking at diet came from abroad—particularly from Germany and Great Britain. In 1860 an English pediatrician, Charles H. F. Routh, published an influential monograph in which he argued that improving artificial infant feeding would do more than anything else to reduce the appalling rate at which infants died.[18] Eight years later, Eustace Smith, another English pediatrician, extended Routh's work by demonstrating that bad nutrition led to weak constitutions, which in turn made infants susceptible to epidemic forms of gastroenteritis, as well as to other infectious diseases. Smith also connected improper feeding to marasmus (infantile atrophy, wasting away, or the failure to gain weight and thrive) and other nutritional diseases of infancy and childhood. "Many thousands of infants and children die yearly in London alone," he wrote, "for the simple reason that they are fed systematically on food they cannot digest."[19] At the same time, German pediatricians and chemists were illuminating the relationship between the chemical components of foods and the physiological requirements of infants.

English and German pediatric thought on the nutritional value and digestibility of artificial infant food as a critical determinant of infant health traveled quickly to the United States, and by the 1870s American physicians interested in preventing morbidity and mortality among the very young were paying increasingly close attention to infant feeding. In 1873 Jacobi published his seminal *Infant Diet* and made the first substantial contribution to what developed into a sizable body of late nineteenth-century American medical literature on infant feeding. The production of that body of literature coincided with, and was an integral part of, the emergence of pediatrics as a medical specialty in the United States. Although physicians' texts on the diseases and management of infants and children had been regularly published in the United States since early in the century, it was not until after the Civil War that pediatrics began to develop as more than a sub-specialty of obstetrics. Like Dewees, most of the early American pediatric writers had been obstetricians whose interest in infants was always secondary to their concern with the reproductive process. When taught at all in medical schools, pediatrics was traditionally covered within courses on obstetric theory and practice. It was not until 1860 that the first American course exclusively on pediatrics was given; and it consisted only of weekly clinical lectures delivered by Jacobi. Not until 1888, when Harvard appointed Thomas Morgan Rotch, did any medical school have a full faculty position in pediatrics. Breaking with obstetrics was thus necessary if pediatrics was to emerge as a medical specialty. This break came slowly and was not completely effected until the early twentieth century.[20] But by the 1870s a number of developments had already appeared that ensured that it would take place.

Among the most important of these developments was the establishment of foundling asylums, infant dispensaries and clinics, and children's hospitals in urban areas during the decades straddling the Civil War. By 1880, New York, Boston, Washington, Philadelphia, San Francisco, Chicago, St Louis, and Cincinnati all boasted one or more children's hospitals and numerous clinics and dispensaries.[21] The institutions made it possible for a significant number of medical professionals to devote the greater part of their attention to the young; and, more importantly, enabled a new generation of pediatric theorists to base their works on the clinical observation of large numbers of patients rather than on their experiences as private practitioners. In writing his textbook, Job Lewis Smith, for instance, drew heavily upon the clinical observations he made as consulting physician to the Ward's Island Infant Hospital in New York.

By 1880 pediatrics had generated enough professional interest and won enough scientific respectability for the American Medical Association to allow the organization of a special section devoted to it. At its first meeting, Jacobi rightly interpreted the creation of the section as a signal that pediatrics had finally gained recognition as more than a subfield of obstetrics. Observing that "pediatric science is no longer, ought no longer be, a simple attachment to obstetrics and the diseases of women," he emphatically declared that "it has nothing whatever in common with these branches."[22] Four years later pediatrics moved further toward specialized identity when William Perry Watson started the *Archives of Pediatrics*, giving the emerging specialty its own journal. And finally, in 1887, forty-three of the most prominent American experts on the diseases of infants and children banded together to create the American Pediatric Society.[23]

To a great extent the emergence of pediatrics as a medical specialty was part of the late nineteenth-century trend toward specialization within medicine and the concurrent development among the American middle class of what Burton Bledstein has called a "culture of professionalism."[24] Yet it was also part of a profound reorientation of attitudes toward children. By the end of the nineteenth century, Americans, like most Westerners, had come to view children and childhood as developmentally unique and thus requiring special treatment. For educators, this view provided a rationale for the development of programs and techniques fitted to the specific capabilities of various age groups. For philanthropists and social welfare workers, it supported age-specific welfare activity.[25] And for physicians, it encouraged the differentiation of expertise not only by disease but also by the age of the afflicted. Earlier pediatric writers, while recognizing that children were not miniature adults, had assumed that the diseases of infancy and childhood were unique, rather than the infants and children themselves. But by the late nineteenth century, this view had changed. Pediatric researchers, particularly in Austria and Germany, began to advance the notion that the developmental uniqueness of the young made the diseases of infancy and childhood seem different. Prominent in promoting this idea was the Austrian pediatrician Theodore von Eschereich. "If the diseases of childhood show such great differences in their number and in the form of their manifestation, as well as in their course and termination," he explained to an American audience, "this can be only due to the fact that between the growing organism of the child and that of the completely developed adult great differences exist in the reaction called forth by disease process variations, which change constantly in the course of childhood."[26] L. Emmett Holt, whose 1897 *The Diseases of Infancy and Childhood* gained him an international reputation and whose 1894 *The Care and Feeding of Children* made him the Dr. Spock of the early twentieth century, frequently advanced the same argument. It was, according to Holt, "not so much that the diseases of early life are peculiar, as that the patients themselves are peculiar."[27]

The idea that infants and children themselves, rather than the diseases they suffered, were special had a profound effect on the way pediatrics developed. Most significantly, it made it unique as a medical specialty. As Jacobi explained in Keating's five-volume encyclopedia: "Pediatrics . . . is no specialty in the common acceptation of the term. It does not deal with an organ, but with an entire organism."[28] Whereas in the rest of medicine, specialization encouraged physicians to narrow their focus to a particular body part, function, or disease, in pediatrics it did just the opposite. From the beginning, then, pediatrics was something of a contradiction in terms: a holistic specialty.

The holistic orientation of pediatrics encouraged pediatricians to take a broad view of their responsibilities and generated within the new specialty considerable commitment to social reform. Perhaps more than any other group of medical specialists, pediatricians actively involved themselves in the social reform movements of the late nineteenth and early twentieth centuries. Yet it also made the definition and legitimization of their specialty somewhat problematic. Whereas other specialists could distinguish themselves from general practitioners by claiming expertise in particular organic functions and disease processes, pediatricians could not. Their expertise was age specific, not organ or disease specific. Additionally, because the therapeutic treatment of many of the major afflictions of infancy and childhood was still quite primitive, the initial focus of pediatrics was largely preventive. As a consequence, the expertise that pediatricians could claim was in the broad and nebulous area of infant and child management.

To define and legitimize their specialty, pediatricians were forced to dem-

onstrate that the successful rearing of infants and children and the prevention of morbidity and mortality among them required specialized medical
knowledge. This, of course, had been the goal of pediatric writers since the
mid-eighteenth century. When William Cadogan published his *Essay Upon
the Nursing and Management of Children*, he made quite clear his belief that
for the sake of the young their rearing should become the "care of men of
sense." "In my opinion," he declared, "this business has been too long fatally
left to the management of women, who cannot be supposed to have the
proper knowledge to fit them for such a task, notwithstanding that they look
upon it as their own province."[29] Buchan, Armstrong, Underwood, and
other eighteenth-century English pediatricians advanced the same argument, as did early nineteenth-century pediatricians on both sides of the
Atlantic. Lamenting that the "scientific management" of infants and children "is almost new to this country," Dewees envisioned his 1825 text as
helping put an end to the "time of ignorance when the care of children is
entirely confined to females."[30]

A major goal of eighteenth- and early nineteenth-century physicians interested in infant and child health was thus the "medicalization" of a set of
activities that traditionally had been the responsibility of mothers and
nursemaids. They therefore sought to convince both the public and other
physicians of the benefits of applying medical knowledge to the rearing of the
young. Late nineteenth-century physicians involved in defining and legitimizing pediatrics as a medical specialty sought to do the same. Yet their task
was somewhat more complicated, for not only did they have to argue that
infant and child rearing required medical expertise, they also had to convince their own profession that such expertise was so specialized that it was
largely beyond the mastery of the general practitioner or other specialists. To
accomplish these two objects, pediatricians increasingly focused their attention on one specific task of infant and child management, contending that its
successful execution was so complicated that it demanded the utmost in
medical skill and learning. That task was infant feeding, and, as pediatric
historian Fielding Garrison rightly observed, it became the central focus of
the specialty in the late nineteenth and early twentieth centuries and provided pediatricians with an area in which they could demonstrate their
specific scientific expertise.[31] Indeed, for Thomas Rotch, who along with
Jacobi and Holt constituted a very visible triumvirate in turn-of-the-century
American pediatrics, perfecting and monitoring infant feeding was the single most important activity of the new specialty. In 1893 Rotch declared
that "the preventive medicine of early life is preeminently the intelligent
management of nutriment," and concluded that "infant feeding, then, is the
subject of all others which should interest and incite to research all who are
working in the preventive medicine of early life."[32]

To justify the preeminence they gave to proper infant feeding, pediatricians argued that it was the one form of prophylaxis that addressed all the life-threatening diseases faced by infants and young children. In their opinion, improper feeding not only led to infectious and noninfectious gastrointestinal problems, but also to such serious nutritional disorders as marasmus, rickets, and scurvy. Moreover, they contended, the improperly fed infant and young child failed to develop, was constitutionally weak and therefore was much less able to resist and survive such deadly infectious diseases as whooping cough, scarlet fever, and bronchopneumonia. As Holt explained in the first paragraph of his long section on infant feeding,

> Nutrition in its broadest sense is the most important branch of pediatrics. In no other field and at no other time in life does prophylaxis give such results as in the conditions of nutrition in infancy. The largest part of the immense mortality in the first year is traceable directly to disorders of nutrition. The importance of correct ideas regarding this subject can hardly be overestimated. The problem is not simply to save life during the perilous first year, but to adopt those means which shall tend to healthy growth and development. The child must be fed so as to avoid not only the immediate dangers of acute indigestion, diarrhoea and marasmus, but the more remote ones of chronic indigestion, rickets, scurvy, and general malnutrition, since these conditions are the most important predisposing causes of acute diseases in early life.[33]

There was, then, medical logic behind pediatricians' emphasis on the importance of infant feeding. And it therefore would be an absurd oversimplification to suggest that the compatibility between promoting scientific infant feeding and achieving professional legitimization was their sole motivation for placing such importance on improving the nature of what infants were fed as the best strategy for preventing infant mortality. Nevertheless, the professional needs of pediatrics were influential not only in highlighting how crucial was infant feeding but also in shaping the way in which the improvement of such feeding was conceptualized and pursued.

When late nineteenth-century physicians and infant health reformers spoke of the need to improve infant feeding, they were generally referring to the need to improve artificial or hand-feeding, that is, all types of feeding other than breastfeeding. In part this focus on artificial feeding reflected widening recognition that American women were weaning their children earlier and feeding their infants by hand more than ever before. Particularly in cities and industrial towns, increasing numbers of working-class mothers were finding employment outside the home and were therefore forced to wean their infants early and raise them by hand. Middle-class women apparently were also weaning earlier and relying on artificial feeding more than they had in the past.[34] At the same time technological improvements in nursing bottles, particularly the development of the India rubber nipple,

made it easier to hand-feed liquids to infants and thus increased the popularity of artificial feeding.[35]

The new concern with artificial feeding also reflected a significant shift in
medical attitudes toward the safety of hand-feeding and the ability of the
average woman to breastfeed. Undergirding much of eighteenth- and early
nineteenth-century pediatric theory had been the unshakable conviction
that maternal breast milk represented the only safe and healthful aliment for
infants. Fully subscribing to the philosophic and scientific naturalism that
infused much of medicine from the mid-eighteenth through the mid-
nineteenth century and influenced by experience with their own patients,
the pioneers of Western pediatrics had been unequivocal in their belief that
hand-feeding was invariably detrimental to the infant and that virtually all
mothers could nurse if they so chose. Hugh Smith, in his popular *Letters to
Married Women on Nursing and the Management of their Children*, charged
that "every mother is designed by nature to foster her own child" and called
the intentional failure to nurse a "strange perversion of human nature."
Similarly, William Buchan, in his even more popular *Domestic Medicine*,
contended that "nothing could be more preposterous" than the idea that
some women were unable to nurse their own infants.[36] Such convictions
prevailed through the early nineteenth century and found reinforcement in
the naturalistic and therapeutically nihilistic popular health reforms of the
period. Writing on infant care, Andrew Combe, a Scottish physician whose
health treatises were widely read on both sides of the Atlantic, expressed the
wisdom of the day when he claimed that an "admirable harmony" existed
between maternal physiology and infant requirements, which precluded the
need for administration of any medicine or artificial food. Likewise, William
Dewees flatly declared that maternal breast milk was entirely sufficient for
infant needs and charged that not one woman in a hundred was physically
incapable of nursing her child. Indeed, for Dewees, the obligation to nurse
was the central one in an array of duties that together made up what he
called "the awful responsibility of motherhood."[37]

By the middle of the nineteenth century, however, attitudes were beginning to change. The age-old notion that the quality of a mother's milk could
be influenced by her physical, moral, and mental state was resurrected as
health reformers began to express mounting concern over the effects of
modern life on female health. In particular, while physicians and other
health theorists continued to contend that in principle maternal breast milk
was the ideal food for infants and that nature had designed women to nurse,
they also began to issue warnings, backed with impressionistic evidence,
that in reality this was not always the case. As early as 1858, William A.
Cornell, a Boston physician who wrote a regular health column for the
Mother's Assistant and Young Lady's Friend, a popular maternal association
periodical, was frequently warning his readers against interpreting too liter-

ally the injunction to breastfeed. In one column, for instance, he told of the case of a young mother who faithfully breastfed her infants only to watch three die of convulsions before she heeded her doctor's advice and hand-fed the fourth.[38]

The impressions of doctors like Cornell found scientific backing in Routh's 1860 *Infant Feeding*. Employing a detailed, if somewhat methodologically suspect, analysis of the mortality returns from the various foundling homes located in Great Britain, Routh took issue with the traditional explanation that the high infant death rates in such institutions were caused principally by the necessity of hand-feeding the inmates. In his estimation, only 3.2 percent of all foundling deaths could be directly linked to artificial alimenta-tion. He also claimed that of those deaths the vast majority were from inadequate nutrition, principally due to faulty assimilation caused by igno-rance of those foods appropriate for infant digestion. Therefore, Routh con-cluded, while hand-feeding did seem to contribute to infant mortality, its contribution owed "not so much to the absence of breast milk, as injudicious feeding."[39] Indeed, he argued that not only was maternal breastfeeding not absolutely necessary for infant survival, it sometimes could be counterpro-ductive. Citing figures from what he claimed was a scientific study of a large number of newborns, he estimated that almost one-fourth of all babies either died or failed to thrive on breast milk.[40]

Routh's opinions were not accepted without challenge. That there was no adequate substitute for breast milk had too long been a central tenet of pediatric thought to be discarded lightly. Nevertheless, by the 1870s a grow-ing number of physicians were reaching the conclusion that although breast milk might in the ideal be the best food for babies, it was not always so in actual practice. Such was the message of Jacobi's *Infant Diet*, which when first published in 1873 made its author a national figure in American pedi-atrics.[41] Although Jacobi would later reverse his position and become a leader in reviving the idea that most woman could and should nurse their infants, he took great pains in *Infant Diet* to caution against romanticizing breastfeeding. "Mother's milk," he advised, "may be unreliable in quantity, or as widely removed in quality from the physiological type of nourishment required by the infant, as could be the most badly prepared artificial food." Though contending that mother's milk is ideally the most appropriate food for infants, he warned that nature rarely lived up to the ideal and that the impediments to the production of nutritious breast milk were numerous. "Many a mother," he observed, "raises at her own breast sickly, bloated, rachitic children, until finally one is born that she is quite unable to nurse: then for the first time appears in the family a noisy, ruddy, muscular child."[42]

Significantly, Jacobi and other American pediatricians began to voice their misgivings about the traditional notion that most women could and should breastfeed their infants at a time when doctors and health reformers were showing marked concern over what seemed an increasing incidence of female sickliness. Through the latter part of the century, commentators on American health frequently remarked on what appeared to them a spreading epidemic of female invalidism. In 1871, for instance, after having completed a journey in which she visited dozens of friends and relatives, Catherine Beecher reported a "terrible decay of female health all over the land."[43] Other writers agreed, so much so that, as the century drew to a close, it had become almost clichéd to remark upon the ill-health of American women.

Applying the pseudoscientific, evolutionary theories of the day, doctors attached to this epidemic of female invalidism a variety of diagnostic labels—from neurasthenia to hyperesthesia—but the upshot of all their diagnoses was that modern life, with its demands on the nervous and mental systems, was in conflict with the biological nature of women.[44] As a consequence of this conflict, it was widely suggested, women's reproductive and nursing abilities were being vitiated and were evolving toward higher refinement but biological uselessness. Doctors were thus increasingly prone to view women, and especially "nervous" upper- and middle-class women, as physiologically incapable of producing the quantity and quality of breast milk required to rear a healthy infant. Noting that healthy nerves were absolutely crucial to the production and secretion of breast milk, Jacobi was emphatic in declaring that "a woman with a markedly nervous temperament is generally unsuitable for the office of nursing, since her milk is liable to become deficient in quantity or perverted in quality."[45] Rotch later made the same point. Remarking on the apparent nervousness and sickliness of American women, he advised that the mammary gland, though "a beautifully adapted piece of mechanism constructed for the elaboration and secretion of an animal food," could easily be adversely affected by nervous debility or other physiological problems. He therefore warned that "when from any cause this sensitive machinery is thrown out of equilibrium its product is at once changed, sometimes but slightly, but again to such an extent that the most disastrous consequences may follow when it is imbibed by the consumer."[46]

Rotch and Jacobi, of course, were at the top of their profession and their discussion of the dangers inherent in indiscriminate breastfeeding was relatively complex and consistent with current scientific understanding of physiology and chemistry. Among less sophisticated physicians and popular health writers, the discussion was often conducted in more prosaic terms. One popular but probably apocryphal anecdote that found its way into many late nineteenth-century health manuals recounted the experience of a nursing mother who watched her husband being attacked by a band of soldiers. Still in a state of nervous excitement, she put her baby to breast. After nursing for a few moments, the infant went into convulsion and soon after died.[47] Whether scientific or prosaic, though, the message behind late nineteenth-century medical advice on breastfeeding was essentially the same: while in theory breast milk was the ideal food for infants, in practice it could be as deadly as even the worst and most inappropriate artificial foods. The impact of that message was twofold. First, it transformed nursing from a natural process to a potentially dangerous one that required medical supervision. Second, it gave impetus to medical efforts to find and make available safe alternatives to breast milk that would as closely as possible approximate the character and quality of that milk when it had not been perverted by physiological complications in the mother.

In pursuing the latter, only a few late nineteenth-century American physicians and infant health advocates recommended wet-nursing, which had traditionally been a favored option among better-off families in which a mother could not or chose not to breastfeed. Because of the growing shortage of servants in the United States, wet nurses were difficult to find and prohibitively expensive for all but the wealthy. Also, long extant fears that wet nurses imparted moral qualities through their milk had recently been revived and given a new dimension by the supposed scientific discovery that venereal disease could be transmitted through a mother's milk.[48] With wet-nursing not an acceptable alternative, physicians thus turned their attention to other substitutes for mother's milk. In particular they looked to cow's milk, which because of its availability held promise as a viable substitute.

Feeding cow's milk to infants was not, of course, new. Along with the milk of other domesticated animals, cow's milk had for centuries been commonly used to suckle infants deprived of the breast. Moreover, although still regarded as generally inferior to human breast milk, it was by midcentury widely considered superior to the various farinaceous mixtures that had also long been used as substitutes for human milk. Among physicians concerned with feeding the young it had become common wisdom that the digestive systems of infants were not sufficiently developed to process the starch that was the chief component of such mixtures.[49] But cow's milk also had its problems. Although believed to be one of the easiest of known foods to digest and commonly fed to invalids as well as infants, it was compositionally different from breast milk and therefore considered less digestible. Indeed, at the same time they began recommending cow's milk as the best artificial food for infants, doctors also began expressing concern that, in undiluted form, it was capable of causing severe bouts of indigestion which could lead to diarrheal and nutritional problems.[50] As a consequence, through much of the latter half of the century, pediatric concern with devising alternatives to maternal nursing was channeled toward discovering how milk from cows could be made similar to breast milk and therefore more digestible.

The first scientific, comparative chemical analysis of human and cow's milk was published in 1838 by a young German, Johann Franz Simon.[51] But it was not until the middle of the next decade that such analyses were provided scientific footing by the research of Justus von Liebig. Building on the work and speculations of the Dutch chemist G. J. Mulder, Liebig refuted the prevailing assumption that all food had essentially the same nutritive value by demonstrating that foods were composed of different proportions of fats, carbohydrates, and proteins, each of which, he contended, met a particular physiological need. Somewhat later, other food chemists added minerals and salts, popularly called ash, to that list.[52] In breaking food down to its constituent elements, Liebig not only provided a method by which the nutritional value of various foods could be measured and compared, but also provided a scientific basis for the concoction of food equivalents. In order to duplicate the nutritional value of a specific food, one had only to concoct a mixture of other foods that, when combined, provided an equivalent proportion of the basic nutritional elements.

One result of the work of Liebig and others in the developing science of food chemistry was to inspire the commercial production of artificial infant foods that manufacturers claimed closely approximated the nutritional value of healthy human milk.[53] In 1867 Liebig himself began marketing in Europe an infant food that he contended perfectly met the nutritional needs of infants when properly prepared and mixed with cow's milk. The following year it was being sold in the United States, having received the enthusiastic endorsement of a number of medical journals.[54] Other manufactured infant foods soon joined Liebig's. Among the most popular were Ridge's Food (an English product that actually preceded Liebig's to the American market), Nestle's Milk Food, Mellin's Food, and Horlick's Malted Milk. Vigorously promoting their milk foods in women's magazines and medical journals, manufacturers frequently exploited medical and popular concern that the pace of modern life was depriving many women of the ability to nurse. While paying lip service to breastfeeding, Ridge's Food advised in an 1882 advertisement,

> The mammary glands have suffered . . . outrages at the hands of the corsetmaker, the dressmaker, and the manufacturer of bosom pads, so that what is left of our mothers is in the majority of cases, only an apology for the ideal which nature designed. . . . In all classes and conditions of modern life, the mother's milk is most frequently neither in quantity or quality adequate to the nourishment of the child, . . . BUT THE BANE HAS AN ANTIDOTE.[55]

The antidote, of course, was Ridge's Food, which the manufacturer promised would enable even the most organically enervated and nervous woman to raise a healthy infant. Although backed up by little if any hard evidence, such promises apparently were convincing to many middle-class parents and their general practitioners. For by the late 1880s the manufacturers of proprietary foods had carved out a sizable American market and many doctors were recommending the mixtures to mothers who could not or would not nurse.[56]

The proprietary food market, however, was largely a middle- and upper-class one. The poor and the working classes generally breastfed, purchased bulk or loose milk, or concocted some homemade version of infant pablum. The small minority who did employ commercially prepared infant foods, tended to use condensed milk. Appearing on the market at about the same time proprietary infant foods did, condensed milk had the attraction of being cheap, filling, unadulterated and capable of keeping for a long time without souring. Moreover, because of its high sugar content, infants readily took to it.[57]

Although initially welcoming the appearance of proprietary foods and condensed milk, pediatricians soon came to look askance at them and by the 1890s were charging that they caused rickets, scurvy, and other nutritional disorders and were in no small part responsible for the continuing high rate of infant diarrheal diseases.[58] Some of the pediatricians' charges were well founded. But many were not, and seem to be rooted as much in professional self-interest as in science.[59] Having staked out infant feeding as a field in which they would battle for professional legitimization as a specialty, pediatricians looked with some alarm at the entry of large commercial concerns into that field. And with good reason, for one of the basic marketing claims of the proprietary food manufacturers was that by following the few simple instructions accompanying the product, anyone could prepare a food that would fully satisfy an infant's nutritional needs. Hence, there was little need for medical supervision. Fully cognizant of the threat posed by the new infant foods and ever the watchdog of professional interests, Rotch complained in 1893,

> It would seem hardly necessary to suggest that the proper authority for establishing rules for substitute feeding should emanate from the medical profession and not from non-medical capitalists. Yet when we study the history of substitute feeding as it is represented all over the world, the part which the family physician plays in comparison with numberless patent and proprietary foods is a humiliating one, and one which should no longer be tolerated.[60]

Despite the complaints of eminent pediatricians such as Rotch, proprietary foods and condensed milk continued to be used fairly widely through the early twentieth century. Indeed, by the turn of the century, prepared infant food had become the mainstay of many general practitioners in their family practice.

Liebig's research, however, did more than simply inspire the commercial production of artificial infant foods. By providing a model of analysis, it established for pediatricians and others interested in infant feeding a course along which they could pursue research and develop their own formulas, particularly for making cow's milk approximate human milk. Such formulas, it is true, had been devised even before Liebig. Aware that human milk was thinner and tasted sweeter than cow's milk, physicians had long advised diluting and adding sugar to the latter. After Liebig, however, such advice took on an increasingly scientific, or perhaps more accurately, pseudoscientific, quality. At the heart of that advice were two assumptions or doctrines that guided medical devising of infant formulas through the early part of the twentieth century. The first of these derived from the continuing conviction that healthy maternal breast milk was without question the most suitable aliment for infants. Doctors therefore sought to create formulas on the principle that the closer such a formula duplicated human milk the better it was. Articulated as early as 1847 by the British pediatrician George Gream, when he advised, "the better types of foods are those which most nearly resemble the mother's milk," this doctrine of similarity held a regnant position in pediatric thought throughout the period under consideration.[61]

The second assumption proceeded from the discovery by analysts that cow's milk had a significantly higher proportion of casein or protein than mother's milk. This discovery led physicians to theorize that it was the difference in casein content which was responsible for the frequent attacks of indigestion suffered by bottle-fed babies. One of the first to advance such a theory was Charles Dulcena Meigs, an obstetrics professor at Jefferson Medical College. In 1850 Meigs published the lectures on pediatrics he gave as part of his course on obstetrics. Discussing the digestive diseases of infants, he cited the earlier work of Simon and suggested that much infant indigestion might be traceable to the casein content of cow's milk.[62] Yet Meigs did not offer any real explanation why this was so, and his suggestion thus remained little more than an interesting hypothesis for the next decade and a half. In the late 1860s, however, a German pediatrician, Philipp Biedert, began publishing the results of his research in milk analysis and provided the basis for the transformation of Meig's casein theory into medical doctrine. In an 1869 publication, Biedert demonstrated that cow's milk was considerably more acidic than human milk, that it contained approximately twice as much casein, and that the casein in cow's milk coagulated into denser curds than it did in human milk, thus making it difficult for infants to digest. Biedert also argued that diluting cow's milk with water to lower the casein content offered only a partial solution to the problem, since the other nutritional components of the liquid were also diluted. He therefore devised a method for mixing infant formula which entailed diluting cow's milk with cream until the percentage of casein equaled that of human milk and then adding sugar until the appropriate level of carbohydrates was reached. The advantage of using cream lay in the fact that one could also regulate the fat content of the formula, thus, ostensibly, making the resultant mixture an exact duplicate of mother's milk.[63]

Biedert's formula, which provided the basis for all subsequent formulas developed in the late nineteenth and early twentieth centuries, required, of course, that the exact percentages of the basic nutritional elements in human and cow's milk be known. As a consequence, for the next several decades, much of pediatric research into infant feeding was concerned with precisely determining those percentages and devising formulas that would make cow's milk constituently duplicate human milk. This concern reached its apogee in the last decade of the century with the development, principally by Rotch, of an immensely complicated method of formula mixing known as percentage feeding.

When Rotch began advocating percentage feeding he was fast becoming recognized as one of America's preeminent pediatricians. After receiving a medical degree from Harvard in 1874 and spending two years studying abroad, he had returned to Boston where he established a practice specializing in infants and children. In 1879 he became an instructor in the diseases of children at Harvard and by 1893 was a full professor. Ten years later, the university created for him the first American chair in pediatrics. A prolific writer, he was the author of countless articles and in 1895 published a pediatric textbook that became a standard in the field. Deeply committed to promoting his specialty, he tirelessly fought for its legitimization, served as the first president of the New England Pediatric Society, and was a founding member of the American Pediatric Society.[64]

Although interested in all aspects of infant and child health, Rotch early became convinced that the great majority of morbidity and mortality during the initial years of life could be traced to improper feeding. Furthermore, like other pediatricians of his day, he firmly believed that although breast milk was the ideal food for infants, the conditions of modern life were making its supply and quality unreliable. "While recognizing the importance of feeding infants during the early months of life means human milk," he observed in 1887, "we must allow that in civilized communities the necessity of supplying the infant with food not directly from the human breast must often arise." Therefore, he concluded, "it manifestly becomes a duty to carefully investigate the different methods of artificial feeding."[65]

In pursuing such an investigation, Rotch began by accepting Biedert's findings—modified and made more accurate in 1885 by Arthur V. Meigs—that prototypical human milk was composed of approximately 87 percent water, 4 percent fat, 7 percent sugar, 0.1 percent ash, and only 1 percent casein whereas cow's milk was roughly 88 percent water, 4 percent fat, 5 percent sugar, 0.4 percent ash, and fully 3 percent casein.[66] In addition, he accepted Biedert's contention that it was the difference in casein content which made cow's milk difficult to digest, and therefore that it was the casein content that had to be most closely monitored and regulated. But he also suggested that the different levels of sugar and fat could affect infant digestion and thus that they too had to be carefully modified. To do so and to make cow's milk approximate human milk in content, Rotch initially recommended the relatively simple system of modification devised by Biedert and perfected by Meigs. But he soon abandoned this system when subsequent research convinced him that not only did human milk vary from mother to mother but also that there was significant variation in infant digestive systems. These convictions led Rotch to conclude that no standard modification of cow's milk could be appropriate for all babies and that if digestible formulas were to be mixed they had to be done to fit the specific physiological needs and digestive capabilities of individual infants.[67] Contending that "what is one infant's food may be another's poison," and that the minutest gradations in a formula's components could determine whether an infant thrived or wasted away, Rotch thus devised an increasingly complex system of formula computation which required algebraic calculation and chemical analysis.[68]

Despite the difficulty of Rotch's "percentage method," it was hailed as a great step forward in infant feeding by many of the nation's pediatricians and especially by those who had taken or were teaching the newly established pediatric courses in medical schools. While a number of older pediatricians tended to agree with Jacobi when he groused, "you cannot feed babies with mathematics, you must feed them with brains," most of their younger colleagues found in Rotch's method a system compatible with their conviction that infant feeding required scientific expertise.[69] One physican, who studied with L. Emmett Holt at Columbia around the turn of the century, recalled that when the eminent pediatrician lectured on percentage feeding, he "enveloped the subject with an esoteric aura. Indeed it appeared the very Eden of Pediatrics, where skill was most needed and the pediatrician reigned alone."[70] Pediatricians and other physicians were also attracted to percentage feeding because it made their services absolutely indispensible to families who wished and could afford to offer their infants the most modern scientific care.

Also lending support to Rotch's system was its apparent effectiveness as a prophylaxis and therapy for infant digestive and nutritional disorders. This was particularly true after Rotch convinced a wealthy Bostonian to supply the funds for establishing laboratories in which infant formula could be carefully mixed to order in sanitary surroundings. In retrospect, it seems probable that whatever success percentage feeding may have enjoyed had less to do with the ability of these laboratories to produce intricately calibrated individual formulas for pediatricians than it did with their ability to supply high quality milk with a relatively low bacterial count. Yet at a time when even the best educated physicians were only beginning to appreciate

the role of bacteria in producing gastroenteritus and were still largely ignorant of vitamins and calories, it was not illogical for them to conclude that
the successes they were having were due to the the complicated and individual formulas of Rotch's system.

By the first decade of the century, however, percentage feeding was
beginning to attract increasing criticism. Some of that criticism was practical
and centered on the incredible complexity and difficulty of the system. In
response, some proponents of percentage feeding devised cards with basic
sample formulas that could be used by the practitioner unable or unwilling
to do the required calculations. Yet even these were highly intricate and did
little to still mounting criticism that percentage feeding had grown so elaborate that, in actual practice, few physicians were willing to use it. At the
same time other critics were beginning to charge that no matter how willing
or sophisticated the practitioner might be, the precise percentages called for
by the system were rarely if ever obtained. In 1902, for instance, A. H.
Wentworth, a physician attached to Harvard's Pharmacological Laboratory, made two important discoveries when he analyzed samples of milk
from various Boston dairies as well as samples of formulas mixed by the local
milk laboratory. The first discovery was the tremendous variability in the
constituent elements of raw milk depending on the source. Also, as often as
not, the bottles of milk prepared by the milk laboratory did not agree with
the formulas that physicians had ordered. These discoveries led Wentworth
and others to argue that the supposed precision of percentage feeding was
largely mythical.[71]

Percentage feeding also came under attack as new European, and especially German, theories of infant feeding began filtering into the United States
in the first decade of the century. Although Biedert's research had provided
the foundation on which percentage feeding was built, European pediatric
researchers had never been as enamored with the mathematical manipulation of infant formulas as their American counterparts. Indeed, percentage
feeding was such a peculiarly American phenomenon that it was frequently
referred to as the American system. Thus, while pediatricians in the United
States were occupying themselves devising ever more intricate ways to
calibrate and control the constituent elements in infant foods, pediatricians
on the continent were conducting research in other areas. One such area
was infant metabolism and the caloric needs of the normal baby. Following
the 1898 publication of Max Rubner's and Otto Heubner's research into
infant metabolism, a large number of German pediatric researchers began
arguing that it was the caloric rather than the chemical content of infant
food which was critical for infant development. This argument directly
challenged the basic contention of Rotch and other proponents of percentage feeding that the amount of food given to an infant was much less a
determinant of infant survival than the chemical proportions of that food;

and was used by those American pediatricians who adopted the German findings to support criticism that percentage feeding was an elaborate, pseudoscientific hoax. Simultaneously, other German researchers were providing American critics with additional ammunition with which to challenge the basic premises of percentage feeding. In particular, a number of American pediatricians found confirmation of their growing disenchantment with percentage feeding in the theory advanced by Heinrich Finklestein that bottle-fed infant indigestion was not due to excess protein but rather to excess fat and to a lesser extent sugar. Although subsequently proven largely erroneous, Finklestein's ideas found ardent supporters in the United States, particularly among a group of Chicago pediatricians, including Isaac Abt and Joseph Brennemann, who were challenging the supremacy in infant feeding enjoyed by Rotch and his Boston- and New York-based followers.[72]

Also contributing to mounting disenchantment with percentage feeding was a revival of interest in encouraging breastfeeding, a revival influenced immensely by the work of Pierre Budin. Like other French pediatricians, and for that matter, like most continental pediatricians, Budin had never been as caught up as his American counterparts with the promise that improving artificial feeding might hold for reducing infant mortality. Convinced that artificial feeding represented more of a problem than a solution, he established in 1892 the first of a number of "consultation de nourrissons" designed to encourage poor mothers to breastfeed their newborns. Budin also carefully documented his work, and in so doing, not only provided persuasive evidence that breastfeeding could lower the incidence of infant digestive disorders but also inspired revision of the notion that few women were capable of successful nursing.[73]

As the second decade of the century opened, then, the influence that the percentage system had exerted on American pediatric theories of infant feeding was on the wane. And with the waning of that influence came the end of what had been a thirty-year obsession among American pediatricians with devising ever more precise and complicated infant formulas. Never again would pediatric theory place such a high premium on minute gradations in infant formulas. In retrospect it seems clear that the legacy of that thirty-year obsession was somewhat mixed. Even if the attempts of pediatric theorists to concoct finely tuned infant formulas had proven scientifically justified, their direct effect on the nation's infant mortality rate would still have been negligible. For such attempts produced formulas that were so expensive as to be out of the reach of all but the well-to-do. This was especially true of percentage feeding which, as Harvey Levenstein has recently observed, was "primarily the plaything of the Fifth Avenue and Beacon Hill physicians, who dominated pediatrics, and their well-to-do clients."[74] Few, if any, of the urban infant poor, who contributed such vast numbers to the yearly infant death tolls, ever had the experience of having the contents of their nursing bottles mixed in scientific laboratories accord' ing to algebraic calculations. Moreover, the emphasis that pediatric theory placed on the physician's control and manipulation of the four basic compo' nents of cow's milk initially tended to impede pediatric acceptance and support of pasteurization, the one form of milk modification which actually did hold promise for reducing gastroenteritis among the bottle'fed infants of the urban poor. Convinced that heating could alter the required proportions of the constituent elements in milk, most American pediatricians opposed pasteurization and sought to guarantee the cleanliness of milk supplies through other less effective methods.

Yet by making infant feeding a medically respectable field of research, the percentage system and other attempts to improve infant foods created an atmosphere in which scientific inquiry into the digestive and nutritional disorders of infancy received sufficient support to produce such significant breakthroughs as the 1915 discovery by John Howland and William Mar' riott that the frequent fatalities among infants with severe diarrhea were connected to the state of acidosis which the disorder produced.[75] Thus, even though much turn'of'the'century pediatric research into infant feeding led down dead ends and to the formulation of pseudoscientific theory, it also produced a number of medically significant results. More importantly, by emphasizing the crucial role that the quality of artificial food available played in infant survival, the late nineteenth'century pediatric preoccupa' tion with scientifically improving infant feeding gave unprecedented atten' tion to what infants were being fed, and in so doing helped transform the way that infant mortality, as a preventable social problem, was concep' tualized and approached. Although public health authorities and concerned physicians continued to view infant mortality as causally connected to urban poverty and to the filthy and overcrowded conditions in which many city poor lived, they came to see that connection as secondary in importance to that between infant death and infant feeding. Thus, the last two decades of the nineteenth and the first decade of the twentieth centuries saw the "milk question," as it came to be known, occupy an increasingly central place in America's ongoing battle to reduce urban infant mortality.

3

Pure Milk for Babes: Improving the Urban Milk Supply

In an 1874 talk before the American Public Health Association, Henry Hartshorne, Philadelphia's veteran sanitary reformer, observed that improper nutriment seemed about to displace foul air and inherited debility as the most commonly cited cause of urban infant mortality.[1] Hartshorne's observation was prophetic. In the last two decades of the nineteenth and the first decade of the twentieth centuries, pediatric promotion of the idea that improper nutriment was the primary cause of the yearly epidemics of infant summer diarrhea exerted a powerful influence on public health. And with good reason. Not only did it provide a specific scientific explanation of those epidemics, it also promised a solution to the dilemma that public health reformers had found themselves facing in their attempts to reduce mortality among urban infants. Made aware by their own statistics that infants of the poor contributed most heavily to the summer death roles, public health reformers had developed an explanation for this that rested on the assumption of an interaction between inherited constitutional weakness and the debilitating effects of a slum environment. The first of the interactive factors they traced to parental debility, which they proposed was the result of both environment and dissolute and unhygienic behavior. The second factor they traced to the filthy, crowded, and inhospitable environment in which poor urban infants were forced to battle for life. Reducing infant mortality, therefore, required significant behavioral and environmental reform. Both of these, however, proved extremely difficult to accomplish, and thus public health officials were left wondering whether infant mortality might ever be reduced.

Therein lay the attractiveness of the pediatric solution. While granting influence to inherited constitution and the physical environment, it defined improper nutriment as the single primary cause. If proper nutriment could be made available then the major cause of infant death could be removed and infant health so improved that the influence of the other causes could be resisted. As Baltimore pediatrician and Johns Hopkins professor J. H. Mason Knox observed, "notwithstanding the weakened condition with which many of these children are born into the world, notwithstanding the squalid environment amid which they must live their lives, that when their nourishment is suited to their needs, they are for the most part able to resist these yearly devastating epidemics."[2]

In directing their attention toward making available proper nutriment to urban infants, public health officials did not ignore that infants died in large numbers from diseases and developmental problems that were not specifically digestive or nutritional. They were well aware that each year bronchopneumonia, tuberculosis, inherited syphilis, whooping cough, and various congenital deficiencies killed thousands of infants. Nor did they abandon their work to control infectious disease and to improve parental health and tenement conditions. Sanitizing the urban environment and improving the health of the general population remained part of their program to reduce infant mortality. Yet they did shift their emphasis. After 1875, improving the quality of urban milk supplies increasingly came to dominate their efforts to save infant lives. The result was a pure milk campaign that went through two overlapping but essentially discrete stages. The first, having its origins earlier in the century but increasingly shaped by pediatric concern with the compositional integrity of milk fed to infants, centered on ensuring the chemical purity of urban milk supplies by protecting them from adulteration, dilution, and spoilage. The second, beginning in the 1890s, involved various efforts to prevent or rectify the microbial contamination of commercial milk.

In shifting the thrust of their battle to reduce infant mortality from improving the conditions in which infants were forced to live to improving the quality of the commercial milk available to them, American public health reformers did not so much discover a new issue as make central one that had long been peripheral. Concern that much of the milk sold in large cities was dangerous to drink had been voiced as early as the 1830s when temperance and other urban reformers first set their sights on outlawing the sale of swill milk; that is, milk produced by cows confined to sheds and fed on the watery waste product left over from the production of distilled spirits. Long common in England and on the continent, feeding swill to urban dairy herds did not become an established practice in the United States until the second quarter of the century, when shrinking urban pasturage and declining distillery revenues made it economically attractive for northeastern city dairymen to purchase swill and for distillers to sell it to them. So mutually beneficial was the arrangement that swill dairying quickly mushroomed. One contemporary observer estimated that by the late 1830s swill milk accounted for 50–80 percent of all milk consumed in America's large northeastern cities.[3] This economic relationship between urban distillers and swill dairying first attracted public criticism of swill milk. The source of this initial criticism was not infant health and welfare advocates but temperance reformers. Infant health did become an issue, but it did so primarily because it was strategically useful for temperance and subsequent reformers to make it one.

Undoubtedly the most passionate and visible temperance campaign against swill milk took place in New York City and was spearheaded by Robert Hartley, future head of the New York Association for Improving the Condition of the Poor. Elected in 1833 as corresponding secretary of the New York Temperance Association, Hartley set himself the task of denying New York distillers the income they derived from selling swill and renting cowsheds to dairymen. In 1842, after spending six years agitating against swill milk, Hartley published a detailed study of swill milk production in which he argued that outlawing swill dairying would not only cripple New York distilleries and mean "6,482,400 less gallons a year to corrupt mankind," but would also reduce mortality among the infants of the city's poor. Indeed, Hartley contended it was widespread consumption of swill milk that was the primary cause of New York's high infant death rate.[4]

Although Hartley's arguments attracted some support among the New York medical and reform community, their departure from prevailing medical theory and obvious temperance intent limited their public appeal and influence. After a constrained public outcry following publication of his study, the issue of swill milk seemed to disappear from the public consciousness. Five years later, however, it was back in the news when the New York Tribune published an exposé of one of the largest and filthiest of the swill milk stables and urged the city to act. This time, however, temperance was a tertiary issue, ranking behind public insanitation and municipal corruption. Goaded into action by the exposé, the New York Academy of Medicine formed a committee to investigate the possible health problems related to consumption of swill milk. Chaired by Augustus Gardner and including John Griscom, the committee charged that the filthy conditions of the stables made them health nuisances. It also speculated that swill milk might contribute to cholera infantum, but could not give a convincing reason why this was so. Perhaps because they did not want to take on the politically powerful distillery industry without more substantive proof and perhaps because they were unconvinced that food rather than filth and foul air was the major determinant of infant mortality, the academy chose neither to act nor even publish the committee report.[5]

Nevertheless, public concern with swill milk was mounting, and the 1850s saw a number of exposés on the problem published.[6] The most widely read and certainly most influential of these was a series of articles appearing in Frank Leslie's Illustrated Weekly Newspaper, beginning in the spring of 1858. Sensing an issue that would capture his readers' growing concern with both public health and municipal corruption, Leslie vividly portrayed in print and illustration the conditions prevailing in swill-cow dairies.[7] Joined by the *Times* and the *Tribune*, his campaign against the swill dealers ultimately forced both the Common Council and the Board of Health to launch investigations. The reports issued, however, were little more than whitewashes. Leslie therefore turned to the state legislature, which in 1862 finally passed a law prohibiting both the sale of unwholesome milk and the maintaining of swill stables.[8] Opponents of swill-milk dairying interpreted the New York law, as well as similar laws soon passed by other states, as sounding the death knell for swill milk The prognosis was correct, but the diagnosis was wrong. While the demise of swill dairying in the Northeast soon followed, it was brought about less by regulatory legislation than by changes in the region's agricultural production.

By the third and fourth decades of the century, northeastern crop farmers—especially those who grew wheat—were facing hard times. Soil depletion had significantly lowered their output per acre and competition from the western part of the state and from the Great Lakes region, which now could be reached by the Erie Canal, was eroding their share of the domestic and foreign markets. In response, many farmers sold off their land and migrated westward. Others, however, remained and turned to dairying. As a consequence, between 1830 and 1870, commercial dairying became a critically important part of northeastern agriculture.[9] Initially, the production of cheese dominated the developing dairy industry, in large part because cheese was less perishable and easier to ship to distant markets than fluid milk. By the 1860s, however, rail transport throughout the Northeast had improved to the point at which it was both economically and technologically possible for cities to import a significant amount of their milk supply from distant farmers.[10] Thus, the supply and quality of imported milk increased while its cost dropped. This development, rather than the regulatory effectiveness of the anti-swill-milk laws spelled the beginning of the end for distillery dairies as the major suppliers of milk consumed by urban infants.

Yet if the rise of the northeastern dairy industry and the concomitant increase of milk imported to cities served to ensure that urban infants would less frequently be condemned to consume milk from cows fed on distillery swill, they did not ensure that such infants would have available to them a healthful and nutritious supply of milk. Many rural cows were sick with tuberculosis or other communicable diseases that ultimately were transmitted to consumers, especially since rural dairymen took few sanitary precautions. They commonly milked cows whose flanks and udders were caked with mud and excrement that often fell into the milk.[11] If they washed milk pails and cans at all, they more often than not used dirty or contaminated water. They also allowed the cans to stand uncooled in barns or at roadside pickup points. Milk handlers did not do much better, initially transporting the milk in open wagons and unrefrigerated railroad cars. Once in the city, milk was often dispensed in loose or bulk form by grocers and street vendors from open cans, into which were dipped common ladles or containers.[12]

Moreover, as milk imported by rail from distant regions came to constitute an ever greater proportion of the urban milk supply, the number of middle-men who handled it on its journey from producer to consumer also in-creased. Heated competition, the irregularities of the milk supply, and the frequency with which milk still spoiled before it reached the city inspired many of these middlemen to stretch their supplies by skimming cream and adding water, and to mask spoilage by adding sugar, molasses, chalk, bicar-bonate of soda, and other adulterants.[13] Also, since the operations of the middlemen were much larger and more centralized than those of the individ-ual farmers from whom they purchased milk, they could and often did set prices that barely covered the cost of production. This in turn led farmers to cheat, by watering their milk, by skimming the cream off the top, and by allowing some of their evening milk to sit overnight so that it could fetch the slightly higher price paid for morning milk, which was thought to have a higher fat content.[14] Indeed, by the time milk reached city retailers, who were also not above sophisticating their wares, it often had only a faint resemblance to the substance produced by cows. It was, therefore, with caustic humor but no great inaccuracy that New York's health commissioner observed that in touring the city he frequently came upon a "decidedly suspicious-looking fluid bearing the name of milk."[15] Preventing adultera-tion and the masking of spoilage by the handlers of milk thus became the principal goal of infant health reformers and public health officials when they focused their attention on improving the urban milk supply as the most effective means of reducing urban infant mortality.

Adding to the attention that health reformers were increasingly giving to sophisticated milk was the concurrent growth of official and public concern over the adulteration of all commercial food products.[16] Although some such adulteration undoubtedly took place and was remarked upon before the Civil War, it seems to have increased dramatically in the last third of the century, encouraged both by the war-inspired reorganization of food pro-duction along industrial lines and by the anonymity afforded producers in the growing urban market.[17] Indeed, by the 1870s concern over the quality of American food was finding wide expression. In 1879, for instance, *Harper's Weekly* lamented that "the adulteration of food and drinks has become almost as general as the use of these articles themselves."[18] That same year, the newly formed National Board of Health created a standing committee on adulteration, and four years later the American Public Health Association declared that sophisticated foods represented one of the four most serious health hazards facing the nation.[19]

The increasing incidence of food adulteration and mounting public and official concern over it did not, however, automatically inspire a concerted effort by public health authorities to initiate and implement programs that would effectively regulate the commercial food supply. While such authorities tended to pay lip service to the need for regulatory measures that would prevent the production and sale of adulterated foods, they showed a notable reluctance to act in that direction. Although the 1870s had been a period of institutional advance for public health—witnessing as it did the creation of several independent boards of health—it had also been a period in which the actual regulatory powers of those boards had been severely curtailed by budgetary cuts necessitated by the depression that began in 1873. Responding to the need to reduce government expenditures in the face of falling tax revenues, New York City slashed the budget of its Department of Health in 1876 from $328,000 to $220,000. Nor was New York alone. Boards of health in Boston, Philadephia, and other major cities also suffered similar cutbacks.[20] Aware that they were facing sharp budgetary cuts and concerned that they would not be able even to maintain existing sanitary efforts, public health officials were rather reluctant to enter new regulatory areas.

Many public health officials also saw entry into the arena of food regulation as posing a threat to the progress they had lately made in acquiring a reputation for scientific expertise that removed them from the vagaries of moral and social reform. By the mid-1870s a new generation of officials was coming to power in municipal and state boards of health. Better trained than the pioneer generations of public health reformers and less inclined to look beyond science for causes and cures to public ill health, they increasingly positioned themselves as expert arbiters between social and moral reformers on one hand and city officials and business interests on the other. As arbiters, armed with increasingly complex sanitary theories, they could operate independently and be considerably more effective than had been their generalist predecessors. Consequently, they tended to shy away from areas of public health in which scientific theory was not sufficiently developed to allow them the maintenance of a pose of disinterested and expert objectivity.[21] Food adulteration was one such area. Although the sophistication of foods was generally conceded to be a problem, little hard evidence existed as to its extent and even less scientific theory was available explaining how and why common adulteration led to increased morbidity and mortality. Indeed, while generally sympathetic to the need for better food regulation, the new generation of public health officials often found themselves at loggerheads with popular food reformers because of the latter's reliance on what they considered to be speculation and hearsay.

The one exception to the general reluctance shown by public health officials to involve themselves in food regulation concerned the production and sale of milk.[22] By the 1870s food chemists and pediatricians had developed a substantial body of scientific theory connecting the chemical composition of milk to the adequate nutrition and survival of infants and very young children. Sophistication, whether through watering or through the addition of adulterants to mask spoilage, obviously altered that composition and could be scientifically proven to pose a distinct threat to infant health. As the 1870s progressed, an increasing number of public health officials were beginning to find substantial merit in the arguments of physicians such as Austin Flint, who contended, "there is reason to believe that infant mortality in cities is attributable in no small measure to the use of sophisticated and artificial milk."[23] Not untypical, for instance, was J. Chesterton Morris, who stood before the American Public Health Association and flatly declared that "if the adulteration of milk could be stopped, urban infant mortality would immediately drop by 20 to 25 percent."[24] It was no accident, then, that the anti-food adulteration bills passed by a number of states beginning in the early 1880s were in effect anti-milk adulteration bills. Massachusetts, for example, passed an anti-adulteration law in 1882 which stipulated that two-fifths of the appropriated funds go toward the safeguarding of milk. Two years later, when the initial $3,000 appropriation was raised to $10,000, the fraction of funds earmarked for milk protection was increased to three-fifths.[25]

Spurred on both by the perception that something specific had to be done to combat infant mortality and by mounting concern with food adulteration, public health officials thus set out to improve and regulate the urban milk supply. Between 1880 and 1895, twenty-three American municipalities passed or strengthened ordinances governing the sale of milk.[26] Yet enforcing such regulations was no easy matter. For one thing, the budgetary cutbacks of the 1870s had left municipal health departments short of personnel and without the manpower to inspect more than a fraction of the milk sold within city limits. For another, much of the watering, skimming, and adulteration of milk took place outside city limits, and therefore outside the jurisdiction of the various municipal health departments. Municipal authorities were thus largely limited to inspecting the supplies of retailers and imposing fines on them if adulteration was detected. Moreover, most of the anti-adulteration bills had provisions requiring that those fined must have knowingly sold adulterated milk. Not surprisingly, retailers often claimed they were the innocent victims of unscrupulous wholesalers. Finally, the technology for inspecting milk was initially quite primitive and easily circumvented.[27] Yet despite the enforcement and technological problems, a number of municipalities began passing milk ordinances in the 1880s which established milk solid percentages and forbade the sale of watered, adulterated, or skimmed milk. Indeed, by 1890 fourteen municipal health departments were regularly collecting samples of milk sold in their cities and arresting or fining violators.[28]

Not surprisingly, the milk ordinances adopted by American municipalities were resisted by milk dealers and retailers who challenged them both politically and in the courts. Moreover, they initially made only a small dent in the widespread practice of adulteration. Nevertheless, the milk ordinances served as a catalyst to a number of developments that ultimately led to effective municipal milk regulation. The court challenges that dealers and retailers mounted against health departments produced a series of federal and state court decisions that eventually established the power of city health officials to regulate the sale of milk within their municipal borders, even if it was produced outside. In 1896, after New York City's Board of Health put into effect a permit system for licensing dealers, its right to do so was challenged all the way to the U.S. Supreme Court. In 1905, the court decided in the city's favor, thereby affirming the legal right of officially constituted boards and departments of health to set standards for commercial milk and prohibit from commercial activity those who failed to meet the standards. The early inspections also established the percentage of solids milk contained as a criterion for compositional integrity. Thus, by 1905, thirty-two states, the District of Columbia, Hawaii, and Puerto Rico had adopted and were enforcing chemical composition standards as a means of improving the quality of their milk supplies.[29] Finally, the early inspections inspired the beginning of an alliance between health departments and large milk interests. In part, this alliance was the consequence of the latter's recognition that fighting milk regulation was proving futile. But it also resulted from their realization that strict enforcement of the regulations could drive into bankruptcy their small and underfinanced competitors. Thus, as the nineteenth century came to an end, the country's large milk producers and dealers began shifting their response to milk regulation from active opposition to selective support as a means of increasing their control and dominance of the urban milk market.[30]

By the first decade of the twentieth century, state and municipal regulations, enforced and promoted by the alliance of large milk interests and health departments, had for the most part succeeded in eliminating most of the more blatant forms of milk adulteration and had produced an urban milk supply that was chemically standardized. But they had not produced one that was particularly safe for infants to drink. Designed primarily to ensure the compositional integrity of milk by prohibiting watering and adulteration, the regulations did little if anything to address the more serious problem of bacterial contamination. Indeed, if watered milk had ever posed a serious threat to those who drank it, it was primarily because the water used was often contaminated. By the end of the century, however, with scientific

understanding of the biological etiology of disease growing more sophisticated, many public health reformers were becoming increasingly aware of
the inadequacy of the regulatory measures they had fought so long and hard
to get enacted. Especially among those with interest and training in the new
science of bacteriology, the conviction existed that the dangers of milk
sophistication had been widely exaggerated and had served to slow appreciation that even undoctored milk could be harmful if it was old and dirty.[31]
Articulating that conviction, New York's William Park declared in 1901:
"The most deleterious changes which occur in milk during transportation
are now known not to be due to skimming of cream or to the addition of
water, but to changes produced in the milk by the multiplication of bacteria."[32] Although the compositional integrity of milk remained a vital issue—
especially among pediatricians—by the turn of the century it was fast being
eclipsed by concern over the bacterial contamination and transformation of
milk.

While the bacterial contamination of milk did not become a significant
issue for public health reformers until the end of the nineteenth century,
suspicion that milk could cause and spread communicable disease had been
voiced for some time. Especially after 1854 when English physician John
Snow demonstrated that many of the victims of cholera in London that year
were subscribers to a single water company, medical researchers and sanitary reformers began to suspect that, along with air, various ingested foods
and liquids could act as mediums for the spread of disease. In 1857, for
instance, William Taylor traced seven typhoid cases in Penrith, England, to
milk from a single dairy; ten years later he did the same for an outbreak of
scarlet fever. Similarly, in 1870, Edward Ballard, then the medical officer of
health of the metropolitan district of Islington and later the MOH to the
Local Government Board (LGB), reported that he had found that the only
common thread linking 170 cases of typhoid was consumption of milk from a
single source.[33] Yet, as was the case in early research into the role water
played in spreading disease, the full implications of the initial investigations
linking epidemics to specific milk sources were not immediately appreciated
and did not dramatically alter prevailing approaches to the prevention of
communicable diseases. Most public health reformers continued to sub-
scribe to anti-contagionist and miasmatic etiologies and thus interpreted the
observed links between water and milk and various disease outbreaks as
further proof that miasma-producing filth, whatever the source, needed to
be eradicated. Hence, they incorporated the purification of water and milk
into their general programs of sanitary reform. The initial discoveries that
epidemics could be traced to water and milk did not, therefore, immediately
challenge existing medical wisdom that etiologically most disease was spon-
taneous and chemical rather than communicable and biological.

By the late 1860s, however, as medicine and public health were con-

fronted with the discoveries of Pasteur and other early bacteriologists, pa-
thologists, and microscopists, that wisdom slowly began to change.[34] In
England, William Farr altered his zymotic theory to incorporate the possibility of infection by organic particles, thereby transforming the scientific
foundation of the theory from chemistry to biology. Similarly, in the United
States, Elisha Harris, future founder and president of the American Public
Health Association and a leading proponent of Farr's original theory, found
the new biological evidence quite convincing and in 1867 observed that
"some of the worst zymotic diseases are accompanied and, perhaps, caused
by minute living organisms . . . that infest particular parts of the human
body."[35] For at least another decade, however, thinking about such disease-
causing microorganisms remained quite confused, with numerous competing theories being advanced. Contributing to this confusion were the limitations of existing research techniques. Despite technical innovations by Pasteur and his co-workers, it remained virtually impossible to obtain pure
cultures and thus to isolate specific bacterium and positively identify them
as the singular causes of specific diseases. In the late 1870s and early 1880s,
however, Robert Koch, until then a somewhat obscure German country
physician, developed techniques for cultivating bacteria in solid mediums
and for isolating them.[36] As a consequence, between 1877 and 1890 the
microorganisms causing malignant edema, typhoid, cholera, pneumonia, tuberculosis, diphtheria, and a number of other diseases were isolated and
identified, and medical researchers were able to develop and put forth a
demonstrable germ theory of disease causation.

This germ theory, of course, did not meet with immediate and universal
acceptance. Not only did it contradict still powerful chemical and anti-
contagionist explanations of disease causation and transmission, it also left
several questions initially unanswered. Demonstrating that specific microorganisms caused specific diseases did not explain the mechanics of microbial
infection. How was such infection produced, how was it transmitted, and
what were the best means of preventing it and treating its consequences?
Several decades would pass before medical researchers provided satisfactory
answers to these questions and quieted debate over the germ theory. Nevertheless, the initial discoveries that specific diseases could be traced to
identifiable microorganisms did have an immediate and profound effect on
public health, spawning the new sciences of bacteriology and immunology
and serving to transfer the locus of much public health work from the field to
the laboratory.

By employing the techniques developed by Koch, sanitarians gained a
replicable and potentially standardizable method of determining pollution
and thus no longer had to rely on vague and often sensory measures of filth.
In short, the microscope came to replace the nose as the sanitarian's chief
instrument of detection. Moreover, the isolation and identification of

disease-causing microbes and the consequent production of antitoxins not only seemed to promise an effective means of controlling communicable disease, it also provided public health reformers with a strategy and ration- ale for sustaining the elevation of their activities above the mire of social and moral reform. If disease could be defined as associated with environment and personal hygiene but specifically caused by the intrusion of microbes, then morbidity could be controlled and mortality reduced without necessitating wide-scale social reorganization or behavioral reform.

Microscopic enumeration of bacteria in various mediums also worked to undermine the still extant conviction that polluted and vitiated air was a primary cause of disease. In less than a decade it was empirically shown that many of the organisms identified as pathogenic were not released into the atmosphere from moist surfaces, were not unduly present in expired air, and for that matter did not survive long when aerated. As a consequence, sani- tarians increasingly turned their attention to other mediums of transmission, particularly water. In 1885 English sanitarians began testing London's water for bacterial count, and two years later German sanitarians began doing the same for Berlin's water. In the United States the first systematic monitoring of bacteria present in a public water supply was conducted by William Sedgwick at the Lawrence Experiment Station established by the Massa- chusetts Board of Health in 1887. Sedgwick, a trained biologist, came to the station in 1888 and over the next four years developed techniques for mea- suring and filtering bacteria in water supplies. Widely copied by other states, many of which sent observers to the Lawrence station, Sedgwick's methods became standard practice in the United States by the turn of the century.[37]

As a carrier of pathogenic bacteria, milk was somewhat slower than water to attract the attention and efforts of public health officials. A commercially produced and marketed foodstuff, it was never as completely under the jurisdiction of boards of health as was water and was therefore not as easily tested. Still, concern that pathogens in milk were also capable of producing epidemic disease gradually mounted, especially after 1881 when Edward Hart read before the International Medical Congress in London a paper on the role that milk played in spreading zymotic diseases. Having meticulously gathered together all existing published investigations linking milk to out- breaks of communicable disease, Hart presented evidence describing fifty epidemics of typhoid, fifteen of scarlet fever, and four of diphtheria—all traceable to milk.[38]

Widely reported in medical and public health journals, Hart's paper inspired a rash of epidemiological studies seeking to link milk to various outbreaks of disease. Even in the United States, where epidemiology was neither as well developed nor as well funded as it was in England and on the continent, researchers began looking into the dangers posed by milkborne diseases. In 1883, for instance, a Pennsylvania doctor, citing the influence of Hart, published a report—the first of its kind in the United States—linking forty cases of typhoid in Allegheny City to a single dairy where workers were infected with the disease and where an overflowing privy stood less than fifty feet from a well that supplied water for washing milk containers. Over the next ten years, numerous other reports were published linking milk not only to typhoid but also to epidemics of scarlet fever and diphtheria.[39] Simultaneously, bacteriologists were isolating and cultivating the germs of bovine tuberculosis, thereby giving substance to long held suspicion that milk might be capable of transmitting that disease to humans.[40]

The general public also was slowly waking to the possible connection between milk and epidemic disease, especially after 1895 when a severe and widely reported epidemic of typhoid broke out in Stamford, Connecticut, infecting 386 of the city's 15,000 inhabitants. Since most of the infected were under ten years of age, health authorities immediately suspected milk as the transmitter of the disease, a suspicion that they subsequently proved. Later that year, similar outbreaks were reported in Providence and Buffalo, and public health researchers in Michigan, New York, and Washington, D.C., began compiling and publishing reports enumerating hundreds of milkborne epidemics.[41] At the same time the popular press discovered that milk could be a carrier of disease, and a number of articles appeared warning of the danger and emphasizing that, unlike waterborne typhoid epidemics, those spread by milk were not largely confined to the poor.[42]

As evidence mounted that milk was frequently a transmitter of infectious disease microbes, public health officials felt compelled to act, but were frustrated by a number of difficult scientific, technical, and operational problems. It was one thing to trace an epidemic outbreak back to a particular milk supply, but quite another to determine prior to such an outbreak whether a supply of milk was contaminated. The effects of dilution, the tremendous number of bacteria present in even relatively fresh milk, and the morphological similarity of a number of milkborne pathogenic and nonpathogenic organisms, made the process of detection extremely difficult and time consuming.[43] Indeed, when possible at all, it required at least twenty-four hours and was therefore relatively useless as a field technique for testing a batch of milk before it reached consumers. Public health officials thus found themselves in the exasperating position of being able to act with certainty only after a milkborne epidemic had begun and had done significant damage. What preventive action they could take was largely limited to testing cows for tuberculosis and to monitoring producers and handlers in the hope of preventing contact between infected persons and the milk supply. But given the tremendous number of dairies, dealers, and retailers involved in supplying a city with its milk, this was never a truly effective solution. Moreover, with typhoid, the milkborne epidemic disease they most worried about, even an outwardly healthy person could be a carrier of infectious microbes.

More significantly, even if public health officials had possessed the capa- bility of effectively controlling milkborne communicable diseases, they would have put only a small dent in the morbidity and mortality of those who suffered most from contaminated milk. Only a small portion of infant morbidity and mortality was attributable to epidemic diseases caused by specific microbes. In 1885, for instance, the proportion of infant deaths in New York City attributable to such diseases was only 7.6 percent, and in 1900, 5 percent.[44] In short, rather than dying from diseases such as typhoid, which could be traced to a specific and known microbe, the large numbers of infants who succumbed each year to summer diarrhea seemed to be dying from gastroenteric response to infection from still unspecified and unidenti- fied microbes.

If public health reformers were unable to identify the specific bac- teriologic causes of summer infant diarrhea, it was not because bacteriolo- gists and other medical researchers had shown no interest in doing so. At least since 1885, when Austrian pediatrician Theodore von Escherich pub- lished a study of the bacterial flora of the infant intestine, American medical investigators had been attempting to isolate and identify the bacterium or bacteria responsible for the summer epidemics. Through the 1890s William Booker conducted a number of influential studies, using infants from Bal- timore's Thomas Wilson Sanitarium. Soon after it was founded in 1901, the Rockefeller Institute of Medical Research also sponsored an ambitious and wide-ranging investigation aimed at discovering the specific bacterial cause of summer infant diarrhea. And between 1902 and 1904, other physicians at the Thomas Wilson Sanitarium explored the relationship between infant ileocolitis, or bloody diarrhea, and the groups of bacilli that Kiyoshi Shiga had in 1898 connected to dysentery.[45]

The results of these and other investigations were, however, anything but definitive. Booker, like Escherich before him, increased medical knowledge of the bacteria that existed in healthy and sick children, but was unable to pinpoint one type as the cause of the summer diarrheal outbreaks. Although he showed a willingness to speculate, he was forced to conclude that "no specific micro-organism is found to be the specific exciter of summer diar- rhoea of infants."[46] The report published by the Rockefeller Institute was similarly tentative, as was that produced by the other Wilson Sanitarium study. Indeed, although after 1910 researchers increasingly pointed to the contamination of food with E. coli bacilli, they never developed any hard proof.

Convinced that the summer epidemics of infant diarrhea were caused by bacterially contaminated milk, yet hampered by their inability to identify or isolate the specific microbe or microbes, bacteriologists and like-minded medical researchers initially focused their attention on the changes that bacterial multiplication produced in milk. Building on Pasteur's demonstration that the souring of milk was caused by living microbes, they speculated that such souring was the result of bacterial contamination, was akin to fermentation or putrefaction, and involved the chemical production of poisonous toxins. They therefore reasoned that the older milk was the more likely it was to be toxic and capable of producing gastroenteric disorders in infants who drank it.

Between 1890 and 1903 Herbert W. Conn, a bacteriologist connected to the Connecticut Agricultural Experiment Station at Storrs, identified a large number of bacteria commonly found in milk, showed that bacterial multiplication attended souring, and demonstrated that if milk was not cooled soon after it was drawn, the bacteria within multiplied rapidly and could number in the millions per single cubic centimeter after twenty-four hours.[47] Prompted by the research of Conn and other bacteriologists, public health reformers began proposing that urban milk be tested for the number of bacteria it contained as a means of detecting whether it was old and dirty and had been handled unhygienically. "Counting the number of bacteria," argued Providence's Charles Chapin, "will tell whether or not milk has been properly cared for. Few bacteria means sanitary conditions and cold milk, large numbers of bacteria mean dirty conditions and milk not properly cooled."[48]

In 1892 William Sedgwick and John L. Batchelder conducted the first such test in the United States. After analyzing samples from Boston's milk supply, they reported that the number of bacteria they found ranged from 708,000 to over 4,000,000 per cubic centimeter. Four years later Maud Frye collected samples of milk delivered to consumers in Buffalo and found that the bacterial count ranged from 48,000 to over 44,000,000. At about the same time Herman Biggs, who had created and was the head of New York City's pioneering Bacteriological Diagnostic Laboratory, initiated research into bacteria in the city's milk. In 1901 one of his assistants, William Park, published an influential paper recounting that research and recommending that municipal health departments be granted the authority to regulate the bacterial count in commercially marketed milk. Two years later George W. Goler, Rochester's health commissioner, made the same recommendation; but like Park's it received little support from municipal authorities and was opposed by the milk industry.[49]

In opposing bacterial testing of milk, industry spokesmen argued with some justification that no accepted and standardized methods existed for such testing and that experts disagreed as to why, in what number, and to whom bacteria in milk was dangerous. Any type of enumeration that could be done in the field was closer to gross estimating than accurate counting. Moreover, since milk, even with large numbers of bacteria, was daily consumed by many adults and children with no apparent ill effect, the mere presence of such numbers hardly seemed justification for declaring a batch of milk dangerous to the public health. Granting the relative validity of indus-try objections, proponents of bacterial testing argued that it represented an inexpensive and comparatively reliable way of determining whether or not milk was old and putrid. They also contended that experience had shown that such milk was deadly to infants who consumed it. Admitting that "our knowledge is yet insufficient to state just how many bacteria must be accu-mulate to make them noticeably dangerous in milk," Park nevertheless advised that "we have only to refer to universal clinical experience that a great number of children in cities sicken on milk supplied in summer, and those put on milk which is sterile or contains few bacteria mend rapidly, while those kept on impure milk continue ill or die."[50] This, of course, was not a new idea. As early as 1879, James Curtis, writing in Alfred Buck's much used reference work, A Treatise on Hygiene and Public Health, conjec-tured that it was not foul air but rotten food, and especially old and soured milk, that was primarily responsible for the epidemics of infant summer diarrhea in the nation's cities.[51] Yet the discovery that such milk was laden with bacteria gave new specificity and authority to this conjecture.

Researchers also soon provided an explanation why bacteria-laden milk had a particularly devastating effect on infants, theorizing that the imma-ture digestive systems of those under one year were exceptionally sensitive to bacteria and their byproducts. Even if the various species of bacteria in a particular milk supply were by themselves not pathogenic and even in great quantity did not represent a danger to older children and adults, their presence in large number was sufficient to cause life-threatening reactions among infants who consumed them. As Milton Roseneau, director of the Hygienic Laboratory of the U.S. Marine Hospital and Public Health Ser-vice, explained,

> So far as numbers are concerned, they need not greatly alarm us, for we know that disease is due to agencies and conditions other than merely the presence of enor-mous numbers of bacteria. By universal consent, however, milk containing exces-sive numbers of bacteria is unsuitable for infant feeding. The tender mucous membrane of infants is very susceptible to bacteria and their products, and a large proportion of the summer complaints of infants has been traced to the use of bacteria laden milk.[52]

The preservation of the nation's infants was thus seen as demanding that safe numerical levels be set, that testing procedures be standardized, and that regulations be created and enforced. Yet the development, standardiza-tion, and implementation of such procedures was relatively slow in coming. Not until 1905 did the laboratory section of the American Public Health

Association establish a committee to undertake the preparation of the first "Standard Report on Bacterial Methods for the Examination of Milk"; and not until 1910 did the committee issue its report.[53] In the meantime, urban milk reformers experimented with and heatedly debated various approaches to ensuring that urban infants had a clean and nutritious supply of milk available to them.

Commonly referred to as the "milk question," the turn-of-the-century debate on milk reform was fueled by a widening perception that a half-century of effort by public health officials to improve the urban milk supply had not been as effective as hoped. Although urban swill dairies had been outlawed, various anti-adulteration regulations passed, and milk inspection initiated by a number of cities and states, the quality of commercial milk available in urban areas remained deplorable, primarily because the methods of production and handling continued to be unsanitary. As William Sedgwick observed in 1892,

[milk] is usually drawn from animals in stables which will not bear description in good society, from cows which often have flaking excrement all over their flanks, by milkmen who are anything but clean. It is drawn into milk pails which are seldom or never thoroughly cleansed, sent to the city, where it is still further delayed and finally delivered to the consumer in a partially decomposed condition.[54]

Yet, while increasingly aware of the importance of improving the hygiene of milk production and handling, those involved in debate on the milk question also recognized the difficulty of doing so. How could urban and state health departments even begin to monitor and regulate the myriad sources from which a city's milk supply typically came and the numerous channels through which it flowed? By the turn of the century, New York City's milk supply, for instance, came from 35,000 dairies situated in five different states, passed through 400 processors and over 12 lines of transportation, and was handled by 150 wholesalers and 12,000 retailers.[55] Indeed, the size of the task seemed mind-boggling. Nevertheless, some milk reformers, joined by those land-grant university scientists involved in the scientific dairying movement, continued to argue that through education, government regulation, and economic incentive, a revolution in the milk industry could be effected. Others, however, disagreed. Although they granted the ultimate necessity of revolutionizing the milk industry, they saw that as taking decades to accomplish. Thus, they argued, solving the milk problem demanded more immediate remedial measures.

One such measure was developed in the 1890s and involved the establishment of milk stations or depots in city tenement districts. The stated purpose of such stations was to reduce the diarrheal deaths suffered by the urban poor. Operating for the most part during the dangerous summer months, the stations provided tenement mothers with free or subsidized milk that was often pasteurized and, initially at least, modified into infant formula. The idea for the creation of such stations had been broached as early as 1881, when Abraham Jacobi had recommended in print that philanthropists set up milk depots "where the poor could buy clean milk at a fair price."[56] Eleven years passed, however, before Jacobi could find a philanthropist willing to act on his recommendation. In 1892 he convinced Nathan Straus, of the New York merchant family, that such a depot would do much to save the city's infants. The following year Straus opened on the Lower East Side the first of his many milk stations. Technically, the Straus station was not really the first milk depot opened in the United States. In 1889 Dr. Henry Koplick set up a milk depot at New York's Good Samaritan Dispensary. But unlike Straus's stations, Koplick's was designed to serve a rather narrow therapeutic function and limited its provision of milk to those sick babies being treated at the dispensary. It was, then, only with the appearance of the Straus station that the philanthropic dispensing of milk to poor urban infants can really be said to have begun. Moreover, Straus, with his money and his zeal for publicizing his work, was the true catalyst for the proliferation of milk stations throughout urban America.

The original Straus station began operation just as the Panic of 1893 was increasing the misery of thousands of impoverished New Yorkers. In its first year, it dispensed 34,400 feeding bottles of pasteurized milk, modified according to a few basic formulas provided by Jacobi and Rowland G. Freeman, another New York pediatrician active in infant welfare work among the poor. Within two years, a half million bottles were being dispensed; within ten, 1.8 million; and within fifteen, over four million. In 1895, to meet the increasing demand, Straus erected a central pasteurizing plant that served as a model for the numerous others he eventually donated to various philanthropic groups throughout the country. He also opened more milk stations in New York and by 1910 was funding the operation of eighteen, eight of which remained open year round.[57] Because of his passionate advocacy of the then controversial and still primitive pasteurization process, his ill-hidden and impatient contempt for its opponents, and his tendency to claim for himself the lion's share of credit for reducing infant mortality in New York, Straus aroused a good deal of hostility, especially from the medical profession. Indeed, so bitter did the attacks become that in 1910 Straus threatened to close his stations and was dissuaded from doing so only by a massive public outcry, that included popular demonstrations, newspaper editorials, and a resolution passed by the Board of Aldermen imploring him to keep the stations open. For the most part, however, Straus and his work attracted more praise than criticism and provided inspiration to a wide variety of philanthropic organizations to establish similar stations throughout urban America. A 1910 survey conducted by the United States Marine Hospital and Public Health Service revealed that milk stations had been opened and were being operated, chiefly by private agencies, in thirty cities. Three years later, 297 stations in thirty-eight cities were providing milk to poor babies.[58]

Municipal health departments also began opening milk stations, although they did it later and to a lesser extent than philanthropies. Rochester was the first to do so. In 1897, with $300 and the services of two volunteer nurses, the health department began operating a milk station during the summer months. Subsequently, it opened three other stations.[59] New York City, however, provided the most substantial government support. In 1906 the need for such support was raised at a conference on milk reform sponsored by the New York Association for Improving the Condition of the Poor (NYAICP), the New York Academy of Medicine, and the Health Department. Soon after, John Spargo, a socialist and child welfare advocate, published a letter in the New York Times calling for the city to take responsibility for funding and operating milk stations. Others in the New York infant and child welfare community quickly took up Spargo's call; and in May 1907 the Board of Aldermen voted funds for the erection of seven seasonal milk stations. The resolution, however, required that the stations be operated with funds provided by private charities. Not satisfied with this limited support, infant welfare advocates continued to lobby the city, and in 1910 the municipal government appropriated $40,000, that allowed the Department of Health to set up fifteen stations the following year. These soon multiplied in number, and by 1914 the department's Division of Child Hygiene was operating fifty-six stations throughout the city.[60]

Becoming a fixture in the swarming tenement districts of America's turn-of-the-century cities, milk stations were a highly visible symbol of the nation's growing determination to reduce its urban infant mortality rate and played a significant role in shaping how that determination would manifest itself in the early decades of the twentieth century. Initially, most of the organizations that followed Straus's example and established milk stations were already existing charities, that took on milk work as an extra burden. Diet kitchens, settlement houses, children's aid societies, and various women's clubs: all, and independently of each other, set up milk stations in poor neighborhoods. Although the varied sponsorship made this charitable activity highly decentralized and occasionally duplicative, it also made it an ideal point of entry for the equally decentralized social welfare community to involve itself in infant health work. Prior to this point, reform activity aimed at reducing infant mortality had largely been dominated by the public health and medical communities. After 1900, however, and especially after 1910, social welfare and charity workers became increasingly involved; and as they did so their ideas and practices exerted a major influence on the way

Americans conceptualized and attempted to ameliorate the problem of infant mortality. Moreover, between 1905 and 1910, when the various charitable organizations supporting milk stations began joining together to form centralized "baby milk funds," they created an organizational network of welfare activists who served as one of the core cadres in what soon evolved into a multifaceted and socially oriented infant welfare campaign.

Yet the actual influence that milk stations had on reducing urban infant mortality must be judged as being from the beginning rather limited. Although they gave away or sold at a reduced price millions of bottles of clean and nutritionally sound milk, they supplied only an infinitesimal fraction of the milk consumed each year by the nation's urban infants. Also, while a few of the poor mothers who visited the stations were steady customers, most were not. Since only a single day's supply was dispensed at a time and often this could be picked up only by the mother, feeding an infant exclusively on milk station milk posed significant logistical problems. Even for those mothers who were not employed outside the home, a visit to a milk station was time consuming and often required arranging for a neighbor or someone else to watch the other children. Indeed, the common pattern seems to have been for tenement mothers to use the milk stations sporadically, or to seek out station milk only if their infants became sick. Consequently, despite the great number of nursing bottles dispensed or sold, only rarely was an urban infant after weaning fed solely the aseptic and nutritionally balanced milk available at the stations. Most milk reformers seemed quite aware of the limitations of milk stations. Although they gave them their avid support, they were forced to concede that even if such stations doubled or tripled in number, they would not solve what remained the critical problem: the inferior quality of the entire urban milk supply. Thus, while milk reformers promoted the proliferation of milk stations in the nation's cities, they also continued to debate how the quality of the milk supply might best be improved.

Although many approaches to solving the milk problem were proposed between 1890 and 1910, two attracted the greatest attention and support. The first was essentially preventive. Its aim was to guarantee a clean and nutritious supply of raw milk by establishing medical milk commissions to oversee production and handling. Proposed in 1893 by Henry L. Coit, a Newark physician, it developed into what was commonly referred to as the certified milk movement and attracted the ardent support of pediatricians and other physicians whose private practices included treating infants. The second was essentially remedial and aimed at purifying the existing milk supply through the application of heat immediately before sale or consumption. Developing into a campaign for home and commercial pasteurization, this approach found its greatest support among sanitarians.

The two approaches, however, were not mutually exclusive. Nor was the division between pediatricians and sanitarians hard and fast. Advocates of purified milk were quick to acknowledge that certified milk was a superior product. Furthermore, not all public health departments and individual sanitarians were in favor of pursuing the expedient of milk purification. Both the Massachusetts State Board of Health and the Boston Health Department long resisted all entreaties that they consider requiring pasteurization. Similarly, New York's Elias Bartley and Rochester's George Goler adamantly opposed purifying milk, arguing that to do so would undo much of the good that preventive milk regulation had accomplished.[61] Nor were all pediatricians opposed to milk purification and in favor of milk certification. Few proponents of pasteurization were as passionate in their support as was Abraham Jacobi. Nevertheless, the division between the two approaches and their advocates was quite substantial and served to polarize turn-of-the-century milk reform.

What we now call "pasteurization"—that is, the process in which milk is heated to a temperature of approximately 145°F (62.8°C), held there for approximately thirty minutes and then rapidly cooled to below 50°F—was not perfected until the early part of this century.[62] But the basic principle and technique date back to the 1860s when Pasteur discovered that if wine and beer were heated to a temperature between 158°F and 178°F, the microbes that caused spoilage would be killed. Not long afterward, European wine and beer producers began heating their products to prevent spoilage and termed the process *pasteurization*.[63] At the same time a number of European physicians, especially in France and Germany, began recommending that cow's milk purchased for infant feeding should be "cooked" or boiled to prevent it from souring and upsetting infant digestion with its acidity. Although Jacobi had long advised that "cow's milk ought to be cooked at once in order to keep it as long as possible from turning sour,"[64] the practice was slow to reach the United States because a number of objections existed to such cooked or sterilized milk. One was that it tasted and looked strange, a consequence of the applied heat caramelizing the milk sugar. Another was based on the widespread belief that boiling or sterilizing milk chemically changed and nutritionally depleted it. In 1886, however, Franz von Soxhlet, a German chemist, developed an apparatus and a method for the purification of milk which purportedly did not substantially alter its taste or chemical composition and which was said to kill most of the bacteria present. Introduced to Americans by Jacobi in 1889, it immediately excited great interest among pediatricians and others devoted to improving infant feeding as a means of reducing infant mortality.[65]

That interest, however, was short-lived. Percentage feeding was coming into vogue and with it the conviction that even the slightest chemical alteration of milk represented a danger to infants. By the latter half of the 1890s, even those pediatricians who were not devotees of percentage feeding, were commonly voicing opposition to purifying milk with heat. As Arthur V. Meigs—a staunch critic of percentage feeding—observed in his 1896 textbook on infant feeding: "The sterilization of milk has been vaunted very much in recent years. . . . But latterly there seems to be a tendency to the general agreement that so high a temperature produces changes which render the milk less desirable as a food for infants, if it is not put in a condition to be positively injurious."[66] Two years later, Rowland Freeman confirmed Meigs' observation, reporting that a survey he took of his fellow pediatricians revealed a "remarkable unanimity of opinion in favor of raw milk and opposed to purified milk."[67] Over the next two decades, pediatric opinion changed, especially as an improved pasteurization process replaced sterilization and boiling. But it changed slowly. Polling the members of the American Pediatric Society in 1912, John Lovett Morse discovered that over half still believed that babies did not thrive well on pasteurized milk and that such milk could lead to infant digestive disorders.[68]

Generally hostile to milk purification, pediatricians saw as the best solution to the milk question the plan devised by Coit for securing and certifying a superior grade of raw milk. After losing an infant son to contaminated milk in 1887, Coit embarked upon what became a lifelong campaign to make safe raw milk available for the feeding of infants.[69] In 1890, he succeeded in getting the New Jersey State Medical Society to establish a committee dedicated to improving the urban milk supply. For two years, that committee, which consisted of forty-one physicians beside Coit, investigated the milk question and lobbied state and municipal governments for stricter and more effective regulation of producers and handlers. The committee's efforts, however, were largely unsuccessful, and Coit became convinced that reform would not come about through government regulation. He thus proposed a plan by which private commissions of physicians would contract with a dairyman and oversee the production of a clean and nutritionally sound supply of raw milk. Coit's plan quickly gained support among Newark area physicians and within four months an Essex County Medical Milk Commision was formed. Less than two months later, a dairy was put under contract.[70]

In accordance with Coit's proposal, the first medical milk commission was voluntary, made up entirely of physicians, and was charged with the responsibility of minutely regulating the production of milk at the dairy with which it had contracted. The contract dictated what the dairy's herds could be fed, how they could be housed, and what methods and implements could be used to milk them. In addition, it prohibited the use of animals proven or suspected to be sick, established strict standards for the cooling and shipment of the milk, set percentages for chemical composition, and required that delivered milk contain no more than 10,000 bacteria per cubic centimeter. In return for satisfying these requirements, the dairy was allowed to advertise its milk as certified and therefore get a price for it that was considerably higher than that of regular commercial raw milk. Within a short time the Essex County Medical Milk Commission was attracting a good deal of attention, especially from private physicians involved in pediatric work. In 1896 the New York County Medical Society established its own medical milk commission, and the following year the Philadelphia Medical Society did the same. Other medical societies soon followed suit, and by 1906 thirty-six medical milk commissions had been founded throughout the nation.[71]

In promoting milk certification, Coit and its other proponents contended that production and handling, closely monitored by milk commissions, offered the best promise for improving the urban milk supply. In actuality, however, the promise of milk certification was much more limited. By publicizing the critical value of hygienically produced milk and by showing that it could be provided to those willing to pay extra, it did spawn among the middle and upper classes a demand for quality milk and, as a consequence, encouraged the construction of at least a few model dairies to meet that demand. Milk certification also provided pediatricians with what they had long desired: a supply of milk carefully regulated for cleanliness and chemical content and therefore suitable for those infants under their care. Constituting the majority of the membership of the medical milk commissions, pediatricians seemed to see their voluntary services as one way to ensure the availability of a supply of milk appropriate for clinical use.

Yet certified milk's accomplishments were also its failures. The rigid criteria necessary for certification and the emphasis that medical milk commissions put on new equipment and new facilitites tended to place the average dairy outside the pale of possible reform and to discourage rather than encourage general improvement in dairying methods. As milk reformer Charles North recalled in 1921,

> The certified milk movement created a powerful impulse towards expensive barns, cow stables, and milk houses, and expensive barn and dairy equipments. Sentiment was strongly towards the idea that only model dairies could produce milk of high sanitary character, and that because model dairies were out of the reach of rank and file dairymen, the rank and file could not be expected to produce a very sanitary milk.[72]

Indeed, not until after 1908, when North and others began demonstrating that the critical factor in producing clean milk was the methods employed rather than the equipment used, did reform of the average American dairy begin. The emphasis on equipment and facilities also made certified milk extremely expensive and therefore severely limited its use. Selling for 60–100 percent more than noncertified milk, it was far too dear for purchase by the average urban consumer, and way out of reach for the poor whose infants made up such a large proportion of the yearly infant mortality. Even at the height of its popularity, certified milk represented only the very top layer of the urban milk supply. Of the 1,500,000 quarts of milk daily consumed by New Yorkers in 1908, certified milk accounted for no more than 16,000.[73] Certified milk may have saved some lives, but it did so primarily among the small class of prosperous urbanites who could afford it.

The development of certified milk also tended to channel the energy of pediatrics away from more general reform of the urban milk supply. By meeting pediatricians' stringent demands for clinical usage, it fulfilled their professional needs and satisfied what had been a major impulse behind their calls for reform of the milk supply. Despite the lip service they paid to improving all milk, most proponents of certified milk placed particular emphasis on its appropriateness for feeding infants under the care of a physician. This is quite clear in Coit's original proposal, which, significantly, was entitled, "A Plan to Secure Cow's Milk Designed for Clinical Purposes."[74] Indeed, in 1898 Coit wrote to a colleague that he was "only committed to [certified milk] insofar as it is a factor in pediatrics."[75] Because of this emphasis, the pediatric advocates of certified milk were rather rigid in protecting to the letter requirements for certification and were, by and large, opposed to any alternative or compromise proposals that would produce milk in any way compositionally inferior to that which was certified. Despite mounting evidence that certified milk would never supply more than a fraction of the public's needs, many pediatricians continued through the first decade of the twentieth century to hold it up as the ideal against which all other proposals must necessarily be found wanting.

If prevailing pediatric theory and the requirements and character of private practice tended to marshal the support of pediatricians behind the production of a qualitatively superior but severely limited supply of raw milk, the responsibility for effecting a widespread diminution of the urban infant death rate tended to push public health sanitarians toward advocating milk purification. Especially for those cheaper grades of milk that were commonly purchased by the poor, milk purification seemed to represent the most promising course. While acknowledging that guaranteeing the availability of pure and fresh raw milk would more effectively reduce infant mortality, sanitarians contended that for the time being this was impossible. Both the cost of producing such milk and the intransigence of the milk industry made it highly unlikely that good raw milk would soon be affordable and available in large quantities. "Pure milk may be better than purified milk," observed public health official Leslie Lunsden, "but can pure milk be obtained in sufficient quantity to supply our large cities, and at what cost?"[76] For sanitarians, the obvious answer was no. They also contended that comparison of purified milk to certified milk was misleading, arguing that the real comparison should be between purified milk and the lower grades of raw milk which constituted the bulk of most cities' milk supplies and were still sold out of open cans and carried home by the consumer in a bucket or similar container.[77] Such milk, the tests by Sedgwick, Park, and others had shown, was old, stale, and incredibly laden with bacteria. Any improvement would thus represent a dramatic gain and undoubtedly save infant lives.

Joining sanitarians in the promotion of milk purification was a small group of philanthropists and pediatricians involved in infant welfare work. Of the former, probably the most visable and influential was Straus, who was the person perhaps most responsible for New York City's adopting a compulsory pasteurization ordinance in 1912. Unflagging in his support of the process, Straus lobbied nationally and internationally for its adoption and impatiently brushed aside the objections of its critics. His message was simple and issued over and over again: "Pasteurization destroys all the germs of disease that may be in the milk but does not impair the taste, digestibility or nutritive qualities of milk."[78] Straus's chief ally in the medical profession was Abraham Jacobi, whose social conscience and medical pragmatism continued to distinguish him from many of his pediatric colleagues.[79] Indeed, Jacobi was a constant thorn in the sides of percentage feeders and those pediatricians who largely limited their concern with the milk supply to supporting the creation of certified model dairies. In particular, Jacobi was fond of castigating Rotch, who had come out against Straus's plan for compulsory pasteurization. In a 1906 essay that appeared in *Charities and the Commons*, as well as in several medical journals, Jacobi condemned those who seemed only concerned with supplying the prosperous with milk, noting that "democratic nature knows no difference in class." Then, taking one of his many swipes at Rotch, he sardonically observed: "It is true that a great Boston pediatrist has blamed New Yorkers for insisting on supplying poor and rich alike, and thereby rendering solution of the feeding problem more difficult."[80]

But Jacobi was not the only pediatrician promoting milk purification. Although support for the process was rare among infant and childhood specialists, it did exist, especially among those who were involved in fighting infant mortality among the poor. Perhaps typical was J. H. Mason Knox, medical superintendent and director of the Wilson Sanitarium for Infants and Children and founder of the philanthropic Baltimore Babies' Milk Association.[81] Committed to improving the health of the urban infant poor, Knox never tired of reproving his fellow pediatricians for devoting too much of their science and clinical efforts to the needs of their prosperous private patients. Writing on the responsibility that pediatrics had to all infants, he complained that too often the chief beneficiaries of advances in pediatric science were the "tiny heirs of comfort and luxury." For them, he noted, special scales and fabrics had been developed. If bottle fed, "a milk of the first quality is procured, which has been produced by carefully selected cows, under conditions bordering on surgical asepsis, and modified in sterile ves-sels with boiled water under the direction of a physician." Yet such babies, he observed, made up only a small percentage of the urban infant population and "don't contribute much to the death statistics." Hence, he concluded, if urban infant mortality was truly to be reduced, it was more critical that good milk be made available to the poor than that the production of milk for the prosperous be improved.[82]

The argument that purification represented the only approach capable of immediately affecting the milk available to the poor was a powerful one and carried considerable emotional weight. Yet as sanitarians and their pediatric and philanthropist allies were well aware, it did not directly address many of the most substantive scientific objections to milk purification. The opposi-tion to milk purification voiced by mainstream pediatrics may have been rooted in the specialty's clinical orientation and practical needs, but it was not without scientific justification, given what was then known about the food value of milk and the manner in which bacteria acted on both the liquid and those who consumed it. Furthermore, though opponents and propo-nents both used science to their own ends, neither was entirely free of the constraints that it placed on their arguments. Admittedly, where one stood on the raw versus purified milk issue might influence what questions one researched or how one interpreted certain discoveries, but it could not and did not entirely dictate either. Bacteriology, food chemistry, physiology, and the other sciences involved had their own methodological and interpretive rules that tended to constrain debate and move it in a particular direction.

During the 1890s much of the research done on milk and its reaction to heat tended to support opposition to purification. Particularly influential was the 1894 discovery by the German bacteriologist Carl Flugge that while heat killed most "adult" microbes, it left alive the spores from which grew the bacteria that were suspected of putrefying milk. Flugge and other re-searchers also showed that heat killed or rendered inert the milk-souring lactic acid bacilli which normally acted as an impediment to the growth of more harmful bacteria. Because of this, they warned, purified milk was an ideal medium for the multiplication of pathogens and was doubly dangerous because even when laden with such harmful bacteria, it lacked the tell-tale sour taste of old and dirty milk. Another related objection raised by re-searchers in the 1890s was the possibility that heated milk, even if relatively low in bacteria, still contained byproducts of bacterial growth which could be harmful.

Opposition to milk purification received further support when researchers, studying the physiology of digestion, discovered that enzymes, the chemical byproducts of bacteria normally found in milk, aided in the absorption of the liquid. Since such enzymes, or ferments, as they were commonly called, were capable of being destroyed by high temperatures, some argued that purifica-tion adversely affected the digestibility of milk and produced nutritional deficiencies in infants who were fed it. Finally, food chemists, throughout the decade, were adding further confirmation to what had long been sus-pected: that heating milk to high temperatures, and especially boiling it, altered some of its constituent elements. Indeed, the American Pediatric Society issued a report in 1898 questioning the safety of purified milk for infant feeding, adding to the other objections that it was probably instru-mental in producing scurvy and rickets in infants.[83]

As the twentieth century opened, proponents of milk purification were thus faced with the necessity of solving at least two fundamental and related scientific problems. Was it possible to heat milk to a temperature that would kill pathogenic bacteria and their toxic byproducts yet not destroy the neces-sary ferments nor diminish milk's nutritive value by altering its chemical composition? And was it possible, after heating, to inhibit the growth of bacteria from heat-resistant spores? In 1904, Conn, who had become a pas-sionate advocate of milk purification, solved the latter of these two problems by showing that the growth of spore-bearing bacteria could be effectively inhibited if milk was rapidly cooled below 50°F immediately after heating. Two years later, Roseneau, also an articulate and committed proponent of milk purification, provided the solution to the first by demonstrating con-clusively that if milk were heated to 60°C and held at that temperature for approximately twenty minutes, all pathogenic bacteria and their harmful byproducts would be destroyed but neither milk's ferments nor its chemical composition would be damaged.[84] These discoveries did not satisfy all the scientific objections to milk purification. The charge that heating milk de-stroyed its anti-scorbutic and anti-ricketic properties lingered for another decade or two until the role of vitamins in preventing these diseases was understood. But the discoveries did provide the basis for the development of an effective process of pasteurization and decidedly tipped the weight of scientific evidence in favor of those promoting milk purification as a solution to the urban milk problem.

The solution of critical scientific problems and the subsequent develop-ment of an effective process of pasteurization were not, however, alone sufficient to remove all obstacles to the adoption of milk purification as a means of guaranteeing a clean and safe urban milk supply. Also problematic was how such purification would be implemented; that is, who would do the purifying. Initially, most proponents of purification, seeing the process as a corrective for an inferior commercial product, had favored home purifica-tion shortly before consumption. The apparatus designed by Soxhlet was for home use, as were a number of others that came on the market during the 1890s. Moreover, even when such apparatuses were not used, the results of heating milk at home were at first believed to be quite encouraging. Freeman reported that thanks to the educative efforts of Jacobi and Straus, many of New York City's tenement dwellers were boiling the milk they fed to their infants. As a result, he conjectured, mortality among such infants was declining. In 1903 Freeman's conjecture was given strong support in a widely read report published by William Park and L. Emmett Holt. After extensively studying feeding patterns in New York's tenements, Park and Holt arrived at the unanticipated conclusion that infants fed on heated or boiled milk died much less frequently from diarrheal diseases than did those who were fed raw commercial milk.[85]

Yet home purification had its problems and these gained increasing acknowledgement as the science and technology of milk purification grew in sophistication. For one thing, home purification, while reducing the bacteria present in purchased milk, did not necessarily make it qualitatively equal to clean fresh milk. Purified old and stale milk was still old and stale milk. For another, except in better off households that could afford the proper heating and cooling equipment, home purification was a decidedly primitive affair. Although not initially much of an issue, this developed into a significant one as it became clear that heating and cooling had to be carefully done if the ferments and lactic acidproducing bacteria in milk were not to be destroyed with the pathogenic bacteria and if subsequent bacterial growth was to be inhibited.

In response to the increasingly apparent inadequacies of home purification, proponents of purified milk began to agitate for compulsory commercial pasteurization. They did so, however, with some hesitancy because they feared that milk processors might manipulate compulsory regulations to their own benefit. It was a fear that was well justified. Since the turn of the century a number of large milk concerns had been voluntarily "pasteurizing" their milk supplies. Their intent, however, was not to purify the milk of harmful bacteria but to increase its shelflife. As a consequence, they employed what was called the "flash method" of pasteurization, a quick and comparatively inexpensive process in which milk was momentarily heated to a high temperature. This killed the lactic acid bacteria and therefore retarded spoilage, but it did not destroy the more dangerous bacteria.[86] Widely condemned by milk reformers, industry use of the flash method did little to allay misgivings about the advisability of requiring commercial pasteurization. Indeed, so strong were those misgivings that when in 1906 and 1908, respectively, Massachusetts and New York City passed the nation's first pasteurization ordinances, their intent was not to mandate commercial adoption of the process but to prohibit processors and dealers from secretly pasteurizing their milk and selling it as fresh.[87]

In 1909, however, Chicago did pass an ordinance which, while not actually requiring commercial pasteurization, had that effect by setting bacterial limits that most commercial milk could not meet unless pasteurized. Equally important, the Chicago ordinance protected consumers from improperly pasteurized milk by prohibiting the use of the flash method. The following year the New York City Health Department passed a resolution advising that only properly pasteurized milk was safe for drinking, and one year later announced its intent to require that all milk sold in the city, except that which was certified, would have to be pasteurized. Other cities soon followed, and although many of the initial ordinances were challenged in court, their legality was ultimately validated. Moreover, following the highly publicized discovery of tuberculin cows at a number of certified milk dairies and the simultaneous implication of certified milk in several septic sore-throat outbreaks, some cities began to require or recommend that even milk produced on model dairies be pasteurized. As a consequence, by 1916 pasteurized milk accounted for 95 percent of Pittsburgh's milk supply, 88 percent of New York's, 85 percent of Philadelphia's, and 80 percent of Boston's and Chicago's. And by 1921 over 90 percent of American cities with populations over 100,000 had the bulk of their milk supplies pasteurized.[88]

It is extremely difficult to assess with any certainty the effect that milk regulation and especially commercial pasteurization had on the urban infant death rate. Infant mortality is causally complex, and its reduction is usually tied to an amalgam of changes in the social and material environment. The implementation of milk regulations and the introduction of pasteurization came at a time when many municipalities were also making significant strides in improving their water supply, sewerage, and refuse removal systems. Moreover, ensuring the quality and purity of marketed milk does little to guard against the significant danger of reinfection in the home. Nevertheless, infant mortality and especially mortality from diarrheal diseases did decline concurrent with the implementation of effective milk regulations and the adoption of commercial pasteurization in America's larger cities.[89] As one demographer has recently demonstrated, summer mortality among infants, which declined slowly between 1890 and 1910, dropped rapidly in the second decade of the century and by 1921 was all but negligible.[90] Furthermore, those cities that led the nation is regulating milk and promoting pasteurization seem to have experienced the earliest and most significant reductions in infant mortality. In 1885, for instance, New York had one of the highest infant mortality rates of any major city outside of the South. But by 1919, it had one of the lowest. (See Table 3.) Given that most of that reduction came from a dramatic decline in deaths from diarrheal diseases, it seems reasonable to speculate that New York's pioneering efforts to regulate the milk supply and require pasteurization had some influence.[91]

Ironically, though, just as the advocates of milk purification were gaining the upper hand and as the milk question appeared well on its way to being

Table 3
Infant Mortality in New York City,[a] 1885–1919

Year	Births[b]	Deaths < 1 year[c]	Infant Mortality Rate[d]
1885	37,543	9,303	247.8
1890	46,176	10,288	222.8
1900	90,801	16,627	183.1
1905	115,422	16,498	142.9
1910	135,873	16,215	119.3
1915	144,138	13,866	96.2
1919	133,027	10,699	80.4

Source: Ernst Meyer, *Infant Mortality in New York City: A Study of the Results Accomplished by Infant Life-Saving Agencies, 1885–1920* (New York: The Rockefeller Foundation International Health Board, 1921), p. 130 (facing).
[a] Manhattan and the Bronx.
[b] Estimated, not recorded, births. Estimates based on New York City Health Department assessment that in 1885 recorded births were 20 percent less than actual births, in 1890 15 percent less, in 1900 10 percent less, in 1910 5 percent less, and in 1919 2 percent less.
[c] Exclusive of still births.
[d] Rates have been recalculated to correct original compiler's mathematical errors.

solved, the importance of that solution was diminishing in the minds of those interested in reducing infant mortality. What had made the improvement of the urban milk supply so central to American efforts to combat infant mortality between 1880 and 1910 was the promise it seemed to hold as a well-defined and comparatively uncomplicated way to lower the urban infant death rate. Confronted with mortality statistics showing that infants of the poor overwhelmingly contributed to city death rates and yet frustrated by their inability to alter both the physical and behavioral conditions of poverty, late nineteenth-century public health reformers had sought an alternative solution and found it in improving the urban milk supply. In so doing they were influenced by both pediatric theory, which emphasized inferior food as the single most important cause of infant mortality, and by the science of bacteriology, which offered an effective interventionist strategy for improving that food. If infants of the poor died in such numbers primarily because of the quality of the commercial milk available to them, then improving that quality could effect a significant reduction in their mortality without necessitating eradication of poverty or reform of the myriad other physical and behavioral problems attending it.

Yet the implementation of milk reform came slowly, especially to midsized and small cities where the fight for clean commercial milk continued well into the 1930s. Public health officials and infant welfare activists, confronted with a barrage of statistics showing that infant mortality was still very high, began to express dissatisfaction with the approach that they had followed for almost three decades. Moreover, the same statistics that revealed the persistence of high infant mortality emphasized that, along

with digestive and nutritional disorders, congenital problems and respiratory diseases were also major killers of infants. Finally, because the pure milk
campaign—and especially milk station activity—attracted the involvement
of social welfare agencies, the community of those taking part in the discourse on infant mortality significantly expanded beyond public health and
medical professionals. Because of these and other developments explored in
the next chapter, the way infant mortality was conceptualized and approached changed once again. Reconceived, infant mortality moved to the
center of late Progressive era social reform and inspired a campaign to reduce
it that, in scope and in interest generated, dwarfed all previous infant health
reform efforts.

4

A Question
of
Motherhood

In 1906 the Association for Improving the Condition of the Poor hired Wilbur C. Phillips, a young Harvard graduate, to be secretary and administrative officer of its recently created New York Milk Committee (NYMC). Phillips's first assignment was to search and evaluate the state of infant welfare in the United States and abroad, paying particular attention to the work being done by milk stations. Although ultimately far less numerous than in America, milk stations had also begun to appear in cities on the continent and in England during the 1890s. In 1893 Gaston Variot started dispensing milk to sick babies at the Belleville Dispensary in Paris and the following year Leon Dufour of Fecamp opened the first French milk station, or "goutte de lait," as he called it. In 1899 St. Helen's Corporation opened the first milk station in England and soon afterward additional stations were opened in Liverpool and other cities. Although finding much of value in the efforts of these stations to supply infants with clean and wholesome milk, Phillips was more impressed by the maternal education program established by Pierre Budin at the Charité Hospital in Paris. Concerned that many infants who were born in the hospital subsequently sickened and died at home and somewhat uncomfortable with the limitations of merely dispensing milk, Budin in 1892 had designed and implemented a program of follow-up instruction for Charité's maternity patients. Called the "consultation de nourrisons" after its main feature, the program required that mothers who gave birth at the hospital return periodically to confer with Budin and to have their infants medically examined. In his conferences or consultations with new mothers, Budin stressed the importance of breastfeeding, provided information on the basics of infant hygiene, and for those mothers unable to nurse, emphasized the value of sterilizing and keeping cool the milk they fed their babies. Three years later Budin began a similar program at Maternité Hospital and in 1898 established one at the Clinique d'Accouchement Tarnier.[1]

Inspired by Budin's work and impressed with the French physician's often stated contention that supplying pure milk to uninstructed mothers was an inadequate approach to combating infant mortality, Phillips concluded that the thrust of American infant welfare activity was somewhat misdirected. Such activity, he noted, consisted almost entirely of increasing the supply of clean milk available for infant feeding, with little if any attention paid to maternal instruction. Indeed, he argued that "the importance of pure milk in reducing infant mortality, although worthy of grave consideration, has, up to the present time, been overemphasized."[2] Consequently, he recommended that the NYMC pioneer a new type of milk station, one that would encourage breastfeeding, provide medical exams, and dispense information on infant hygiene along with milk.[3]

The leadership of the NYMC responded enthusiastically to Phillips's recommendation and agreed to fund the operation of seven of this new type of milk station. In preparation for their June, 1908, opening, a staff of nurses was hired to supervise operations and to make instructional visits to the homes of poor families with recently born infants. Twenty-nine volunteer doctors were recruited to assist the station nurses, examine infants brought in, and provide consultations and classes on breastfeeding and infant hygiene. After some persuading, neighborhood churches and synagogues agreed to provide lists of parishioners with new babies and to donate rooms for lectures, demonstrations, and classes.[4]

The opening of the NYMC milk stations signaled the inauguration of a new and third phase in the American effort to reduce infant deaths, a phase in which infant mortality was redefined and reconceptualized, and in which the focus of infant welfare activity shifted from milk reform to maternal reform. As was true with the previous shift in focus—from general environmental sanitation to milk reform—this one did not entail a complete abandoning of prior concerns and activities. Public health reformers and others interested in reducing the infant death rate continued to press for improvements in the commercial milk supply and to support philanthropic and municipal efforts to dispense pure milk to poor urban infants. Yet, increasingly, such "milk work" was seen as an inadequate response to infant mortality unless it was part of a larger program of maternal reform. As early as 1908 Charles Chapin, in his "Municipal Sanitation" column in the *American Journal of Public Hygiene*, noted that "the conviction is growing that in order to preserve infant life something more has to be done than distribute clean milk. Good milk for bottle-fed babies is a necessity, but the education of mothers in the care of children will do more than all else to reduce infant mortality."[5] Within two years, L. Emmett Holt could thus be assured of a sympathetic response when he flatly declared that "infant mortality will not be solved by purifying milk and establishing milk stations."[6] So too could American demographer Edward Bunnell Phelps when in 1912 he statistically demonstrated that milk stations were not having a significant impact on the urban infant death rate and called for "universal education which will develop more intelligent motherhood and through the home reduce infant mortality."[7] It was a call that was apparently being heeded. A survey that same year of the work being done by voluntary infant welfare associa- tions concluded that there was a definite "shifting of emphasis in many of the societies from the milk problem to the education of mothers."[8]

What explains this shifting of emphasis? The general impetus probably came from mounting frustration over the inability of three decades of milk reform to effect a significant diminution of the infant death rate. Although, ultimately, sanitizing the commercial milk supply probably did play an im- portant role in reducing infant mortality, it had not at this point proceeded far enough so that its impact was readily apparent. Widespread pasteuriza- tion was not yet in place and what milk regulations had been implemented had for the most part improved higher grades of milk rather than the "loose" milk that was the staple of the poor. Moreover, although infant milk stations had been established in many cities and were dispensing millions of bottles of milk, they were still far too few in number to supply more than a tiny fraction of the milk urban infants consumed. Finally, and quite significantly, what gains milk reform had actually produced seem to have been masked by municipal and state adoption of new reporting and classification procedures and by the publication of more comprehensive statistics.

In the first decade of the century a number of American cities reorganized and tightened their registration and reporting procedures and adopted the international classification system of causes of death initially designed in the early 1890s by Jacque Bertillon, chief of the Bureau of Municipal Statistics of Paris. Two relevant consequences appear to have followed from these vital registration reforms. The first was the production of a "statistical" increase in the infant mortality rate in some cities. Following reform of its system of death registration and reporting, New York City saw its recorded infant mortality rate rise sharply from 1903 through 1906, before again resuming the gradual downward trend it had followed from the late 1880s. Other cities experienced a similar phenomenon.[9] The second consequence was the production of a similar statistical increase in infant deaths attributed to diarrheal diseases and digestive disorders. This occurred because Bertillon's classification system redefined cholera infantum as gastroenteritis and con- solidated most diarrheal deaths under one nosological category, thereby statistically increasing the number of infant deaths attributed to that cause. In Philadelphia, for instance, registration records show a significant rise in infant diarrheal deaths following the city's 1904 adoption of the new classifi- cation system. New York City's death records show a similar increase. During the first few years of the century, the proportion of all infant deaths in the city attributed to digestive problems had hovered around 26 percent.

In 1904, however, when city officials first began using the new classification system, infant diarrheal deaths jumped to 29.3 percent and climbed thereafter, peaking at 35.9 percent in 1910.[10] (See Table 4.)

A caveat is necessary here, as it is also quite possible that the recorded rise in diarrhea-related infant deaths had a substantive basis. It could have reflected one of those periodic upswings in virulence that characterize an endemic infection's interaction with a host population. Indeed, this seems quite likely in regard to the 1910 peak, since England and France also experienced a significant rise in such deaths during that or the following year.[11] Whatever the reasons, in the first decade of the twentieth century those Americans concerned with reducing the infant death rate were confronted with seemingly irrefutable evidence that little headway was being made. Small wonder, then, that they came to conclude that milk reform was not the panacea for infant mortality that it had seemed to be.

Also lending impetus to the shift to maternal reform was the concern of many physicians that milk work left largely unaddressed most of the other causes of infant mortality. Although convinced that digestive and nutritional disorders accounted for the greatest proportion of infant deaths, turn-of-the-century physicians were well aware that respiratory diseases and, to a lesser extent, specific infectious diseases killed sizable numbers of infants. While uncertain of the precise etiology of most of these diseases and as yet not possessed of effective therapies, physicians were nonetheless convinced that many diseases of infancy could be prevented if parents followed certain rules of infant hygiene and management. Educating mothers thus seemed to offer a promising strategy for lowering the incidence of infant death from pneumonia, bronchopneumonia, whooping cough, influenza, and other diseases.

Finally, the shift to maternal reform was in large part motivated by a new appreciation among physicians and public health officials of the value of

Table 4
Diarrhea-related Deaths for Infants Less Than One in New York City, 1902–1910

Year	Infant Deaths from All Causes	Infant Deaths from Diarrhea	Percentage of All Infant Deaths
1902	15,526	4090	26.3
1903	14,413	3769	26.2
1904	16,125	4726	29.3
1905	16,522	4945	29.9
1906	17,188	4943	28.8
1907	17,437	5314	30.5
1908	16,231	5118	31.5
1909	15,976	4254	26.6
1910	16,212	5807	35.8

Source: S. Josephine Baker, "Reduction of Infant Mortality in New York City," American Journal of Diseases of Children 5 (1913): 155.

breastfeeding, along with something of a change in opinion as to the ability of most women to nurse their infants. Several decades of pediatric and public health concern with what infants were fed had produced a significant body of literature charting the correlation between feeding practices and rates of infant death. Holt's and Park's examination of infant feeding in New York's tenement houses is an example that comes readily to mind. But there were many others, equally or more influential. In particular, during the last decade of the nineteenth and the first decade of the twentieth centuries, a number of French, German, and English studies appeared, offering evidence that much of the bacterial contamination of milk took place in the home and suggesting that breastfeeding and improved maternal care might be the only effective antidote.

Canvassing families in which infants were reported to have died of summer diarrhea, German researchers at the end of the century discovered that only a tiny fraction of all such infants in Groz, Berlin, and a number of other cities had been breastfed. French researchers made similar discoveries. An analysis of the types of feeding given to the 550 Parisian infants who died from diarrheal diseases during a two-week period in the summer of 1898 revealed that only 57 had been breastfed exclusively, while the remaining 493 had been artificially or mixed-fed.[12] English investigators also found a similar correlation between feeding practices and infant mortality. Investigating the circumstances in which over 6,000 infants died in Liverpool, E. W. Hope concluded that artificially fed babies less than three months of age were fifteen times more likely to die than breastfed babies. Similarly, George Newman, MOH of Finsbury and future chief medical officer to the Ministry of Health, found that of those impoverished infants in his district who died during 1902 from diarrhea, only 20 percent had been breastfed.[13]

Strictly speaking, these studies did not really prove anything. Unaccompanied by data on incidence of breast versus artificial feeding, statistics on mortality by type of feeding are meaningless. Nevertheless, public health officials and infant welfare activists interpreted them as providing incontestable proof that maternal nursing offered substantial protection against infant diarrheal diseases. And to a great extent they were probably correct. As later medical research has shown, breastfeeding significantly lowers the incidence of acute digestive disorders among infants for at least three major reasons. First, breast milk is more easily digested. Second, it is comparatively aseptic and therefore unlikely to transmit any of the pathogens that can cause acute diarrhea. And third, because of the lower buffering power of human milk (due to the lower casein and phosphate content) and the presence in it of the iron-binding protein, lactoferin, it acts to impede the growth of E. coli bacteria.[14]

In addition to illustrating the preventive power of breastfeeding, the studies also seemed to point to the importance of domestic and infant hygiene. Because they often involved house-to-house canvassing and were therefore not simply based on aggregate mortality data, these studies provided health investigators with the opportunity to gather certain types of information that they had previously lacked. In particular, these studies allowed for the collection of data on rates of gastroenteric morbidity. This led to a startling discovery. Summer diarrhea was not only a disease of infancy, as mortality records had seemed to indicate, but a disease that apparently afflicted all ages. In most of the homes where an infant diarrheal death had occurred, parents and older siblings had also suffered bouts of diarrhea. Only infants had died, however, and thus only they showed up in the mortality statistics.[15]

Along with the data on the apparent preventive effectiveness of breast-feeding, the discovery that homes where infants died of diarrheal diseases were usually the sites of multiple infection led medical researchers and health officials to reevaluate existing assumptions on the nature and causes of summer diarrhea. Specifically, they came to regard it as an infectious disease spread primarily but not exclusively by domestic fecal contamination of food, and especially milk.[16] No one was more influential in promoting this new conception of infant diarrhea than Arthur Newsholme, chief medical officer to Great Britain's Local Government Board between 1908 and 1918. Especially after 1910 when the LGB began publishing annual reports on infant mortality, Newsholme exerted an immense influence on infant welfare both in Great Britain and in America. With the possible exceptions of George Newman and L. Emmett Holt, no one was cited with greater frequency and respect by American infant welfare activists than was Newsholme.

Newsholme first began to suspect the importance of domestic contamination when he was serving as the medical officer of health in Brighton during the 1890s. From an analysis of records kept by his sanitary inspectors of the method of feeding of all babies of the Brighton working class who died of diarrheal diseases, Newsholme gradually arrived at the conclusion that domestic contamination of food and milk was a far more critical factor in producing epidemics of summer diarrhea than any contamination that might take place on the farm or in transit. First articulating his suspicions in the annual reports he published as Brighton's MOH, he gave wide publicity to his views in his 1899 inaugural address as president of the Incorporated Society of Medical Officers of Health and in a number of articles that he published over the course of the next few years. Although initially giving as much weight to public as household insanitation, Newsholme eventually came to see the latter as more important, since infant mortality remained high despite significant advances in improving the general sanitary environment. Moreover, as he observed in his 1894 report, in 72 percent of the cases in which infant deaths from diarrhea occurred, no violations of the general sanitary code could be detected. He therefore insisted that "the chief means of preventing diarrhoea will remain with the householder, and they com-prise the minutiae of domestic cleanliness, care in the preparation of infants' food, avoidance of stale food, extreme cleanliness of bottles, etc."[17]

Newsholme's views were not accepted without some opposition, especial-ly since so much concern existed over the bacterial contamination of milk on the farm.[18] Yet he was able to counter his critics with an impressive statistic: one showing that in Brighton, at least, diarrhea-related mortality among infants fed on condensed milk was as high as that of those fed on cow's milk. Since experiments had shown that condensed milk was almost sterile before opening, Newsholme argued that its contamination had to take place in the home. And if condensed milk was subject to domestic contamination, there was every reason to believe that cow's milk was too. Concluding that the chief causes of diarrhea-related infant mortality were "defects of domestic sanitation and lack of cleanliness in methods of infantile feeding," News-holme argued that educating mothers in the basics of infant and home hygiene and convincing them to breastfeed for aseptic reasons would do more to lower the infant death rate than any other single activity.[19] His argument was soon echoed by a host of other physicians and reformers, who were beginning to abandon their earlier belief that only a small fraction of women had the physiological ability to nurse their infants. Even in the United States, where that belief had been strongest, a change in opinion was clearly manifest by the first decade of the century. Reversing his earlier position, Jacobi began insisting that "one hundred percent of women can be made to nurse, even the 'flower of fashion of the land.' "[20]

As a result of this new emphasis on the critical importance of breastfeed-ing and proper hygienic management of the home, the influences of maternal employment came under close scrutiny. Armed with the evidence purpor-tedly showing that artificial feeding and domestic insanitation were major factors in producing infant deaths, public health officials and infant welfare activists charged that women employed outside the home could not possibly provide their infants with the type of nursing and the domestic environment required to guarantee their survival.[21] That working mothers neglected their infants and thus doomed them to early death was not, admittedly, an entirely new charge, and had been occasionally heard throughout the nine-teenth century.[22] But it was not until the last decades of the century that such charges reached a crescendo level and motivated governments to act. Thus, in order to allow for maternal care in the critical period of early infancy, Austria included in its 1885 Factory Act a provision prohibiting the employment of women for four weeks following confinement. Five years later Germany amended its 1878 factory laws to do the same. Great Britain followed in 1891, prohibiting a factory owner from "knowingly" employing a woman within four weeks after she had given birth. Similar laws were

enacted in Norway (1892), in Denmark (1901), in Italy (1902), and in France
(1909). In the United States, however, concern over maternal employment
was considerably less pronounced and no such national legislation was
passed. Indeed, when a congressionally mandated study of maternal working and infant mortality in six Massachusetts cities was published in 1912, it
reported that no clear relationship between high infant mortality and mothers working was discernible, and instead pointed to the foreign birth, illit-
eracy, and ignorance of mothers as primary determinants.[23]

Perhaps nowhere was the reorientation of thinking on infant mortality
more succinctly captured than in George Newman's immensely influential
Infant Mortality: A Social Problem (1906). Widely read and quoted on both
sides of the Atlantic, Newman's book took issue with the assumption that
reforming the commercial milk supply and improving general environmental
conditions would necessarily lead to a reduction in the infant death rate. A
careful and highly sophisticated demographic and medical analysis of the
socioeconomic and pathogenic determinants of infant death, it characterized
infant mortality as a complex social problem with numerous interrelated
causes. Many of these, Newman admitted, were environmental conditions
that seemed to attend poverty. He was also careful to note that communities
with large numbers of poor families generally suffered higher infant mortality than did more prosperous communities. Yet he cautioned against concluding that poverty per se, or the conditions that it inspired, directly caused
infant mortality. For Newman, too many exceptions had been recorded to
support such a conclusion. Citing studies of infant mortality among the
inhabitants of slum sections in Liverpool, Manchester, and Finnsbury, he
noted that Italian and Irish immigrant families had much lower infant death
rates than did native English families living in the same areas. Similarly, he
noted that in Ireland and Scotland it was not uncommon for the infant
mortality to be comparatively low even in extremely impoverished communities, despite miniscule household income, wretched housing, and nonexistent public sanitation.[24] Indeed, the abundance of exceptions led Newman
to observe: "Poverty is not alone responsible, for in many poor communities
the infant mortality is low. Housing and external environment alone do not
cause it, for under some of the worst external conditions in the world, the
evil is absent. It is difficult to escape the conclusion that this loss of infant life
is in some way intimately related to the social life of the people."[25]

By social life of the people, Newman primarily meant habits and customs.
And of these, the ones he believed most responsible for infant mortality
were the habits and customs surrounding infant nurture. Noting that human young, like all animals, "are profoundly susceptible to their upbring-
ing," Newman concluded that "more than any other single agency, infant
mortality depends on infant rearing."[26] In support of this conclusion Newman cited the success enjoyed by Budin in reducing infant mortality through

promoting breastfeeding among poor mothers and observed that a decade of
public health surveys seemed to offer irrefutable proof that breastfeeding
and hygienic infant care could go a long way toward countering whatever
deleterious external conditions might exist. For Newman the infant's relationship to general environmental conditions was problematic and indirect
and mediated by the quality of its nurture. In short, standing between the
infant and the environment was its mother. In a statement that became the
maxim of infant welfare work on both sides of the Atlantic, Newman asserted, "the problem of infant mortality is not one of sanitation alone, or
housing, or indeed of poverty as such, *but is mainly a question of motherhood*" (italics in original).[27]

In suggesting that infant mortality was essentially a problem involving
maternal nurture, Newman and other early twentieth-century infant health
reformers refocused attention away from the environment and toward the
individual, away from external conditions and toward personal behavior
and health. As English infant welfare activist George McCleary later observed: "Infant mortality, it became clear, was a matter not so much of
environmental hygiene but of personal hygiene."[28] Yet in defining it as such,
infant health reformers did not entirely dismiss the influence of environment. In their opinion, external socioeconomic and sanitary conditions
might not have a direct influence on the infant, but they did have a direct
effect on the mother; and along with knowledge of hygiene significantly
affected her ability to carry, bear, and raise a healthy infant. Consequently,
the new maternal orientation of infant welfare theoretically supported the
design and pursuit of a two-pronged effort to improve motherhood. The first
entailed establishing programs of social and medical welfare for expectant
and new mothers so that they might enjoy good health, medical attendance
and supervision, and freedom from economic worry and the necessity of working during the critical months immediately prior to and after birth. The second entailed promoting maternal health, proper feeding, and hygienic infant
care through instruction. Requiring the coordinated efforts of public health
officials, medical professionals and social welfare workers, both prongs—
again theoretically—were equally important. But theory is one thing and
practice another. In the initial stages of the international fight against infant
mortality, maternal hygienic education occupied center stage. Like milk
reform before it, educating mothers seemed to hold promise as a panacea for
infant mortality that could avoid the critical and problematic issue of poverty and make unnecessary more fundamental socioeconomic reform and the
provision of social and medical welfare. But also like milk reform, the promise it held was illusory. The extent to which this was recognized and accepted as the campaign developed and the degree to which the various Western
nations developed and implemented social and medical welfare measures
ultimately came to distinguish the way that each chose to confront the

problem of infant mortality. Indeed, the infant protection strategies adopted by the Western industrialized nations were all ideologically pronatalist, predicated on a certain family ideal, and they placed the burden of responsibility on the mother. Where they differed, and continue to differ, is in the amount of support they give to the mother in bearing that responsibility.[29]

Lending urgency to the new program of maternal reform was a profound awakening of international interest in the problem of infant mortality. Although concern over infant mortality had been building through the second half of the nineteenth century, it had been doing so primarily among public health officials, concerned physicians, and a select few urban reformers and philanthropists. While certainly not a well-guarded secret, that 15–20 percent of all infants were perishing before their first birthdays had not in any significant way dominated public consciousness in the nineteenth century. This changed rapidly, however, around 1900. Indeed, the first two decades of the twentieth century witnessed a virtual explosion of public concern over infant mortality and the consequent emergence of an international infant welfare movement of truly immense dimensions.

Given that health statisticians had long been illustrating the extent of infant mortality in the industrialized West, it seems important to ask why widespread interest in the problem only surfaced after 1900 and did so at such a rapid pace. Yet providing an answer to that question is not an easy task. For, as is true of the diverse collection of "progressive" reform movements that swept through the West in the decades straddling the turn of the century, the specific catalysts and character of infant welfare defy easy classification. Nevertheless, among the participants in early twentieth century infant welfare something of a consensus existed that at least three general social developments played an important catalytic role.[30] Although certainly not constituting an exhaustive list, these three provide at least some insight into why the reduction of infant mortality surfaced as a major social issue when it did.

The first development cited is the concern over national deterioration that gripped the industrialized West in the last decade of the nineteenth and the first decades of the twentieth century. Conceptually shaped by emerging concepts of political economy and by the convergence of several strains of post-Darwinian evolutionary theory, alarm over the quantity and quality of population found specific expression in concern over falling birthrates and was dramatized by increasingly high rates of rejection for military recruits and by the publication of statistics purporting to show rising mental and physical degeneracy.[31] France appears the first to register such concern and to connect it to infant mortality. According to at least one historian, France became obsessed with its declining birthrate following its humiliation in the Franco-Prussian War and as a consequence turned increasing attention to saving infant lives as a means of building the demographic strength it felt necessary to counter the expansionist designs of its eastern neighbor.[32] Whether or not this is a valid assessment, it was common wisdom among early twentieth-century infant welfare activists that one of the major reasons that France pioneered infant life-saving activity was that it earliest and most precipitously suffered the effects of depopulation due to declining birthrates. While not wishing to question "those who glory in the increase of solicitude for the welfare of children as evidence of the growth of pure altruism," John Spargo observed in 1908 that he could not

> escape the conviction that there is much significance in the fact that France, the nation which feels most keenly the perils of a diminishing birth-rate, leads the world in those vast social experiments which aim, in the words of Sir John Gorst, 'to make the most of such children as we have brought into the world.' It is because of the very narrow margin of births over deaths that France values her babies more than any other country.[33]

In England concern over falling birthrates and national degeneration also inspired interest in reducing infant mortality and was later cited by Newsholme as one of the primary catalysts for the heightened concern with infant death that surfaced in the first decade of the century.[34] Although commencing a sharp downward trend later than in France, English birthrates fell just as precipitously, declining over 28 percent between 1876 and 1901. By the turn of the century anxiety over the falling birthrate, combined with concern over the poor quality of recruits for the Boer War, provoked sufficient public and official alarm over national degeneration to inspire the creation of an Inter-departmental Committee on Physical Deterioration. Publishing its report in 1904, the Committee castigated English women for failing to do their procreative duty and professed great concern over what it purported was a dangerous increase in physical debility. Devoting considerable attention to infant mortality, it suggested that eliminating the causes of infant death would not only increase population but would also increase national efficiency, since diseases in infancy yearly enfeebled thousands and condemned them to sickly and unproductive lives.[35]

In the United States concern over national degeneration also served to heighten interest in preventing infant mortality, although it is difficult to determine how much of the connection made between the two was merely the consequence of American infant welfare activists plugging into a discourse initially shaped in England and on the continent. When American infant health reformers got beyond generalities they tended to show less concern with declining birthrates than their English and continental counterparts. Indeed, what concern was expressed usually centered on the disparity between the birthrates of the Anglo-Saxon stock and those of the newly arrived immigrant groups. Nevertheless, American infant welfare activists did conceptualize infant mortality as a problem of national efficiency and spoke of reducing it in terms of conserving national resources and improving the race. Moreover, they placed such preservation and efficiency at the center of preventive philanthropy and reform, suggesting that battling infant mortality was a requisite for the maintenance of national strength. As the NYMC observed in 1911: "In the modern conception of charity, preventive work takes a prominent place. Conservation of natural resources naturally begins with the protection of infancy."[36]

Also commonly cited as heightening interest in the reduction of infant mortality was the tremendous outpouring of public and official concern with child welfare that marked the last decade of the nineteenth and the first decades of the twentieth centuries. Although what came to be known as the child welfare movement began to develop somewhat earlier, not until the end of the century and the advent of progressivism did it blossom into a full-fledged reform movement aimed at granting the child a special protective relationship to the state.[37] For as Robert Wiebe observed, if the social welfare program of American Progressive reformers had a central theme— one that united the various campaigns for improvement of health, education and urban life, and dominated much of the interest in labor legislation—it was protecting the child.[38] Initially, attempts to guarantee such protection centered on ensuring the child that it would not suffer cruelty and exploitation by parents and employers, but increasingly they also came to include ensuring life itself. When prominent American Progressive Edward T. Devine declared in his *Misery and Its Causes* (1910), that "the ideal we place before us is a protected childhood," he was conceptualizing such protection as extending not only to older children but also to those in infancy who faced the constant threat of death.[39] Indeed, for many Progressives, reducing the continuing high rate of infant mortality came to represent the same type of basic requisite for achieving an advanced level of civilization as outlawing child labor.[40]

The third reason commonly cited as precipitating a new and heightened concern with infant mortality in the first decade of the century was an awareness that the infant death rate was remaining constant, or, at least, was not declining at the pace of the general death rate. Although the apparent resistance of infant mortality to reduction had been known and had been provoking concern and frustration for at least two decades, it received renewed and intensive illustration after 1900. Indeed, it is not inaccurate to say that infant mortality was rediscovered.[41]

Aided by the centralization of authority for statistics gathering in independent national agencies and no doubt inspired by the end of one century and the advent of another, turn-of-the-century government and private statisticians compiled an unprecedented wealth of social and vital statistics summarizing and analyzing the major economic, social, and demographic trends that occurred during the previous fifty to a hundred years. When the data collected began to be published, they illuminated a great range of social problems and provided inspiration and statistical legitimization for reform movements designed to ameliorate them. This certainly seems to have been the case with infant mortality. In Germany, for instance, when a comprehensive mortality survey was published in 1905, it revealed that fully 20 percent or 400,000 of the two million infants born in that nation each year failed to survive infancy. Receiving wide publicity in both the medical and popular press and provoking debate within the government, this illumination of the extent of infant death in the nation led to a three-week exposition in Berlin the following year and inspired the founding of a national institute dedicated to the study and prevention of infant mortality.[42]

In England a similar heightening of interest took place when the register general, employing statistics from the 1900 census, included in his 1904 report an extensive analysis of the rates, trends, and causes of infant mortality. Particularly shocking was the report's illustration that after declining somewhat in the 1870s and 1880s, the infant death rate had climbed again so that for 1896–1900 it was at the same level it had been for 1851–55.[43] (See Table 5.) Published soon after the release of the report of the Interdepartmental Committee on Physical Deterioration, the register general's report provoked considerable public outcry in Britain, contributed to the inauguration of a wide-ranging infant welfare movement, and helped catapult the problem of infant mortality to the forefront of public consciousness. In the years that followed, recalled George McCleary, "infant welfare became not only popular but fashionable. It had 'news value' for journalistic purposes, and was a favourite subject for addresses at drawing-room meetings."[44]

In the United States, turn-of-the-century publication of comprehensive

Table 5

Infant Mortality and Crude Death Rates, England and Wales, 1851–1900

Year	Crude Death Rate	Infant Mortality Rate
1851–1855	22.6	156
1856–1860	21.8	151
1861–1865	22.5	151
1866–1870	22.5	156
1871–1875	21.9	153
1876–1880	20.8	144
1881–1885	19.4	138
1886–1890	18.8	145
1891–1895	18.7	150
1896–1900	17.6	156

Source: George F. McCleary, "The Infant Milk Depot: Its History and Function," *Journal of Hygiene* 4 (1904): 329.

comparative and national infant mortality statistics may have had an even greater impact on infant health reform than it did on the other side of the Atlantic. Such statistics had never before been systematically collected or regularly published. Indeed, the perception of infant mortality rates and trends held by even the most statistically sophisticated nineteenth-century American public health reformers had largely been based on the registration reports published by a few large cities and northeastern states. This began to change in 1896 when the census office, employing data gathered during the 1890 census, published a report on the vital statistics of American cities with populations over 100,000 and calculated comparative infant mortality rates. However, because those rates were based on birth estimates derived by adding the recorded number of infants who died during the census year to those enumerated as living, they were unevenly inflated and recognized as relatively meaningless. Boston, for instance, was shown to have an infant mortality rate of 261 while Pittsburgh, which was commonly regarded as the less healthy of the two cities, was shown to have a rate of only 172.[45]

The 1900 census did somewhat better. In 1880 the federal government had created a death registration area, consisting of Massachusetts, New Jersey, the District of Columbia, and several cities considered to have efficient death registration systems. By 1900 that registration area had expanded by eight more states and by many more cities, and included 40.6 percent of the national population.[46] The vital statistics report, published in 1902, provided infant mortality rates for eight registration area states and all cities and towns in those states with over 5,000 inhabitants. It also provided rates for the District of Columbia, and for over a hundred cities outside the registration states. Although again calculated by employing birth estimates, the rates were considerably less inflated and were generally accepted by the public health community as reasonable approximations. More importantly, the 1902 report provided ample demonstration of what a number of public health analysts had begun to suspect: that infant mortality was not a problem limited to the nation's largest cities. Indeed, of the fifteen cities where the infant mortality rate was calculated to be over 200, only three— Baltimore, Washington, and Memphis—had populations over 100,000. Virtually all the rest were northern industrial and textile towns, or were mid-sized cities located in the South.[47] (See Table 6.)

Four years later, the Twelfth Census mortality data were substantially supplemented when the Bureau of the Census, created in 1902 by Congress as an independent and permanent federal agency, published the first of its annual reports on the causes, rates, and trends of mortality in the United States.[48] Covering the years 1900–1904, the report provided in-depth analysis of deaths by cause and age for ten registration states, for the District of Columbia, and for 153 cities outside the registration states. Aside from enumerating the number of infants who had died in the various registration

Table 6

Infant Mortality in 1900 for Selected American Cities (According to the Twelfth Census)

City	Infant Mortality Rate	City	Infant Mortality Rate
Mobile, AL	271.2	Buffalo, NY	137.0
San Francisco, CA	136.2	New York City, NY	170.5
Los Angeles, CA	154.1	Rochester, NY	101.5
Denver, CO	146.6	Charleston, NC	322.7
Bridgeport, CT	155.9	Wilmington, NC	202.8
Washington, DC	232.7	Cincinnati, OH	155.3
Jacksonville, FL	234.3	Cleveland, OH	163.6
Atlanta, GA	258.8	Portland, OR	87.2
Savannah, GA	299.7	Louisville, KY	155.6
Chicago, IL	134.0	Mahonoy, PA	211.0
Indianapolis, IN	153.7	Philadelphia, PA	162.1
New Orleans, LA	197.9	Steelton, PA	214.5
Boston, MA	173.0	Providence, RI	190.2
Fall River, MA	260.2	Woonsocket, RI	209.2
Lawrence, MA	216.4	Memphis, TN	213.9
Lowell, MA	240.5	Nashville, TN	201.1
Baltimore, MD	205.3	San Antonio, TX	178.5
Detroit, MI	176.5	Alexandria, VA	216.1
Minneapolis, MN	95.2	Lynchburg, VA	252.5
Kansas City, MO	165.1	Norfolk, VA	236.4
Omaha, NB	137.5	Richmond, VA	250.0
Newark, NJ	164.0	Seattle, WA	95.5
		Milwaukee, WI	167.6

Source: U.S. Department of Interior, Census Office, *Twelfth Census of the United States, 1890* (Washington, D.C.: Government Printing Office, 1902), 3: 286–564.

states and cities and confirming that infant mortality was shockingly high throughout the nation, the report also was the first national study to employ the International System of Classification of Deaths and thus the first to provide standardized and comparative statistics on the major causes of infant death. Those statistics showed that a large proportion of all infant deaths was due to three causes: digestive or diarrheal disorders, congenital problems, and respiratory diseases. (See Table 7.)

The publication of new, comprehensive, and national mortality statistics after 1900 did not, of course, alone awaken interest in infant welfare reform. But by making available comparative data on rates and causes and by illustrating the extent of mortality among infants, it did serve to focus discourse on its reduction and to heighten interest in devising strategies to save society's youngest members. In Europe that heightening of interest soon inspired the formation of national and international organizations devoted to the study and prevention of infant mortality and in the calling of conferences to examine the problem and to discuss strategies for its amelioration. In 1902 the Ligue Française contre Mortalité Infantile was founded in France, and the following year a similar organization was formed in Belgium. In 1905 the first international conference on infant welfare was held, when

Table 7

Enumerated Causes of Infant Deaths in Registration Area, 1900–1904

Cause	Deaths at All Ages	Deaths under One Year
All causes	2,378,020[a]	507,476
General diseases	726,908	43,055[b]
Diseases of the nervous system	302,876	58,757[c]
Diseases of the circulatory system	250,257	5,821
Diseases of the respiratory system	368,844	82,754[d]
Diseases of the digestive system	321,093	135,288[e]
Diseases of the genito-urinary system	179,127	2,689
Diseases of the skin	7,114	162
Diseases of the locomotor system	4,303	1,006
Congenital problems	131,542	129,953[f]
Ill-defined causes	85,956	35,051

Source: U.S. Census Bureau, Mortality Statistics, 1900–1904 (Washington, D.C.: Government Printing Office, 1906), pp. cxcvi, cc–cci.

[a]Exclusive of maternal deaths in childbirth.

[b]Includes 1,285 deaths from dysentery.

[c]Includes 31,387 deaths from convulsions that could have been due to the effects of acute diarrhea.

[d]Includes 54,724 deaths from pneumonia and bronchopneumonia.

[e]Includes 120,384 deaths from gastroenteritis, of which 111,603 or 92.7 percent occurred during July, August, and September.

[f]Of which 17,251 were from congenital malformation, 49,376 were from prematurity, and 63,326 were from congenital debility.

France hosted the initial meeting of the Congrès Internationale des Gouttes de Lait. Two years later a second international conference was held in Brussels under a new name, Congrès pour la Protection de l'Enfance du Premier Age, and an International Union for the Protection of Infant Life was formed.[49] In the year between the two international conferences, English infant health advocates banded together to form the National Conference on Infantile Mortality and to hold a highly publicized initial meeting at Westminster. In 1908 the Dutch National League was founded and the following year the German Union for the Protection of Infants was created. In addition, by 1912 national committees had been formed in Spain, Switzerland, Luxembourg, Italy, Rumania, and Russia as well as in Norway and Denmark.[50] All these organizations held annual conferences that served to publicize further the problem of infant mortality and to emphasize the urgency of its reduction. More importantly, they provided infant welfare activity in each country a national, institutionalized base, which it previously lacked.

In the United States interest in infant mortality as a national problem was also developing. In 1907 the New York Academy of Medicine, in combination with the NYAICP and the New York City Health Department, sponsored a conference on infant mortality and milk reform which led to the formation of the New York Milk Committee. Attended by public health officials, social workers, and physicians from a number of adjoining states, the conference received considerable publicity from the national press. The following year, the American Academy of Political and Social Science sent letters to health officials of ten major American cities asking them to answer a set of questions on infant welfare work. The academy published their responses in its *Annals* as a symposium on infant mortality.[51] But not until November, 1909, when the American Academy of Medicine (AAM) held a two-day meeting in New Haven on the prevention of infant mortality, did the first truly national American conference take place.

Organized in 1876 to advance the reform of medical education, the AAM had recently broadened the focus of its concerns and had committed itself to promoting what it termed a sociologic approach to medicine.[52] Within the AAM, the chief architect of the conference was Helen C. Putnam. A Providence, Rhode Island, physician and graduate of Women's Medical College of Pennsylvania, Putnam had recently been elected president of the academy and thus enjoyed the distinction of being the only woman to head an American medical association whose members were predominantly male.[53] At the AAM's thirty-third annual meeting, held in Chicago the previous year, she had gained passage of a resolution calling for the appointment of a committee "with power to organize and conduct for the Academy a Conference on the Prevention of Infant Mortality to be held in the winter of 1909–10."[54] A planning committee was soon formed and, with the help of an advisory committee that included some of the most prominent figures in American obstetrics, pediatrics, nursing, social work, education, and public health, a program was defined, papers commissioned, and a date and site settled upon.

Putnam apparently conceived of the New Haven conference when she journeyed to England in 1907 to attend the Second International Congress on School Hygiene and became acquainted with the new, maternally oriented definition of infant mortality popularized by both Newman's book and by the 1906 Westminster conference. The notion that infant mortality was a social problem to be dealt with largely by promoting maternal health and hygienic education seemed eminently logical to her in light of recent medical research. It was also fully consistent with the approach to public health to which she had long been committed. Like Arthur Newsholme, with whom she spoke at length while in England, she had a long and abiding interest in the field of educational hygiene.[55] In writing the proposal that she submitted to the executive council of the American Academy of Medicine, she stressed the need for a conference that would treat infant mortality as a multifaceted social problem, would emphasize the need for hygienic instruction, and would examine the ways in which medical professionals and philanthropic and public health agencies might assist expectant and new mothers mediate between their developing and newborn infants and harmful socioeconomic and environmental conditions.[56]

The view that infant mortality was essentially a question of motherhood and therefore a complicated social problem requiring the combined efforts of medical professionals, public health officials, philanthropists, and social workers found faithful reflection in the division of the New Haven conference program into four discrete sections. The first concerned itself with the medical prevention of infant mortality and was chaired by J. H. Mason Knox, an instructor of pediatrics at Johns Hopkins University and medical superintendant and director of the Thomas Wilson Sanitarium for Infants and Children.[57] The second section focused upon the philanthropic prevention of infant mortality and was chaired by Edward T. Devine, editor of *Survey*, general secretary of the Charity Organization Society of New York and one of the most visible and influential social welfare advocates of his day. The third section, devoted to the institutional prevention of infant mortality, was chaired by Homer Folks, who earlier that year had been the vice-chairman of the First White House Conference on the Care of Dependent Children and who, as secretary of the New York State Charities Aid Association, was one of the leading spokesmen in the Progressive child welfare movement.[58] The final section was on the educational prevention of infant mortality and explored ways in which the rate of infant deaths might be reduced by public health programs that promoted hygienic knowledge and behavior among expectant and new mothers. Heading that section was Charles-Edward Amory Winslow, director of M.I.T.'s Laboratory for Sanitary Research and leading advocate of the individual and educationally oriented approach to health reform that came to be known as the "new public health."[59]

For an initial gathering, the New Haven conference proved remarkably comprehensive. The thirty papers presented in the four sections broached and discussed virtually all the issues that occupied American infant welfare activists during the following two decades. Uniting virtually all the conference papers was a common theme—that if infant mortality was to be reduced, American mothers had to be educated. As Clark University biologist Charles F. Hodge observed at the end of the proceedings, "in most of the papers presented at this conference ignorance has been assigned as cause and education and special instruction the universal cure for infant mortality."[60] Nothing, however, that was said or discussed in the presented papers was quite so important as the action taken by a number of conferees who remained through Saturday and attended a meeting at which they voted to organize the American Association for Study and Prevention of Infant Mortality (AASPIM). With that action, what had been an inchoate movement, consisting of the uncoordinated and little publicized efforts of various individuals, urban health departments, and voluntary agencies, gained a national forum and a promotional organization.

As had been the case with designing the conference itself, the infant welfare activists gathered at Yale could draw on European precedent in shaping the structure and mission of the association they formed. The decade after the turn of the century witnessed the creation of several European national organizations devoted to promoting infant health and to coordinating the efforts of voluntary and municipal agencies working to improve motherhood and reduce the death rate of infants. But it was not only to Europe that the creators of AASPIM looked for inspiration and example. In 1904, with the organization of the National Association for Study and Prevention of Tuberculosis (NASPT), a new type of voluntary health association had made its appearance in America. Prior to that year American voluntary health organizations formed at the national level had for the most part been like the American Public Health Association or the American Medical Association: professional associations that focused on a wide range of health matters or primarily concerned themselves with defining and standardizing professional ethics and education, providing a forum for the exchange of professional information, and improving the sociocultural authority and economic status of their members.[61] NASPT, on the other hand, was a voluntary health organization formed to combat a specific health problem. Its founding in 1904 marked the beginning of a two-decade period that saw the formation of similar associations dedicated to the prevention of insanity, infant mortality, blindness, cancer, heart disease, deafness, paralysis, and venereal disease.[62] Conscious that NASPT was pioneering a new approach to health reform, the organizers of AASPIM used it as a model, adopting its name, structure, and constitution to their purposes. Moreover, like NASPT's founders, they conceived of their association as more than a strictly medical organization, and not only elected Homer Folks and C.-E. A. Winslow vice-presidents, but also required in their bylaws that at least one-third of the elected directors be nonphysicians.[63]

AASPIM held its first annual meeting at Johns Hopkins University in November 1910. In his welcoming remarks as president-elect, Charles R. Henderson, one of the early members of the University of Chicago's Department of Sociology, articulated the purposes and goals of the new association. AASPIM, he declared, in its effort to reduce infant mortality and promote a higher standard of maternity, would dedicate itself to accomplishing five specific but related tasks. First, by encouraging statistical studies of infant mortality, it would try to determine the extent and seriousness of the problem, and by publicizing the findings of experts, to awaken the nation to the necessity of immediate action. Second, by publicizing, encouraging, and coordinating their work, it would promote the creation of a network of voluntary philanthropic and health associations devoted to improving maternal ability to carry, bear, and rear healthy infants. Third, by arousing public sentiment and lobbying legislatures and government officials, it would work for the establishment of municipal, state, and federal infant and

child health bureaus. Fourth, by providing a national organizational structure, it would seek to bring together the various public health officials,
physicians, nurses, philanthropists, and social workers who were involved
in different aspects of infant welfare work. And finally, through holding
annual meetings and publishing the proceedings, it would serve as a forum
and clearinghouse for research into the causes and remedies of infant mortality.[64]

In undertaking the five tasks it set for itself, AASPIM initially gave
highest priority to encouraging statistical studies that would accurately
reflect the rate of infant death in America. In his presidential address to the
first annual meeting, J. H. Mason Knox proposed that the collection of
accurate data was the point at which preventive infant welfare must begin.[65] In one respect this concern with data collection reflected the unshakable faith that many Progressive era reformers had in the power of factual
description to inspire reform efforts. As Edward Bunnel Phelps told those
gathered at the 1910 conference, "the fundamental basis of all rational reform is first proving a deplorable condition exists."[66] Yet it also reflected a
realization that national birth records, necessary for computing infant mortality rates, were horribly incomplete and unreliable. Even after a half-
century of agitation by American demographers and public health officials,
many American states and municipalities registered births either haphaz-
ardly or not at all. In contrast to the statistical bureaus of European countries, which by the first decade of the twentieth century were issuing voluminous and accurate reports on birthrates and trends, the U.S. Census
Bureau had not yet begun to publish accurate annual tabulations of births.
Indeed, it was not until 1915 that it finally created a birth registration area—
and then for only the 31 percent of the nation's population residing in the ten
states that along with the District of Columbia made up the area.[67]

Although they could and did draw heavily on English and continental
records and studies, most American infant health activists felt that the lack
of reliable American birth statistics impeded their efforts to dramatize the
seriousness of the problem and develop effective remedies. In 1912 Julia
Lathrop, newly appointed as the first chief of the United States Children's
Bureau, complained to AASPIM members that it was impossible to know
the extent or even the causes of infant mortality in America without an
accurate picture of how many children were being born each year and where
they were being born.[68] During the next decade, Lathrop and the Children's
Bureau did much to rectify the situation, effectively lobbying for better and
standardized registration and conducting statistical case studies from which
it was hoped generalizations could be extrapolated. In the meantime, by
writing to every commissioner, president, or secretary of municipal and
state boards of health, AASPIM conducted a lobbying campaign designed to
promote the enforcement of existing registration laws.[69]

It was not, however, only to gain an accurate picture of the extent of infant mortality in the United States that AASPIM worked to improve birth registration. Especially at the beginning, its primary motivation seems to have been a conviction that quick and accurate registration of births was a critical prerequisite for an effective program of maternal instruction. As public health and philanthropic infant welfare work shifted from supplying milk to making educational visits to new mothers, early and accurate notification of births became increasingly important. If such visits were to be made and to do any good, births had to be reported and reported relatively quickly. AASPIM and other infant welfare groups thus worked to improve birth registration so as to facilitate the maternal educational work of the visiting nurses attached to health departments, dispensaries, and philanthropic organizations.[70]

Another part of AASPIM's campaign to determine and publicize the extent and seriousness of infant mortality in the United States involved arousing public awareness of the problem and generating public support for its amelioration. At the association's first meeting, William H. Welch, the prominent American pathologist, medical educator, and advocate of sociologic medicine, stressed the need for this, arguing that in a democracy reform cannot be imposed from the top but must come about as the consequence of public enlightenment.[71] Knox echoed Welch, warning the assembled delegates that "we cannot go further than an enlightened public sentiment will approve." He also drew a parallel to NASPT's efforts to educate the public as to the seriousness of tuberculosis and urged that a "special campaign for babies" be immediately mounted. After all, he noted, the lives yearly claimed by tuberculosis amounted to less than half of the annual toll of infant deaths.[72]

The primary purpose of such a campaign, it was agreed, should be convincing the public not only that a tremendous number of infants died each year, but that many of those deaths could and should be prevented. To accomplish this, AASPIM, under the direction of the association's executive secretary, embarked on a multi-pronged educational effort. To reach the public through the popular press, it supplied material to newspaper and magazine writers and regularly sent out news notices to the Associated Press, to Progressive periodicals such as the *Delineator*, and *Survey*, and to women's magazines such as the *Ladies Home Journal*. To reach professionals in medicine, public health, and social work, it urged various professional journals to encourage and publish studies on all facets of infant mortality. It also mailed out thousands of circulars and personal letters in the hope of reaching every state and municipal official, social worker, philanthropist, and medical professional who might be enlisted to join the fight against infant mortality. In 1910 alone, almost 40,000 pieces of mail issued from AASPIM's Baltimore office.[73] Finally, AASPIM put together a traveling exhibit. After an initial showing at the Fifteenth International Congress on Hygiene and Demography, the exhibit eventually traveled through every state, drawing large crowds at state fairs and sanitary exhibitions. Consisting of photographs, illustrations, charts, and text, it forcefully drove home two points: that approximately every two minutes an American baby died, and that at least half of this staggering waste of infant life could be prevented.[74]

AASPIM's chief purpose in waging a campaign to inform the American public as to the extent and seriousness of infant mortality was to inspire collective action aimed at reducing the number of babies who perished each year. Accordingly, it actively encouraged the creation of voluntary organizations devoted to that task and supported and publicized the work of such organizations as were already in existence. Unlike NASPT, which organized a national network of state chapters modeled on itself, AASPIM chose to serve as a coordinating body for a wide variety of voluntary organizations whose main point of juncture was a common interest in lowering the infant death rate. AASPIM took this course because by the time it was founded a number of voluntary associations had already entered the field of infant welfare. These included diet kitchens, children's aid societies, milk depots, and children's dispensaries and clinics. The task before AASPIM, then, was not the initiating of a national network, but the coordinating of one that already existed and contained highly divergent organizations. More importantly, however, AASPIM's conception of itself as a coordinating body sprang from the view that as a problem of motherhood, infant mortality had numerous causes and therefore required the combined efforts of medical, public health, and social welfare agencies. AASPIM thus courted a wide variety of voluntary organizations hoping to convince them to become affiliated members. At the end of the first year, thirty-three associations had signed on; two years later nearly seventy had. By 1914 the number of affiliated associations under AASPIM's coordinating umbrella had reached 140.[75] AASPIM used these associations as conduits of information, as sources of data on specific local conditions and programs, and as lobbying organizations to effect action on the municipal and state level. The associations used AASPIM as an umbrella organization that gave them a certain amount of legitimacy and national visibility by publishing accounts of their work.

Although voluntary agencies formed the core of the campaign against infant mortality, few of those involved in that campaign felt that voluntarism alone would be sufficient to combat the annual loss of infant life. Progressive era reformers widely agreed that private voluntary efforts were insufficient to meet the welter of social and economic problems common to an advanced industrial society. Not only did such efforts seem distinctly inadequate in the face of new forms of social pathology, they also seemed terribly inefficient, wasting energy and resources through the duplication of programs. Only government, it was argued, had the authority, resources, and centralized bureaucratic organization to pursue and coordinate effective reform and regulation. This theme was sounded repeatedly by those in-volved in the American campaign to reduce infant mortality, and as a consequence AASPIM actively lobbied for the creation of municipal, state, and federal agencies that could bring the power and resources of government to bear upon saving the lives of infants. At the same time, however, it had few illusions that its task would be an easy one.

Although most states and major municipalities had long accepted respon-sibility for safeguarding the health of their inhabitants, few had shown any inclination to devise programs—other than those involving milk regula-tion—that were specifically aimed at reducing morbidity and mortality among the young. In 1909, when AASPIM was founded, no state health department had yet created a division or bureau of child hygiene. City governments were also inactive. A 1910 report published by the United States Marine Hospital and Public Health Service revealed that municipal health departments were directly involved in only two of the twenty-eight American cities where preventive infant mortality work was being done.[76] One of these cities was Rochester, which under the leadership of George Goler had established municipal milk stations 1897. The other was New York, which in 1908 had created within the health department a division of child hygiene under the direction of S. Josephine Baker.[77] Thus, with some justification AASPIM's executive secretary declared in 1910: "the [munici-pal or state] health department which definitely recognizes its responsibility to its future citizens is the exception rather than the rule."[78]

To counter this state of affairs, AASPIM engaged in an intensive lobbying campaign aimed not only at health departments but also at state legislatures and city councils. With the aid of Baker, George B. Young (Chicago's com-missioner of health), and Thomas Darlington (head of New York City's Department of Health), a committee drew up and mailed out a plan that presented in detail how divisions of child hygiene could be organized. Sup-ported by other child welfare and child labor organizations, AASPIM's lobbying campaign gradually produced results. By 1918, when AASPIM was transformed into the Child Hygiene Association, twelve states and most major municipalities had established some form of governmental agen-cy or bureau responsible for promoting and safeguarding the health of in-fants and children.[79]

Posing an even more difficult challenge for AASPIM was the federal government. Even if they hadn't shown great interest in devising measures designed specifically to prevent morbidity and mortality among the young, states and municipalities had at least accepted responsibility for public health and welfare. Not so the federal government. When AASPIM was organized, the involvement of the federal government in infant and child health, as well as civilian health in general, was extremely limited. Admittedly, the federal government had accepted responsibility for overseeing food inspection and quarantine measures and was now conducting epidemiological and sanitary research through its Hygienic Laboratory. But these activities hardly constituted major involvement in safeguarding the nation's health. Moreover, although in 1902 Congress had added the words "public health" to the title of the thirty-two-year-old Marine Hospital Service, it had not significantly expanded the agency's functions or authority. Indeed, complaining that the federal government seemed more concerned with protecting crops and livestock than its citizens, Progressive health and child welfare activists had for some time been lobbying for the creation of a federal health department and a children's bureau.[80] Although late on the scene, AASPIM commited itself to supporting the establishment of both, reasoning that each in its own way could be instrumental in lowering the infant death rate.

Encouraging AASPIM's involvement in the campaigns to create a national health department and a federal children's bureau were several of its founding members or directors who were leading those campaigns. Lillian Wald, who along with Florence Kelley is generally given credit for conceiving the notion of a children's bureau, was a participant in the 1909 New Haven conference and a member of AASPIM from the beginning.[81] Julia Lathrop, the bureau's first chief, was also an early member and soon became a director. Another founding member and influential voice in the association was Irving Fisher. A Yale professor of political economy, Fisher had in 1907 been elected president of the Committee of One Hundred of the American Association for the Advancement of Science and had assumed responsibility for leading a lobbying effort that culminated in 1910 with the introduction in Congress of a bill that would establish a national department of health.[82] At AASPIM's first meeting, he secured passage of a resolution supporting that bill and convinced the association to lobby individual House and Senate members. The rationale he presented, and the one which AASPIM adopted as its own, was that the creation of a federal health department would serve to reduce infant mortality not only by improving regulation of interstate commerce in milk, infant foods, and medicines, but also by sponsoring research into the causes of infant mortality and distributing information on effective means of prevention.[83] Unfortunately, the following year Congress voted the bill down. But that defeat was soon followed by what was viewed among those in AASPIM as a great victory. In 1912, Congress finally approved the creation of a children's bureau and required that it involve itself, first and foremost, in the study and prevention of infant mortality. It was also not lost on AASPIM members that in creating the Children's Bureau, the federal government took its first major step into the arena of social welfare.

Along with its efforts to convince state, municipal, and federal authorities to accept responsibility for reducing mortality among infants, AASPIM's work to promote better birth registration, awaken the public to the extent and seriousness of infant deaths, and foster the creation of infant welfare associations played an important part in making infant mortality an issue of critical significance on the agenda of Progressive health reform. Yet, AASPIM did more than play a role as an organization for legislative lobbying and public education. It also helped bring together the various professional and reform groups interested in preventing infant mortality and provided them with a forum in which to articulate, define, and debate strategies for reducing the American infant death rate. Admittedly, in bringing together these groups, AASPIM was never able to provide the American campaign against infant mortality with the degree of centralization enjoyed by its European counterparts. But it did provide at least a modicum of centralization by serving as a single forum for discourse between the medical professionals, public health officials, and social welfare and charity workers who constituted the core cadre in the fight to reduce infant death. AASPIM thus forced the three segments of the infant welfare movement to deal with each other and to define at least a rough consensus of opinion as to the primary causes of infant mortality and the most effective ways to reduce it. The function AASPIM served as a forum for discourse and interaction between the various groups involved in the infant welfare movement also makes its published transactions a revealing record not only of the internal dynamics of the discourse but also of the major ideas that were developed, debated, and shared. The transactions also provide illuminating insight into the context in which that discourse took place.

As was the case in England and on the continent, the American discourse on infant mortality was conducted as part of a somewhat larger discourse on national deterioration, depopulation, and race suicide. This was apparent in the prominent role that both eugenics and the ideology and rhetoric of social efficiency and their advocates played in the discourse. Charles B. Davenport, perhaps the best known American eugenicist of the time, took an active part in that discourse, beginning with the 1909 AAM conference. So too did Fisher, who was an influential proponent of the idea that eugenics was logically consistent with the concepts of political economy and who organized the American Eugenics Society in the early 1920s.[84] Indeed, the program of every annual meeting of AASPIM contained a section on eugenics and social efficiency. Finally, the language and ideas of both were pervasive throughout the other sections.

That eugenics should occupy a major place in the discourse on infant mortality is hardly surprising. During the first third of the century, heredi-tarian theory and concern with national efficiency, particularly as they found expression in the pseudoscience of eugenics, were critical parameters of the conceptual and linguistic universe that informed virtually all dis-course on the application of science to social improvement.[85] Given its subsequent scientific debunking and the horrific and barbarous extremes to which it was taken in Nazi Germany, eugenics has been thoroughly dis-credited and is commonly dismissed today as little more than an attempt to lend scientific rationalization to race, ethnic, and class prejudice. But for many of those involved in the various social reform movements of the early twentieth century, the pseudoscientific nature and ominous potential of eugenics were not readily apparent. Eugenics was granted great respect and was seen as holding potential for facilitating the application of advances in the biologic and social sciences to the systematic improvement of human welfare. Even those disturbed by some of the implications of eugenics, shared many of its basic assumptions, aims, and concerns.

Sympathy toward eugenicist ideas was certainly common among Ameri-can Progressive infant welfare advocates. Indeed, they tended to view them-selves as involved in both a philanthropic effort to save infant lives and a scientific endeavor to advance human welfare by improving the mental and physical quality of humanity. As a consequence, reconciling the two en-deavors was an important preoccupation. In his address opening AASPIM's first annual conference, Henderson suggested that the main challenge facing infant welfare workers was finding a way to unite "philanthropic impulses" with a "scientific vision of the progress of the race." The dictates of human-itarian philanthropy, he told his audience, require that "we cannot neglect to save the life of any infant, no matter how feeble or unfit." Yet he also warned that such philanthropy carried with it the risk of increasing the proportion of unfit and feeble for whom society had to care, thereby destroy-ing national efficiency.[86] To solve this seeming dilemma infant welfare activ-ists advanced two principal arguments. Both were summed up by L. Emmett Holt in his 1913 presidential address to AASPIM members. Holt passion-ately disagreed with the radical eugenic contention—advanced by Karl Pearson and others—that a nation's strength and efficiency are maintained by a high infant death rate weeding out the unfit.[87] "Most of those regarded as unfit in infancy," Holt argued, "were healthy at birth and are merely victims of a bad environment, improper feeding and neglect—conditions which it is quite possible to remove."[88] For Holt, these were also the major causes of infant mortality, and thus preventing infant deaths by removing their causes would work to decrease rather than increase the number of surviving young who were unfit and enfeebled. This was the first argument, and it was aimed to counter the objections to ameliorative health reform that evolutionists had been raising since Darwin in *The Descent of Man* had expressed reservations about society's expanding ability and willingness to increase the capacity of the unfit to survive.[89]

The second argument advanced by Holt also had a history stretching back at least to Darwin. In the same passage in which he had expressed his reservations about health reform, Darwin had offered one way to "check" the "undoubtedly bad effects of the weak surviving and propagating their kind." This was to ensure "that the weaker members of society do not marry so freely as the sound."[90] From Sir Francis Galton's 1901 Huxley Lectures before the Anthropological Institute of London through David Starr Jordon's *Human Harvest* (1907) to Charles B. Davenport's AAM conference paper, "Fit and Unfit Matings," it was this "check" that eugenicists most ardently advanced as a means of halting racial deterioration. And it was this "check" that Holt offered as an alternative to allowing the hereditarily unfit to die in infancy. "We must," he told his fellow AASPIM members, "eliminate the unfit by birth, not by death. The race is to be most effectively improved by preventing marriage and reproduction by the unfit, among whom we would class the diseased, the degenerate, the defective, and the criminal."[91] Nor were Holt's opinions atypical. Less extreme than those held by some of the eugenicists in AASPIM, they were echoed by virtually all the major figures in the association. Even Jacobi was an ardent proponent of preventing marriage between those deemed morally, physically, and mentally degenerate. Moreover, at the 1911 annual meeting, AASPIM passed a resolution urging that all states adopt legislation authorizing "even surgical procedure" to ensure "the prohibition of procreation to the racially unfit."[92]

Aside from requiring that the movement conceptualize and justify its reform efforts in terms of racial improvement and social betterment, the eugenics current that ran through it also reinforced the initial tendency of Progressive infant welfare to focus its attention on improving postneonatal infant care. For an important eugenic argument was that deaths during the neonatal period (the first month) were chiefly attributable to hereditary weakness and therefore unpreventable. Increasingly aware that such deaths accounted for a significant proportion of infant mortality, yet having available to them little if any medical knowledge to explain the cause, infant welfare activists tended to agree. George Newman, for instance, contended in his 1906 study that neonatal mortality could be little affected by public health or medical measures since neonates who died were "not so much diseased as merely unfit and either not ready or not equipped for a separate existence."[93]

William H. Welch advanced a similar contention in an address delivered at the first meeting of AASPIM. Acknowledging that neonatal death was a serious problem, he nevertheless advised that reform activity focus on postneonatal deaths, since mortality in the first month of life was little understood and probably unpreventable. This meant, he continued, that of the

three recognized major causes of death—gastrointestinal disorders, respiratory problems, and constitutional debility following from prematurity, im-
maturity, and congenital malformation—only the first two should occupy
the serious attention of AASPIM because the cause of both was readily
apparent and capable of effectively being removed. That cause, Welch asserted, was maternal ignorance, particularly in regard to the feeding and
care of infants.[94] Welch was to a large extent preaching to the converted; if
one idea informed the AASPIM discourse it was that maternal reform, and
especially maternal education, represented the one best way to save infant
lives. Indeed, it is doubtful that few if any of J. Mason Knox's listeners
disagreed when, in calling upon AASPIM members to initiate a "special
campaign for babies," he declared: "The pivotal point is the mother. She is
the natural caretaker of her baby. She must be instructed in the absolute
necessity of providing it during its dependent years with such food and
surroundings as are compatible with health and life."[95]

The conviction that maternal education could effect an immediate and
significant reduction in the infant death rate focused the American discourse on infant mortality and provided an organizing principle around
which the various agencies and societies involved in infant welfare could
coalesce. Commenting on the reports submitted for 1912 by its affiliated
associations, AASPIM's executive secretary noted that their most "striking
feature" was a clear indication of a shift in emphasis from treating sick babies
and providing milk to examining well babies and educating mothers. This
she took to be evidence that preventive maternal education was now commonly accepted as the most promising method of combating infant mortality.[96] A similar conclusion had been reached that same year by the New
York Milk Committee in a report it released evaluating the lessons it had
learned operating its infant welfare stations. While observing that it remained committed to improving the quality of milk available to the poor, it
was emphatic in declaring that "in the education of the mother in the care of
herself and her baby, we have the strongest weapon for fighting infant
mortality."[97]

Faith in the efficacy of maternal education also served as the basis for a
working consensus among AASPIM's medical professionals, public health
officials, and social welfare and charity workers. Focusing on the individual,
and particularly on the mother, was consistent with the direction in which
each of these groups was developing in the beginning of this century. Many
American public health officials, for instance, found great appeal in Newsholme's contention that *the preservation of life in infancy is more closely a
question of intimate personal hygiene* (italics in original).[98] For it was consistent with a reorientation of focus that public health reform was undergoing.
During the first two decades of the century, public health officials on both
sides of the Atlantic began to redirect their attention away from the environ-

ment and toward the individual, away from sanitary engineering and toward individual instruction. The result was the emergence of a "new public
health" based on the premise that sanitary engineering had accomplished
much of what it was capable of and that further improvements in health
would depend upon convincing individuals of the importance of personal
and domestic hygiene.[99] As one of the English proponents of this direction in
public health observed,

> In this new departure of carrying sanitation into the home I believe we not only
> have an important but almost the only means of further improving the health of
> the people. Sanitary authorities, by providing water supply, drainage and decent
> housing, have done much. In the future, however, the most important advance
> will come from the appreciation by the people themselves of good health.[100]

In the United States similar sentiments were being expressed, particularly
by Charles Chapin who began arguing for a new individually oriented
public health in the first decade of the century.[101] Admittedly, full adoption
of the new approach to public health did not occur until after the First
World War.[102] Yet the initial move in that direction took place earlier and
thus provided a receptive climate for the shift in infant welfare work from
environmentally oriented milk reform to individually oriented maternal
reform.

Maternal educational reform was also consistent with the orientation and
professional needs of the physicians involved in AASPIM. Although the
organization attracted socially conscious doctors from a number of fields, it
drew most heavily from two specialties: pediatrics and obstetrics. For the
former, the need for maternal education had been a consistent theme in its
development and legitimization as a specialty. Moreover, it represented a
point of juncture at which pediatricians could rejoin public health officials
with whom their relations had been strained over the milk question. For
similar reasons, maternal education was attractive to the obstetricians who
were members of AASPIM. Arguably the least esteemed specialty in medicine at the time, obstetrics was in the process of reforming and legitimizing
itself by improving the quality of obstetric training and by promoting the
idea that pregnancy and the birthing process were pathological conditions
that required skilled supervision and assistance. According to J. Whitridge
Williams, professor of obstetrics at Johns Hopkins and a member of
AASPIM's Board of Directors, such reform could come about only if women
realized that the post-parturient health of themselves and their infants was
critically influenced not only by the skill of their birth attendant but also by
the degree to which they followed medical advice during pregnancy.[103]
Promoting prenatal maternal education thus became an important activity
of the obstetricians in AASPIM and increasingly became an object of the

various infant welfare agencies connected to the association.

Maternal education also found support among the social welfare workers and charity officials who had become involved in infant welfare work as philanthropies and charity agencies began funding and operating milk stations, fresh air retreats, and infant dispensaries. The shift to maternal reform coincided with a reorientation of urban child welfare work from the relief and rescue of children to the preventive reform of the family. Viewing the family as the basic unit of social organization and thus as the logical focus of preventive work, child welfare workers after 1900 sought to improve the lot of children, not by removing them from their families as their predecessors had, but by reorganizing the family home so that it better fit their needs. As one speaker at the 1901 National Conference of Charities and Corrections declared, "The old cry of 'Save the Children!' must be superseded by the new cry of 'Save the Family!' for we cannot save the one without the other."[104]

Social welfare's new emphasis on saving the family through reorganizing the home placed a premium on educating mothers, particularly poor, immigrant mothers. Although professing respect for immigrant customs, American social welfare and charity workers sought to modernize and Americanize the immigrant mother in the hope of facilitating her and her family's adaptation to the urban industrial environment. This orientation toward individual reform was especially true of the generation of social workers who after 1900 were trained by the newly organized schools of social work in the individual adjustment techniques of "case work." Convinced that immigrant life would improve significantly with the adoption of the scientific management of the home, they sought to instruct immigrant mothers in nutritious cooking, domestic sanitation, proper ventilation, and the hygienic care and feeding of infants and children.[105] It was thus fully consistent with the direction in which American philanthropy and social work was developing for the National Conference on Charities and Corrections in 1912 to conclude in its initial report on infant mortality that the prevention of infant death meant the education of the mother. Quoting extensively from George Newman, the NCCC stressed that the reduction of infant mortality depended not on the state, the municipality, or the philanthropic agency, "'but upon the health, the intelligence, the devotion and the maternal instinct of the mother.'"[106]

The stress on maternal education also found reinforcement and cultural legitimization in developments outside medicine, public health, and philanthropy. In particular it was consistent with a heightening of interest, especially among the middle class, in all things related to the rearing of children. Nurturing the young, noted Ida Tarbell in her 1912 *The Business of Being a Woman*, "has become the passion of the day."[107] And indeed it had. For although the late nineteenth and early twentieth centuries witnessed a feminist movement that sought to expand the acceptable role of women beyond the rather narrow confines of the Victorian home, they also wit-nessed the development of a cult of motherhood. Finding expression in the organization of child study groups and mothers' associations and in the proliferation of periodicals and books devoted to child care, keeping of the home, and mothering in general, the cult of motherhood made child rearing a national obsession and spawned intense debate on what skills mothers re-quired to perform this sacred task. Although opinion varied, one principle generated wide agreement: maternal education was necessary because the complexity of modern life made the rearing of children far too difficult a task for mothers to carry out successfully without the help of experts.[108]

By the second decade of the twentieth century, the cult of motherhood was increasingly centered around the care and rearing of infants. Julia Lathrop noted this development in a talk she gave at AASPIM's third annual meeting. A few years earlier, Lathrop told her audience, a popular Chicago newspaper columnist had approached her editor with the idea of writing a column on babies. Her idea, however, was rejected out of hand on the grounds that no interest existed. Yet today, Lathrop observed, such columns were in virtually every major newspaper and interest in babies was everywhere.[109] Lathrop was not exaggerating. The second decade of the century saw middle-class women flocking to well-baby classes, organizing baby health shows, and purchasing Holt's *The Care and Feeding of Children* in such numbers as to make it a bestseller. The *Woman's Home Companion* sponsored "best baby shows" and the National Federation of Women's Clubs successfully attempted to have a national baby week proclaimed in 1916. Indeed, according to Katherine Graves Busby in her caustic 1910 analysis of the "American female," interest in babies and the desire to learn all one could about their care and rearing was fast becoming one of the most pronounced characteristics of middle-class women.[110]

Subscription to what has been called the "ideology of instructed mother-hood" thus served as the basis for consensus among the various professional and reform groups involved in AASPIM and gave the early infant welfare movement considerable unity.[111] Yet that unity would prove to be some-what fragile, for the consensus on the efficacy of maternal education was built on the assumption that it could counter the influences of poverty. Even at the outset some members of AASPIM questioned the validity of this assumption. Responding to Welch's 1910 address calling for maternal educa-tion to promote breastfeeding and infant and domestic hygiene, Robert Bruere of the NYAICP protested that although such education was no doubt needed, his experience had convinced him that "low wages [and] insufficient family budgets account for a considerable percentage of infant deaths." It was therefore hardly sufficient, Bruere continued, to convince women to breastfeed and to instruct them in infant and domestic hygiene if their poverty made unavailable the nourishment necessary for the first and the time necessary for the second.[112] Others among the social and charity worker contingent raised similar objections, especially after 1915, when Children's Bureau studies again made the causal significance of poverty a critical and divisive issue in the American discourse on infant mortality. At AASPIM's sixth annual meeting, Sherman Kingsley, head of Chicago's United Charities, observed that within social philanthropy he had begun to hear rumblings of discontent with the association's almost exclusive empha- sis on maternal education and suggested that however valuable such educa- tion might be, it represented an incomplete reform strategy since it ignored the fundamental connection between family resources and the ability of mothers to guarantee their own and their infants' health.[113]

The reservations expressed by Bruere and the rumblings detected by Kingsley were evidence of an essential paradox at the heart of Progressive charity and social work. In theory such work was predicated on the convic- tion that those who suffered social ills did so not because of individual weaknesses and flaws, but because of the weaknesses and flaws inherent in American social and economic organization. This was the fundamental mes- sage of Devine's *Misery and Its Causes*, as well as of the hundreds of other analyses published by Progressive social theorists. But in actual practice, Progressive social workers often pursued a case-work approach that fre- quently ignored the socioeconomic and structural causes of social ills and focused instead on individual and family adjustment. Theory and practice were thus often at odds, with the former always undermining conviction in the efficacy of the latter. This conflict between theory and practice, between analyses of the problem and the reform strategies actually adopted, came to a head at the end of the second decade of the century. But in the years immediately following the founding of AASPIM, the conflict was muted and masked by the hope that maternal education might be the long-sought remedy for infant mortality. Inspired by that hope, American infant welfare activists mounted a wide-ranging and multifaceted campaign to instruct the nation's mothers in the hygienic care and feeding of their infants.

5

Better Mothers,
Better Babies,
Better Homes

The maternal reform campaign mounted by infant welfare activists during the second decade of the century was multidimensional and eventually came to focus on the middle class as well as on the urban poor. It was also a campaign waged by a varied collection of individuals and organizations, including state and municipal public health departments, district nursing associations, philanthropies, settlements and child welfare alliances, the federal government through the Children's Bureau, middle-class women's clubs, reform-minded pediatricians and obstetricians, and the popular press, particularly women's magazines. Although no high command unified all the participants, a certain degree of unity did exist. AASPIM provided a common forum for discourse among the various groups involved and served as a clearinghouse for information. So too, subsequently, did the Children's Bureau. Moreover, because of the voluntaristic tradition of American social and medical welfare and because of the continuing reluctance of municipal, state, and especially federal legislators to appropriate sufficient funding for infant welfare work, public and private agencies frequently worked together, pooling resources, facilities, and personnel.

Consistent with the perception that infant mortality was a problem most serious among the urban poor and that its principal and most readily preventable causes were digestive and nutritional disorders, the initial phase of the maternal education campaign centered on encouraging poor mothers to nurse their infants and on instructing those who could not in hygienic and scientific methods of artificial feeding. Critical to this effort was the transformation of infant milk stations into infant welfare stations or well-baby clinics. Beginning with the NYMC's incorporation of maternal education and infant examinations into the activities of the milk stations opened in the summer of 1908, medical supervision of infants and the instruction of their mothers became an increasingly important part of milk station work. A 1911 survey by the U.S. Marine Hospital and Public Health Service showed that educational efforts were being made by all but one of the forty-three agencies sponsoring milk stations in thirty American cities, although in a number of cases instruction was limited to advising mothers how to care for the milk that was dispensed. Four years later, not only had the number of stations dramatically increased, but so too had the emphasis on education. A 1915 investigation by the U.S. Children's Bureau revealed that 205 agencies were operating 539 infant welfare stations in 142 cities. All agencies reported that they considered their primary function to be assisting mothers—through advice, supervision, and education—to care for their infants and especially to protect them from developing life-threatening digestive and nutritional disorders. Indeed, in the stations of 95 agencies no milk was dispensed.[1]

The chief catalyst for this shift from milk work to maternal education was the growing conviction that domestic insanitation and maternal ignorance of the hygiene of infant feeding were the critical causes of summer diarrheal epidemics. Based on medical research into the correlation between infant survival rates and domestic cleanliness and type of feeding, that conviction found additional support after 1907 in accumulating evidence that flies acted as vectors in the contamination of food with pathogenic bacteria.[2] Merely dispensing milk increasingly came to be seen as an inadequate response to infant diarrheal deaths. "It is useless," declared a 1913 Children's Bureau publication, "to send pure milk into a dirty home to be handled by an ignorant, dirty mother or older child. It is necessary to reach the mothers, not only to teach them how to care for their baby's milk, but also to convince them of the necessity of cleanliness."[3]

Criticism from the medical profession also contributed to the transformation of milk stations into well-baby clinics or infant welfare stations. As evidence mounted that bottle-fed infants were six to ten times as likely to die as those who were breastfed, many doctors expressed the fear that infant milk stations might be counterproductive and actually serve to increase infant mortality by encouraging mothers not to nurse. In France this fear seems to have been especially pronounced and was responsible for the "gouttes de lait" early adopting the practice of requiring mothers to attempt breastfeeding before they could receive dispensed milk. In England the fear was also frequently expressed, and not only slowed the opening of milk stations but also early led to their incorporating consultations like those devised by Budin. Similar concern was expressed by German physicians, with the consequence that only a small number of the 303 infant health centers in operation by 1910 actually dispensed milk. In the United States the charge that milk stations discouraged breastfeeding was somewhat more muted than in England and on the continent. Perhaps, as one English welfare activist suggested, this was because American physicians seemed most enamored with the idea that science could make artificial feeding safe.

Nevertheless, the criticism was raised often enough and with sufficient ardor that milk stations gradually changed the way they operated. Not only did they begin requiring medical certification that a mother could not or ought not nurse her infant, but they also ceased the practice of setting up shop and waiting for mothers to come to them. Hiring nurses to canvass neighborhoods for new mothers and to encourage them to breastfeed, the new infant welfare stations made the provision of milk a last resort.[4]

Physicians also criticized milk stations for operating as if all babies at a particular age had the same nutritional requirements and digestive capabilities. Although by 1910 many doctors involved in infant care had become somewhat disillusioned with the complexity of percentage feeding, they still subscribed to the basic principle on which percentage feeding rested: that the sensitivity and developmental variety of infant digestive systems required that formulas be individually prescribed. Because of cost, however, the early infant milk depots had been forced to rely on three or four basic formulas that were dispensed according to the age of the infant. This, critics charged, was making the baby fit the milk rather than the milk fit the baby, and posed the danger that milk stations were contributing to rather than combating infant digestive disorders. Indeed, in Boston, where the influence of Rotch and the percentage feeding school was strongest, medical opposition delayed the opening of privately funded milk stations until 1909 and kept the health department out of milk station operation altogether.[5] The NYMC pioneered a way around this criticism by requiring all mothers seeking milk to bring their babies in so that they could be examined by a physician who would prescribe an individualized but relatively simple formula. To keep costs down, the NYMC stations did not prepare the formulas themselves. Rather, they dispensed whole milk and other formula ingredients and had the mothers accompanied home by a nurse who would show them how to mix the formulas and would instruct them on other aspects of infant and domestic hygiene. In addition, mothers were expected to return to the stations each week to have their babies examined and weighed, and, if needed, to receive new formula prescriptions.[6]

Promoting home modification and maternal instruction also blunted another criticism that was occasionally made of milk stations: that in dispensing milk they were merely providing material assistance and thus offering "outdoor" relief in response to conditions attending poverty. This was a serious charge. For if one principle had guided American philanthropy for over three-quarters of a century, it was that direct relief in the form of material assistance discouraged self-improvement and promoted pauperism and other types of social dependency. While Progressive era charity and social workers tended to acknowledge that the poor were often victimized by social and economic arrangements over which they had little control and were therefore somewhat less inclined than their nineteenth-century predecessors to blame them for the conditions they suffered, they showed no less healthy a fear that "outdoor" relief would undermine the poor's ability and willingness to help themselves. At the same time, however, they had little if any faith in the efficacy of the "indoor" or institutional relief that the nineteenth century had offered as an alternative. Instead, they proposed to save families and build up homelife, mostly by instruction, but also by providing limited assistance.[7] Admittedly, at what point such limited assistance became counterproductive was a divisive issue among Progressives. But especially among those involved in infant welfare work, it was felt that the provision of milk to poor mothers, especially when it was coupled with instruction in home modification and infant hygiene, was well within the boundaries of the permissible. Lillian Wald, for instance, defended the home modification program of her Henry Street infant welfare station by describing it as fully consistent with "our principle of building up the homes wherever possible."[8]

Adoption of home modification did not blunt one criticism against infant welfare stations, however. This criticism was early and consistently heard from rank-and-file physicians, particularly those who serviced the immigrant poor. In the crowded medical marketplace of turn-of-the-century urban America, competition for patients was intense, and was especially so among those physicians without medical and social connections. As a consequence, such physicians were quick to protest any municipal or philanthropic activity that they perceived as threatening to reduce an already inadequate pool of patients by offering free or subsidized medical care. Historically wary of charity clinics and dispensaries, they greeted the appearance of infant welfare stations with little enthusiasm, especially since such stations did not limit their services to the destitute. After New York's Bureau of Child Hygiene opened a number of infant welfare stations in Brooklyn's Brownsville section, thirty-one physicians signed and sent a petition to the mayor protesting that the city was robbing them of their livelihoods by providing free medical care.[9] Backers of infant welfare stations answered such protests by assuring skeptical physicians that station work was supervisory and educational and therefore did not intrude into the domain of the private practitioner. Yet in actual practice, it was often difficult for the stations to maintain a strict separation between supervision and education on one hand and treatment on the other. Confronted with an acutely sick infant in a family with no regular private doctor, station nurses often called in a volunteer physician, even if the family was capable of paying for private medical attendance. As Chicago's Sherman Kingsley observed, while "great care is being taken not to encroach on the legitimate field of the private practitioner," infant welfare workers were not about "to allow the baby, in the very midst of doctors, nurses, social workers, dispensaries, and hospitals, to die without help or adequate care."[10]

Infant welfare workers, moreover, were often vocally disdainful of the type of physician who practiced in urban tenement districts. Lillian Wald maintained that while a few were exceptionally skilled and dedicated, many were venal and ignorant. Her opinion apparently was shared by many visiting nurses, since they frequently complained that the typical tenement district doctor was ill-trained and mercenary and tended to prescribe large doses of patent medicines and nostrums for the simplest complaints.[11] Physicians involved in infant welfare were equally disdainful. Although more concerned than nurses or social workers with preserving the privatized character of medical practice, they were almost exclusively from the elite segment of the medical profession and showed a marked willingness to turn aside that concern in regard to their socially and medically inferior colleagues. Philadelphia's S. W. Newmeyer ridiculed tenement area physicians for raising the "sacred cow of the physician-patient relationship," contending that in their case it was already abrogated by their ignorance, callousness, and carelessness. "The question as to whether the so-called family physician is in attendance," he declared in 1910, "when he has shown himself incompetent to manage the care, is no reason why we should shout 'Hands Off!' and let the child die."[12] Coupled with the tendency of infant welfare doctors and nurses occasionally to offer treatment to infants, such disdainful dismissals of their skills and economic concerns did little to allay the fears of rank-and-file physicians, and their resentment of philanthropic and municipal infant welfare work continued to fester. For the time being, however, it was countered by the support of the medical elite who saw infant welfare stations not only as doing good for infants, but also as providing critical clinical experience to university-trained physicians.

Following a widely publicized 1911 demonstration by the NYMC of the effectiveness and cost efficiency of its instructional and home modification program, infant milk stations throughout the country began adopting the method. By 1915, only one of the 110 agencies dispensing milk in America's cities gave out nothing but modified milk, while sixty dispensed whole milk only and forty-nine supplied both whole and modified milk. Home modification, however, required that mothers be instructed and supervised and that babies be regularly examined and weighed so that formulas could be individually prescribed. To do the latter, doctors were necessary, and by 1915 over 790 were participating in infant welfare station work. While a small number of these were the paid employees of private agencies and public health departments, most were volunteers. Contributing a few hours weekly, these volunteer physicians examined infants, wrote formula prescriptions and held consultations with mothers. In return, they not only received the personal satisfaction of being part of a humanitarian effort but also gained valuable clinical experience in early childhood medicine and formula prescribing. This last was no small attraction to physicians fresh out of medical school, and in part explains why infant welfare stations were able to enlist the services of so many volunteer doctors. At a time when hospitals were not yet providing significant postgraduate training, volunteer service at a privately funded clinic, dispensary, or health station often represented the only opportunity for new doctors to do a residency in a specialized field. The respected New York pediatrician and infant welfare activist Rowland G. Freeman observed in 1909 that attracting volunteer physicians to work at infant welfare stations examining infants and prescribing individual formulas was not at all difficult because "there was always a large supply of young doctors eager to get experience."[13]

More important than doctors, though, were the nurses employed by the agencies that funded and operated infant welfare stations. By 1915 there were almost 900 of them working during the summer and over half that number working during the winter. For the most part full-time employees, such nurses were the field troops in the campaign to educate urban mothers. They managed the everyday operations of the stations, canvassed neighborhoods for newborns, and climbed innumerable filthy and dimly lit stairways to visit and instruct tenement mothers in their homes. They also often served as social workers, assisting families to take advantage of the myriad but confusing array of private charitable agencies that operated in the early twentieth-century city. Of equal importance with the instructional work of the infant welfare station nurses was the work carried on by visiting nurses employed by district nursing associations, dispensaries, and other charitable organizations. Especially concerned with reaching those mothers and infants who for one reason or another were not enrolled in infant welfare station programs, such nurses numbered over one thousand by 1915 and could be found in over half of all American towns and cities with more than 10,000 inhabitants.[14]

Especially through the first decade of the century, but also well into the second, the maternal education campaign pursued by infant welfare stations and visiting nurses was largely funded and conducted by a variety of private agencies and organizations. These included: baby's milk and baby's welfare associations; settlements and city missions; women's civic leagues, auxiliaries, and clubs; private dispensaries, clinics, and hospitals; poor relief and reformation associations; children's aid societies; and diet kitchens. Indeed, by 1915 hundreds of private agencies in almost 300 American cities and towns were conducting some form of educational infant welfare work. Even a few businesses provided funds or hired nurses. In 1909 the Metropolitan Life Insurance Company, acting on a suggestion by Wald, began a nursing service for its policy holders and their families, a major part of which included instruction and supervision of new mothers. By 1914 that service had reached into 1,700 cities and towns. In addition, the company printed and distributed over one million copies of an instructional booklet on infant and child care.[15]

Urban settlements were in many ways typical of the type of privately funded organizations that became involved in infant welfare work. Proliferating in American cities between 1900 and 1915, settlements devoted themselves to assisting the poor, especially the immigrant poor, adapt to the realities of an urban industrial environment. Although committed to avoiding stereotyping the immigrant poor and based on firsthand experience of the actual conditions that affected their lives, settlement work was nevertheless informed by the traditional fear of outdoor relief, and was therefore primarily educative and concerned with the acculturation of the immigrant.[16] While initially pursuing a program of cultural uplift, settlements soon changed the focus of their instructional activities and began offering courses containing practical information. Particularly popular were courses aimed at immigrant mothers that provided information on cooking, shopping, and infant and child care. Indeed, although settlements promoted a wide variety of reforms, they came to give particular precedence to educating immigrant mothers and advancing infant and child welfare. Organizing mothers clubs, settlements sought to better the condition of neighborhood women and their offspring by providing information that might help the immigrant mother adapt to the urban environment.[17]

The particular concern that settlements showed for educating immigrant mothers and for facilitating their adaptation to life in the United States was characteristic of much of the maternal education that constituted the main activity of American Progressive infant welfare reformers. While such reformers frequently spoke in general terms about the need to educate the urban poor, what they meant was the need to educate the immigrant urban poor. Although convinced that all mothers were woefully ignorant of safe and hygienic infant care practices, American infant welfare advocates showed particular concern for the ignorance of the immigrant mother. At its most generous, that concern was rooted in the conviction that infant care practices, which had been safe and practical in the rural villages from which many of the immigrants came, were not only impractical but dangerous in the American urban environment. At its least generous, the concern flowed from suspicion that the late nineteenth- and early twentieth-century wave of immigration from southern and eastern Europe brought to America a particularly ignorant, backward, and superstitious group of people. As William Guilfoy, New York City's registrar of records, observed in 1912: "It must be admitted that the necessity of instruction was not as pressing as it was 20 years ago, as it has been since the vast immigration from south and east continental Europe."[18] Similarly, the director of New York's milk stations complained before AASPIM that

The Italian mother who ties a string of coral beads around her badly-fed baby's wrist to make him get red blood . . . ; the Polish mother who packs her baby's soiled clothes in the bottom of a tub, sets him on them, and sozzles him with this water, from the bath; the Jewish mother who tries the formula that saved Mrs. Bobscheffsky's child on her own child,—to its extinction—, all require infinite patience and re-instruction.[19]

Just as it had with earlier American sanitary reform, this overriding concern with unacculturated immigrants added a particular orientation to early twentieth-century American infant welfare activity. In particular, it tended to submerge the socioeconomic and class dimensions of infant mortality and lend powerful reinforcement to the idea that infant mortality was a product of maternal ignorance and improper care and, thus, could be effectively combated by instruction. Moreover, it supported the comforting illusion that infant mortality—at least, excessive urban infant mortality—was not a problem intrinsic to American social organization, but, rather, an imported problem that would be greatly ameliorated once the new wave of immigrants was acculturated. This illusion, of course, was not unique to infant welfare. The belief that many of the social problems besetting urban America could be significantly addressed by acculturating immigrants was one which was central to American progressivism. Indeed, as George Rosen observed, the Progressive's campaign to reduce urban infant mortality through maternal instruction has to be understood as significantly shaped by the "Americanization movement which had its beginnings at the end of the last century, reached its peak during the First World War, and ebbed away during the 1920s."[20]

A second and related consequence of the concern focused on the immigrant was the establishment of an American pattern—persisting to this day—of analyzing infant mortality along ethnic and racial lines. Whereas by 1911 English sociomedical investigators had adopted a system that divided the populations they were studying into five socioeconomic classes, their American counterparts showed more interest in discovering racial and ethnic differentials. Considerable effort was thus made to determine infant mortality rates by race and ethnicity of the mother; much was made over the observation that Jewish babies died less frequently than Italian babies, and that black babies died most frequently of all.[21] To a certain extent the attention that American sociomedical investigators gave and continue to give to racial and ethnic infant mortality differentials was and is justified by the pluralistic nature of American society. Moreover, it has led to an appreciation that the consequences of racial and ethnic discrimination can manifest themselves in different rates of infant survival. Yet at the same time, it has supported racist and nativist interpretations of those rate differences that ignore intra- and intergroup economic status, and has justified policy that targeted certain groups of the poor while ignoring others.

Apparently assuming that all immigrant groups, as well as urban blacks, were equally poor, many Progressive infant health advocates tended to regard the different levels of infant mortality they experienced as proof of the importance of innate and acquired characteristics and customs. That blacks suffered the highest mortality was thus seen not as a consequence of their greater poverty, but as a result of their being the most racially and culturally backward and most neglectful of their children.[22] In his magisterial "Race Traits of the American Negro" (1896), Frederick L. Hoffman demonstrated convincingly that infant mortality among urban blacks was almost double that of their white counterparts. But he dismissed environment and poverty as causes for the difference, ridiculing "those who believe in the all powerful effect of the 'milieux.'"[23] "It is not in the *conditions of life*," asserted Hoffman, "but in *the race traits and tendencies* that we find the causes of the excessive mortality" (italics in original).[24] Nor was Hoffman alone in his convictions. Progressive health reformers spent much time discussing poverty and environment, but they did so always with an eye toward what they considered to be distinctive racial and ethnic customs and traits. Indeed, even when a few analysts, like Robert Morse Woodbury, pointed out that once family income was adjusted for, the statistical differences between the various racial and ethnic groups flattened out, their assertions met with more resistance than acceptance.[25]

English and continental infant welfare advocates also had their prejudices. They too viewed the higher infant mortality suffered by the poor as evidence of mental, physical, and cultural inferiority, and also pursued a reform program that sought to remake the poor in their own middle-class image. Yet their view was essentially shaped by the organizing principle of class and as such could not ignore the fundamental importance of socioeconomic status. They might argue that maternal ignorance rather than privation was the primary cause of infant mortality, but even conservatives, like Arthur Newsholme, could not avoid recognizing that "the *ignorance* of the working-class mother is more dangerous, because *associated with relative social helplessness*" (italics in original).[26] American infant welfare activists, on the other hand, while conscious of socioeconomic differences, were in addition conscious of race and ethnicity. The distinction is subtle but important. For it allowed American infant welfare reformers to plug into the international discourse on infant mortality yet to conceptualize the problem and shape their own response to it somewhat differently than their English and European counterparts.

The critical role played by private agencies, like settlements, in initiating and carrying out specialized infant welfare work and maternal education was not specific to America. There were, however, significant differences in the voluntaristic foundations of the European and American early infant welfare movement. Most notable of these was the degree to which voluntary infant welfare activity was subsidized, coordinated, and ultimately taken over by the government, particularly the national government. Especially in France and in Germany, voluntary infant welfare associations had from the beginning received some assistance from local and national government. Moreover, that assistance was soon increased and institutionalized by law or decree. After a 1905 German ministerial decree directed local authorities to unite with voluntary agencies to combat infant mortalty, a dramatic increase in state and national subsidies followed. By 1914 virtually all of the 742 infant welfare centers operating thoughout the empire were run by local officials and operated with public funds. Similarly, in 1909 when the Kaiserin Auguste Victoria Haus was opened as a center for studying and promoting the prevention of infant mortality, it received a hefty subsidy from the national government. When the voluntary Union for the Protection of Infants was organized that same year, the government also committed itself to paying all its operating expenses.[27] In France, the same pattern of increasing and substantial governmental subsidization and involvement in infant welfare activity was also evident. Subsidies that had been paid since before the turn of the century to voluntary agencies working to protect infant life were significantly increased following the 1900 creation of a publically funded national commission to provide assistance to private infant welfare work. Moreover, in 1909 a ministerial decree provided for substantial government support of all infant welfare agencies that did not discriminate by religion and encouraged breastfeeding.[28]

In Great Britain, government funding of infant welfare work developed somewhat more slowly. Because wariness of outdoor relief remained as a powerful legacy of nineteenth-century poor law reform, there was considerable reluctance to devote tax money to what tended to be regarded as a type of poor relief. Nevertheless, just as both national and local governments had early committed themselves to financial and other involvement in the promotion of public health, so too did they commit themselves to similar involvement in the promotion of infant welfare. In 1899 when the nation's first milk depot was opened, it was funded and run by a municipal health department. Between 1900 and 1905, municipalities began hiring and deploying trained nurses to visit new mothers in their homes and to provide them with instruction on domestic and infant hygiene. By 1912 the Local Government Board was subsidizing the work of some private organizations, an arrangement that was formalized and expanded in 1914, when Parliament voted to cover 50 percent of all the approved expenses of voluntary agencies conducting infant welfare work.[29] Moreover, in Great Britain and on the continent, World War I witnessed a tremendous expansion of public sector involvement, so that by the end of the war governments were either operating or providing funding for the bulk of infant welfare activities.

Compared to what was happening on the other side of the Atlantic, American government entry into infant welfare was both slow and attenu- ated. The federal government did not become directly involved in finan- cially assisting the promotion of infant health until 1921, when a program of matching grants to states was established by the Sheppard-Towner Act. And although state and municipal governments became involved earlier, they did so in a halting and uneven manner. While local officials in the United States had long been concerned with infant mortality, and especially so after the infant death rate became an accepted index of community health, as late as 1908 the specialized infant welfare work engaged in by the health departments of even the largest American cities was minimal at best and primarily limited to the inspection and regulation of commercial milk supplies. While all ten of the large municipal health departments polled that year by the American Academy of Political and Social Science reported that they were vigorously pursuing milk regulation and inspection, only one, Rochester, reported operating milk stations. Furthermore, although some effort was being made in six cities to provide education on infant hygiene to new mothers, in all but one city such effort was limited to the dispensing of printed circulars.[30]

What was true of city health departments was more so of state health departments. As of 1908 no state health department had as yet involved itself in any form of infant welfare work beyond milk control. Indeed, although state and local government involvement in infant welfare in- creased over the next decade, it did so slowly and unevenly. By 1915 only four states had created divisions or bureaus of child hygiene to conduct and coordinate multifaceted maternal reform and infant welfare campaigns. By 1918 only twelve states had. Municipalities did somewhat better. By 1915, eighteen cities had children's bureaus and by 1918 over fifty did.[31]

As had been the case with milk reform, New York City led the way, not only by being the first to establish a bureau of child hygiene within its health department but also by pioneering many of the educational techniques later adopted by other cities. The force behind New York's public health cam- paign against infant mortality was S. Josephine Baker. An 1898 graduate of the Medical College of the New York Infirmary for Women and Children, Baker joined the health department in 1901 as a school medical inspector. The following year she switched to the summer corps of physicians which the department had employed part-time since 1876 to visit and treat sick tenement infants during the hottest summer months. Assigned to Hell's Kitchen, Baker soon discovered that infants died in wholesale numbers amid the wretched squalor of the tenement district, and that most tenement mothers were tragically ignorant of even the basics of infant hygiene. She also learned that many of her colleagues considered the job a sinecure and never actually sought out or visited sick infants in their assigned districts.

Moreover, she soon concluded that those like herself who did, seemed to have little effect, since once an infant was sick it was often too late. These discoveries gradually inspired in her a conviction that what was needed to save New York's infants was a special office or division within the health department, staffed by dedicated doctors and nurses, and committed to keeping infants well rather than simply treating them once they fell sick.[32]

Over the next several years, as she was appointed to successively more important positions within the health department, Baker persistently lobbied her superiors for the opportunity to put her convictions into effect. Finally, in 1908 Health Commissioner Thomas Darlington provisionally created a Bureau of Child Hygiene and appointed her its chief. With as yet no staff and no money, Baker immediately set about to design and carry out a demonstration in maternal education which would convince the Board of Estimate and Apportionment that money should be appropriated for well-baby care. After determining which districts of the city had the highest infant mortality rates, she convinced the head of school medical inspection to lend her school nurses (free for the summer) to take part in an educational experiment. Using the previous day's birth reports provided by the city registrar, Baker's nurses visited all new mothers in the districts, encouraged them to breastfeed, and instructed them in the basics of infant hygiene. Returning periodically throughout the summer, the nurses kept tabs on the infants under their charge and made arrangements for those that fell sick to be treated at dispensaries or clinics. The result was that 120 fewer babies died in those districts that summer than had the previous one.[33]

Made official and permanent in August of 1908, New York's Bureau of Child Hygiene ultimately became the most expensive bureau in the Health Department and took responsibility for the young from birth through adolescence. In the beginning, however, its budgets were small and it concentrated most of its efforts on keeping the city's babies alive during the dangerous summer months. To do this Baker invented, perfected, or adapted several methods of baby-saving that were copied by health departments throughout the country. Among the most important of these was the use of trained nurses to visit tenement mothers in their homes, examine their babies, and instruct them in infant hygiene. Although Baker did not innovate the use of visiting nurses to provide home instruction to new mothers, she was responsible for demonstrating on an unprecedented scale their effectiveness in infant welfare work and for contributing to their development as the most significant individual participants in the early twentieth-century battle against infant mortality. Equally important, in originating the practice of using school nurses for summer infant welfare work, Baker provided America's perennially underfunded municipal health departments with a relatively economical means of engaging in home visiting on a large scale. As a consequence, Chicago, Detroit, Indianapolis, Cincinnati, Jersey City, and a number of other cities soon followed New York's lead and began using their own school nurses in summer campaigns of maternal education. Of the 427 non–infant welfare station nurses employed by municipalities for the sum-mer of 1915, almost 75 percent were school nurses.[34]

The job of such nurses was relatively straightforward, even if it was monumental. Each was assigned a district within the city and made respon-sible for all babies born there between the end of May and the beginning of September. Learning of a birth either from departmental records or from house-to-house canvassing, a nurse visited the new mother, examined the infant, provided encouragement and instruction in regard to breastfeeding, emphasized the necessity of making certain that any other food given was fresh and clean, and gave general advice on bathing, clothing, and other aspects of infant hygiene. If the mother could not breastfeed, the nurse urged her to visit an infant welfare station where her baby would be examined by a physician and a formula would be prescribed. Continuing to visit through-out the summer, the nurse monitored the baby's progress and provided ongoing advice to the mother. If the baby became ill, she assisted in getting it attended, either by a private or a dispensary physician. While political patronage was not unknown to affect the appointment of such nurses, most seem to have been dedicated and to have taken their responsibilities se-riously. Unlike the summer corps of physicians, they were full-time employ-ees and were not splitting their time between infant welfare work and private practice.[35]

The nurses' training emphasized that mothers wanted practical advice rather than sermons and considerable effort was made to find nurses who spoke the language of the neighborhood. Nevertheless, some friction be-tween mothers and visiting nurses probably existed. Like other infant wel-fare workers, visiting nurses sought to acculturate immigrant mothers by introducing them to a scientific infant care, considered both more hygienic and more American. Certain essentials of that care, however, rested on a view of the maternal-infant relationship that was a product of industrial, middle-class culture and thus not shared by immigrants from preindustrial, peasant societies. In particular, scientific infant care assumed that mothers had the time and inclination to devote themselves almost exclusively to caring for their infants. The advice and work of the visiting nurses, there-fore, often conflicted both with traditions and customs brought over from the old country and with the realities of life in an urban immigrant slum.

One area of contention was infant feeding. Visiting nurses sought to instruct mothers in a science of infant feeding that rested on a doctrine of regularity. Aimed at building good habits and preventing under- and over-feeding, that doctrine held that infants should be fed by the clock, no more than once in every three to four hours. But scheduled feeding ran counter to immigrant custom, and in many cases was impossible for the overworked and busy immigrant mother. Such mothers tended to feed their infants when they could, a practice that appalled infant welfare workers. In a study of twenty-four families on New York's west side, one maternal reformer complained,

> [The baby] is fed irregularly. When the mother "goes out for the day," she nurses the baby at mealtimes and during the night. Irregular artificial feeding supplements her nursings. In the case of the non-wage earning mother, the nursings are equally irregular. The child is nursed when it cries or whenever the mother thinks it necessary, day or night. The clock is not consulted.[36]

Other areas of contention involved the use of solid food and pacifiers, swaddling, leaving the infant in the care of an older sibling, general cleanliness, and the amount of room the baby should have all to itself.

Yet it would be a mistake to dismiss the advice and work of the visiting nurses as misguided and ineffectual attempts to remake the immigrant mother into a middle-class housewife and to transform the tenement apartment into an approximation of the orderly middle-class home. It would also be a mistake to think that immigrant mothers were unwilling participants in their own reform, participants whose only power lay in resistance. The recorded comments of those involved in health visiting indicate that tenement mothers were not, as was occasionally charged, overly wedded to traditional customs and resistant to change. Most nurses reported that when the efficacy of a new method of feeding or infant care was sufficiently demonstrated and its adoption was at all possible within the constraining conditions of tenement life, immigrant mothers seemed eager to learn and embrace it. Josephine Baker recalled that once mothers saw that their babies were flourishing despite the hot weather, they became eager disciples of the type of practical baby care advice which the bureau nurses gave out.[37] Moreover, many immigrant women seemed to embrace what they found useful and discard what they did not. As a resident physician at Hull House in charge of instruction on infant hygiene, Alice Hamilton was often infuriated that most of the women she dealt with seemed to pick and choose what part of her advice they would follow. Yet years later she came to realize that in doing so they were exhibiting intelligent discretion.[38] Indeed, as Elizabeth Ewen observes in her study of women's lives on the lower east side of New York: "the tension between immigrant women and the representatives of industrial culture were not over the need to change the external conditions of motherhood, but over how and what knowledge was to be incorporated into the rhythm and patterns of daily life."[39]

Although some of the lessons offered by visiting nurses in domestic hygiene and home management were clearly more suited to the native middle-class home than to the immigrant tenement apartment, not all were.

To mothers whose infants died in such numbers each summer from diarrheal epidemics, advice that purchased milk should be heated to kill germs, should be kept cool as possible, and should be guarded from flies was more than just culturally uplifting instruction. So too was advice on the importance of sterilizing diapers, sheets, and bottle nipples. Moreover, visiting nurses often worked in conjunction with mothers to save the lives of seriously ill infants by combining home visitation, welfare assistance, and referral to a dispensary. The results of their efforts were both immediate and apparent. Not untypical is the following case history, recorded by an NYAICP visiting nurse attached to the infant's and children's dispensary at Bellevue Hospital in New York.

July 15—Mother came to the dispensary with her sick baby. The mother has been nursing the baby and the doctor says child has not been getting enough nourishment. . .

July 16—Called. Found family living in two rooms on the ground floor, one of which was a shoemaker's shop. There are eight children, six of whom are living at home. The back living room is very dirty. . . . The mother is very sickly and nervous. Her milk is not sufficient for the baby. I ordered milk and showed mother how to prepare it for her six month's old child. . .

July 17—Called to see if mother had prepared milk properly. Baby's neck is swollen and much worse. Instructed mother to bring baby to the dispensary this afternoon.

Same date—Saw baby at dispensary. Doctor told mother to alternate breast feeding with a prescription of milk. Nurse showed mother how to make prescription.

July 18—Mother said that milk, which I had ordered, had not come. Gave her tickets to the Diet Kitchen. . . . Having seen to it that she got milk from the Diet Kitchen, I instructed her to feed her baby alternately from a bottle and at her breast. The baby is to have a feeding every three hours.

July 20—Mother brought baby to the dispensary. Neck had been dressed in the surgical clinic. Baby is looking better. Mother says it is fine. She also says milk agrees with it.

July 24—Called at home. Baby is better. House is still very dirty. Mother says she is hungry. I gave her milk tickets for herself and for the baby, and instructed her to drink milk. I also promised her that a relief visitor would come from the Association.

July 31—Called. Found visiting housewife from the Association. House was being cleaned and the washing done. Baby was sleeping in front of the house in its carriage. It seemed much better. Temperature 100°. Mother stated, however, that its bowels had not been quite right. Gave instructions for baby's care.

Aug. 5—Called. Found mother and baby both better. Mother says baby does not want anything to eat and she thinks it is sick. Examination shows baby is well, but that it has lost its appetite on account of the heat.

Same date—Mother brought baby to the dispensary. Doctor says baby is get-ting along alright. Does not need any additional treatment. But mother is to continue former instructions.

Aug. 8—Called. Mother and baby are looking better. Baby is doing very well. House was in better condition than nurse has ever seen it before. Baby is now getting along upon its mother's milk. No extra food is required. I shall keep the family under observation until the mother and baby are both perfectly well.[40]

The Bureau of Child Hygiene also led the way in establishing on a large scale a network of municipally funded infant welfare and milk stations. In 1908, when the bureau was created, Rochester was the only city operating milk stations. Everyplace else they were funded and run by private agencies. In New York, seven philanthropic organizations ran fifty-one stations, twenty-five of which were open year round.[41] In 1910, however, in response to relentless pleas from Baker, the city appropriated $40,000 so that the bureau could open fifteen stations the following summer. The appropria-tion, however, came with the proviso that the effectiveness of the stations be proven. To accomplish this, Baker joined with the NYMC (which had raised $165,000 to open thirty stations that summer) in its 1911 demonstration of the effectiveness of its program of home milk modification and maternal instruction. Like the NYMC's Wilbur Phillips, Baker was convinced that supplying milk without training mothers was an inadequate response to infant mortality. She frequently argued in person and in print that "the solution of the problem of infant mortality is 20 per cent. pure milk and 80 per cent. training of mothers. The infant milk stations will serve this wider usefulness when they become educational centers."[42] The demonstration apparently had an effect on city officials for the stations were made perma-nent.

Playing no small role in New York's growing financial commitment to milk stations and other infant welfare activities was Baker's ability as a flexible, shrewd, and effective political operative. Although ideologically sympathet-ic to Progressive good government reform, she forged close ties to a number of powerful Tammany Hall figures and used those ties to get what she wanted. She also was not afraid to engage in confrontation politics. In 1912, when the private funding for the NYMC stations ran out, she threatened to close the bureau's infant welfare stations as well unless the city provided support for those established by the NYMC. Since, as she pointedly noted, the wives of thousands of voters had come to rely on the stations, the threat carried some weight: and the city appropriated enough money not only to keep all the existing stations open but also to establish ten new ones. By the summer of 1912 the bureau was operating a total of fifty-five infant welfare stations.[43] Between the stations it ran and its corps of visiting nurses, the bureau had under supervision 34,000 of the 50,000 city infants who Baker estimated had "mothers who are ignorant of the simplest methods of baby care, and who are unable to pay for such advice or for medical treatment in case of illness."[44]

Along with establishing its own infant welfare stations and hiring its own visiting nurses, the bureau acted to coordinate the activities of private agencies and in so doing provided a model of effective cooperation between a municipal health department and private philanthropies. By the summer of 1911 six philanthropic organizations were operating a total of sixty-four infant milk or welfare stations in New York. In May of that year they were organized by the NYMC into the Association of Infant Milk Stations. One year later they were reorganized by the bureau into the Babies Welfare Association and began receiving funding from the city. By 1915 the association, now entirely coordinated and substantially funded by the bureau, had grown to include seventy-nine infant welfare stations, six research agencies, ninety-two day nurseries, twenty-two institutions and homes for children, seventy-seven dispensaries, thirty-five fresh-air associations, and fifty-four relief agencies.[45]

Other cities followed a similar course of cooperation with private organizations. In the summer of 1909, a number of charitable agencies in Philadelphia banded together to conduct a summer campaign to save the city's babies. The health department assisted by making its health officers available to canvass for sick infants. The 1909 summer campaign began a cooperative arrangement that by 1913 had the department's Division of Child Hygiene coordinating summer infant welfare work involving a "baby alliance" of over 200 private organizations. These included day nurseries, settlements, visiting nurse associations, relief agencies, private hospitals and dispensaries, fresh-air funds, milk depots and infant welfare stations, various women's clubs, and local chapters of the National Congress of Mothers. In addition to the ongoing instructional, supervisory and relief efforts, classes were held throughout the city for new mothers, as were contests where mothers with the healthiest-looking babies were awarded prizes. Both English and foreign language newspapers also ran columns on baby care.[46]

In Chicago, the Department of Health, along with the United Charities, organized an Infant Welfare Committee in the spring of 1909 to combat summer diarrhea among the city's infants. Chaired by the head of the health department and including representatives from settlements, visiting nurse associations, city missions, hospitals and dispensaries, and churches and synagogues, the committee sent volunteer nurses and doctors in search of new mothers and their infants, raised funds for the opening and operation of new milk stations, and carried out an educational program through news-

papers and public lectures. The following year, the committee was transformed into a permanent Infant Welfare Society and continued to coordinate work between the health department and private agencies. In 1912,
however, much of the coordination was taken over by the city when it
created a Division of Child Hygiene.

This pattern of cooperation between municipal health departments and
philanthropic and social service agencies was common throughout the United States. Indeed, such cooperation was especially crucial in smaller towns
and cities because the funding their health departments received was often
minimal at best. Writing on the shortcomings of public health administration in 1911, a Springfield, Illinois, health officer reported that, with the
exception of Chicago, not one of the state's forty-four cities with populations of 3,000 or more, "pays sufficient salary to warrant a competent man in
devoting all his time to the health department."[47] Similarly, a special health
commission created by New York's Governor Sulzer reported in 1913 that
while public health funding varied widely throughout the state, with the
exception of New York City and a few other large municipalities, "in nearly
every case it is inadequate and in many cases ridiculous."[48] Such lack of
funding made small city health officers who wished to combat infant mortality particularly dependent on private charity. Speaking before the American Public Health Association in 1911, an Orange, New Jersey, health official reported that his experience had made him realize "the important fact"
that in small cities cooperation between health departments and private
agencies was imperative in infant welfare work because such "agencies are
not infrequently doing work which probably should be done by the health
department, but through the parsimony or false economy of the city fathers,
cannot be undertaken at the present time."[49]

The refusal of many smaller city governments to appropriate adequate
funding for infant supervision and maternal education also illustrates another important feature of the early infant welfare campaign in America:
that it was national only in a limited sense and was profoundly shaped by
local political, economic, and social configurations. In cities such as New
York and Milwaukee and in states such as Massachusetts and Michigan—
where skillful public health administrators were able to forge effective reform coalitions and elicit monetary support from the economically and
politically powerful—infant welfare, like public health reform in general,
achieved significant dimensions. In other cities and states, however, it did
not. Admittedly, this was not unique to the United States. In England local
political and economic arrangements also exerted considerable influence on
the extent to which municipalities and townships pursued and committed
funds to infant welfare and maternal education. Yet, at least in comparison
to the United States, the weight of local influence was significantly counter-
balanced by oversight and funding from the Local Government Board.

In the United States, however, there was no federal subsidization, coordination, or regulation of infant welfare activity. As a consequence such activity was left to individual states and municipalities, and great discrepancies existed. Through the middle of the second decade of the century, the bulk of infant welfare work was centered in large cities and within New England, and the east north-central, and middle atlantic states. As late as 1915, 43 percent of the 551 infant welfare stations in operation and 49 percent of the visiting nurses were located in eight large cities. Moreover, the fourteen states that comprise the above three geographical regions contained 83 percent of all infant welfare stations and 97 percent of all full-time summer visiting nurses.[50] Indeed, in the entire South, only forty-one infant welfare stations were in existence in 1915; and of these, twenty were in Washington, D.C., and Baltimore.[51] Despite the tendency of infant welfare activists to describe their maternal education effort as a campaign to save all American babies, obviously precious little of that effort was benefiting small-town or rural white infants and even less rural black infants.

Indeed, geographic inequalities in the delivery of public health services, combined with the prevailing conceptualization of infant mortality as an urban immigrant problem and an anything but subtle racism, worked almost entirely to exclude black infants from the early part of the infant welfare campaign.[52] Not until 1916 did the NYAICP pioneer the first attempt to deal with black urban mortality by conducting an infant welfare demonstration in a black neighborhood. Not until the 1921 enactment of the Sheppard-Towner Act did southern states even consider trying to reduce infant mortality among their black populations. This tendency to ignore, or pay only cursory attention to, black infant mortality was particularly tragic because black infants seem to have suffered the highest death rate of any group of American babies. Although his interpretation of the causes of black infant mortality was fundamentally racist, Hoffman had correctly observed in 1896 that "an excessive infant mortality, such as we meet with among the white population in all parts of this country, has at times been the concern of the philanthropist and the economist, but nowhere else do we meet with such frightful infant mortality as we find prevailing among the colored population of the large cities, both North and South."[53] Indeed, using a ratio of infant deaths to infant living, he showed that infant mortality among blacks in four southern cities was 47 percent compared to 24 percent for whites.[54] Moreover, between 1915 and 1920, inclusive, black infant mortality in the newly established and expanding birth registration area was on average roughly 65 percent higher than white infant mortality and 60 percent higher than that of other non-whites (principally Asians and Native Americans). Also, the death rate of black infants between the third and eighth month—that period of infant life when preventable gastroenteric disorders take their greatest toll—was almost 100 percent higher.[55]

To a certain extent, the Children's Bureau tried to make up for the lack of public health funding for maternal education and infant welfare work outside of major cities by publishing in 1914 the first edition of its classic advice manual, *Infant Care*. Mailed free of charge to anyone who requested it and distributed to constituents by congressmen, the pamphlet seems to have been especially valued by rural and small-town women who had little access to informed medical advice and certainly did not receive visits from infant welfare nurses. One Wyoming woman who wrote to the bureau requesting a copy of the pamphlet explained that she was "twenty-six miles from a doctor, five miles from a telephone and a quarter of a mile from my nearest neighbor."[56] From *Infant Care* women received basic advice on such matters as bathing, clothing, and bedding, on how to lift an infant and on how to care for its eyes, mouth, and ears. They also received detailed instructions on both nursing and artificial feeding as well as descriptions of the symptoms of various infant diseases.

State health departments also attempted to target mothers outside cities by conducting statewide maternal education campaigns. By 1915, twenty-six states were publishing and distributing pamphlets or circulars on infant feeding and hygiene. Thirty-three had traveling exhibits, lantern slide shows, or films that were sent around to county fairs and towns and small cities. And twenty-nine sent health officers around the state to lecture on infant care to any organized group who made a formal request. That such general educational efforts could compensate for the lack of direct infant welfare services is, however, highly doubtful, especially since they were spotty in their coverage. Like small cities, many states provided their health departments with rather paltry budgets. Indeed, as late as 1917, per capita spending on public health in the United States was only twenty cents, although most experts at the time considered fifty to seventy-five cents to be the absolute minimum needed.[57]

Even in large American cities, funding was frequently a problem. New York may have been the model that other large American cities wished to emulate, but its experience was hardly typical. In St. Louis, despite the pleas of health officials, the city council steadfastly refused to appropriate funds for the creation of a bureau of child hygiene, for the hiring of visiting nurses, or for the opening of infant welfare stations. The same situation existed in New Orleans, although the city did make a contribution to the operating expenses of the private Infant Welfare Association. In Pittsburgh, where the health department had succeeded in getting funding in 1909 to divide the city into six districts with each district having a milk station and a visiting nurse, a new city administration abruptly killed the program the following year. Similarly, officials of Boston's Division of Child Hygiene complained that the appropriations it received were tragically insufficient. Even in New York, the city most committed to the principle that "public health is purchasable," Baker had to become an expert on manipulating the various administrations who occupied city hall simply to meet her operating expenses. For infant welfare work was not inexpensive. Even though it left medical treatment to private physicians or charitable clinics and limited its services to education and supervision, the New York Bureau of Child Hygiene spent $203,283 in 1914 to run its infant welfare stations and keep its visiting nurses in the field. Baker, then, was not merely being magnanimous when she frequently claimed that without the assistance of private agencies, the reduction of infant mortality in New York City would not have been as dramatic as it was.[58]

In addition to promoting the use of public health nurses in infant welfare work, pioneering the establishment of municipally funded well-baby stations, and demonstrating the effectiveness of municipal cooperation with private agencies, Baker and her Bureau of Child Hygiene devised a number of unique educational strategies. Among the most widely copied of these were the Little Mothers' Leagues, composed of poor and immigrant girls twelve years of age and older. Baker conceived of the leagues in 1910 after reading in John Spargo's *Bitter Cry of Children* that poor working mothers often left toddlers and even infants in the care of the eldest daughter, frequently a child herself. Charging that the young girls' ignorance was a "fertile source" of infant mortality, Spargo had condemned the practice and had urged that it be prohibited. Baker was more pragmatic. Recognizing the economic necessity that motivated it, she sought to lessen the danger of the practice by providing the girls of New York's tenement districts with training in infant care.

Enlisting the aid of school principals, Baker had bureau nurses and doctors give in-school lectures on infant care during the spring of 1910. When school let out for the summer, neighborhood leagues were formed which met for instruction and demonstrations once a week. To keep the girls interested, the bureau deputized them as volunteer aids of the department of health, provided them with official certificates of membership, and gave them silver badges if they attended at least six meetings. In the summer of 1910, 71 leagues were formed. In 1911, the number was 183 and included a membership of approximately twenty thousand girls.[59] The girls were instructed on all aspects of infant care, from bathing to feeding to the need for proper clothing and sufficient fresh air. In addition to believing that such instruction would improve the quality of care the girls gave their younger siblings, the bureau hoped that by instructing daughters they would also reach mothers, especially immigrant mothers. As was true of those Progressive educators who sought to Americanize immigrant families by acculturating their children, the bureau was convinced that the immigrant school child represented particularly fertile ground for reform. This conviction was apparently shared by others, because by 1915 Little Mothers' Leagues had been organized in forty-four American cities with a combined membership of almost fifty thousand young girls.[60]

By 1914 the bureau had over 200 nurses and 130 physicians working for it during the summer months and a budget of well over a quarter of a million dollars. It had also compiled a substantial record of achievement that seemed to demonstrate the effectiveness of a well-funded, municipal public health campaign of maternal instruction. In 1907, the year before the bureau was created, the infant mortality rate in New York had been 144.4. In the bureau's first year of operation, it plummeted to 127.9. Six years later it was 94.6, the lowest infant mortality rate of any major city in the United States or in Europe.[61] Much of that reduction had been in deaths from diarrheal diseases, and Baker and her bureau, which had adopted as its motto Better Mothers, Better Babies, Better Homes, were convinced that this proved the correctness of their emphasis on maternal education of poor mothers in infant and domestic hygiene. At the same time, however, they were becoming increasingly aware that reducing diarrheal deaths in the city's slums solved only part of the problem. As Baker observed at the time in a review of the bureau's work: "while these results have justified our expectations, we are keenly alive to the importance of further efforts along other lines."[62]

One of the lines along which Baker felt further effort needed to be made was the reduction of mortality among institutionalized infants. Although improvements in the sanitary environment of infant institutions had substantially reduced the 80–90 percent mortality that had been common in the nineteenth century, institutionalized babies still suffered a death rate far in excess of that suffered by babies within private families. Indeed, no matter what institutional officials seemed to do, the death rate of their charges continued to hover around 50 percent, over three times the rate of infant death even in the worst city slums. Given that institutionalized infants were housed in a controlled, aseptic environment and received much better medical supervision than the average city infant, charity and public health officials concluded that there could be only one explanation for their disproportionate mortality: the absence of individualized maternal care. That conclusion suggested two courses of action. The first was to deemphasize institutionalization and to assist impoverished, widowed, abandoned, or otherwise disadvantaged mothers in keeping their infants. This was a course of action consistent with the growing conviction among child welfare activists that institutional care was detrimental to the physical and intellectual well-being of the young. Homer Folks, for instance, argued before the Fifteenth International Congress on Hygiene and Demography that "the real and only remedy for this situation is not to provide better care for the so-called foundling, but not to receive him into our care at all. Leave him with his mother: assist the mother if need be, and you will thereby, in the great majority of the cases, substitute breast feeding and individual home care for artificial feeding or wet nursing after a period of artificial feeding, and you will at one sweep enormously reduce infant mortality."[63]

The second possible course of action was to overcome traditional misgivings about providing material assistance to families and to pay foster mothers to take infants who would otherwise be institutionalized. This was a course charted by Henry D. Chapin and the Speedwell Society, an organization founded in 1902 to board out sick institutionalized infants. It was also the course followed by Baker's bureau. First on its own and then with the aid of the Russell Sage Foundation, the bureau established a program in which experienced tenement mothers were paid ten dollars a month to take foundlings into their homes and care for them. The result was that the mortality rate among New York's foundlings was cut in half, an achievement which made Baker an ardent proponent of the idea that "old fashioned, sentimental mothering" was the most critical factor in infant welfare.[64]

Another area in which Baker felt more work could be done was in bringing infant welfare information to the general public. In 1911 the bureau had sponsored the nation's first infant welfare exhibition, a collection of demonstrations, lectures, and displays on milk modification, bathing, maternal nursing, domestic sanitation, clothing, and other facets of infant hygiene. Drawing relatively large crowds and receiving considerable publicity, it was soon copied by other cities. The following year the Philadelphia Health Department, in conjunction with private infant welfare organizations, held a similarly educational "baby show." Containing exhibits on eugenics and heredity, breastfeeding, artificial foods, general infant care, and other related subjects, the show lasted for nine days, cost $14,300 to put on, and attracted over 67,000 visitors. By 1915, Providence, Buffalo, Kansas City, Indianapolis, Seattle, and several other cities had also hosted exhibitions, and the Children's Bureau had published an instructional manual for communities wishing to do so.[65]

One purpose of such exhibitions was to inform the public of the seriousness of the problem of infant mortality and to generate support for the expenditure of public funds to combat it. But the exhibitions also had another purpose, to bring maternal education to the middle classes. Although infant welfare activists remained convinced that infant mortality was highest among the urban poor and continued to channel most of their effort in that direction, they began to express concern about the infant death rate among those who were neither impoverished nor wealthy. Initially, such concern was motivated by recognition that while infant mortality was most serious among the poor, it was not confined to that class. After 1915, however, it was fueled by statistics, first gathered by cities and then by the Children's Bureau, suggesting that infant mortality was also very high among those who stood between the impoverished and the prosperous. The reason for this, many infant welfare activists came to agree, was that while the well-off mother could purchase quality medical and advisory care for herself and her baby and the poor mother had access to it through charity, "the middle-class mother, neither rich nor poor, can seldom afford such care and is too proud to ask for it free."[66]

Aside from promoting the staging of infant welfare exhibitions, the desire to reach the middle classes also gave birth to the idea of devoting a whole week to publicizing the seriousness of infant mortality and to providing public instruction in its prevention. Chicago was the site of the first such baby week. Embarrassed and concerned by statistics showing that Chicago had the highest infant death rate of all major American cities, the health department's Divison of Child Hygiene and the Infant Welfare Association organized in the spring of 1914 an elaborate week-long campaign to heighten public awareness, educate mothers, and raise funds to open forty more infant welfare stations. With the aid of advertising agencies, a publicity blitz was mounted. Posters were placed in downtown store windows and other prominent places; newspapers ran display ads; coupons were inserted in theater programs; movie houses ran stills between features; milk dealers put circulars around bottles they delivered; and local clergy sermonized from the pulpit. Exhibitions, demonstrations, and lectures on infant care were also held throughout the city. New York City soon followed Chicago's example, conducting a baby week campaign in June of that year. Costing $80,000, it had the expressed purpose of convincing middle-class mothers that they too needed instruction, should take advantage of infant welfare stations, and should look to the Bureau of Child Hygiene for advice.[67]

The idea was quick to catch on. By the following summer, so many communities had adopted it that the *Survey* reported, "baby week is a celebration in American towns and cities as familiar nowadays as old home week."[68] Indeed, so positive was the response to local baby weeks that in the fall of 1915 the General Federation of Women's Clubs and the Children's Bureau announced that they were joining in a common effort to promote a national baby week to be held in the spring of the following year. Through its magazine and publicity department, the GFWC mobilized the more than two million American women associated with its national, state, and local chapters. Other women's groups, such as the National Congress of Mothers, also got involved. The Children's Bureau produced a set of instructions on how to hold a baby week, compiled packets of pamphlets on baby care, and sent them out to the 4,234 communities that requested information.[69]

Held March 4–11, 1916, National Baby Week involved millions of American mothers and their infants and was celebrated throughout the country. Although the exact program varied from community to community, certain features were nearly universal. One was an emphasis on education. Along with organizing lectures and demonstrations on the "do's and don't's" of baby care, local baby week committees distributed a mountain of literature on infant and domestic hygiene. A second common feature was a celebration of motherhood as a sacred vocation and as one explicitly connected to the national welfare. Like military heroes, mothers with infants in arms paraded down main street to the applause of flag-waving townspeople. A third common feature was the almost complete absence of any reference to the socioeconomic determinants of infant mortality. While most infant welfare activists still believed poverty to be a major cause of infant mortality, one could not tell this from the activities that took place during baby week. If those activities carried a single message, it was that good mothering saved baby lives and that the good mother was one who cared enough about her infant to devote all her time to it and to give it informed care and a hygienic environment. Indeed, many communities had "best mother contests" in which the winner was determined by an evaluation of her knowledge and devotion.[70]

The message that motherhood was a sacred and nationally valuable vocation and that the quality of mothering was determined by devotion and knowledge was one that struck a resonant chord in middle-class America and goes a long way toward explaining the popularity of baby week campaigns. Although it is risky to generalize about such a large and diverse segment of the American population, most women's historians agree that by the second decade of the century, many middle-class American women were seeking both reassurance of the value of their traditional role as nurturers of the young and expert advice in carrying out that role. Since late in the nineteenth century, various social commentators had been reviling middle-class women as increasingly frivolous and devoid of social usefulness. Some charged them with being physical invalids, beset with nervous disorders, and too selfish and unfit to produce enough healthy children to replenish the race. Others complained that the industrial revolution and the advance of science and technology had robbed household work of most of its previous functions and of its productive value and had created an idle class of socially useless women with too much time on their hands. Heightened by turn-of-the-century eugenicist alarms over race suicide and feminist critiques of the intellectually and physically debilitating consequences of women's confinement to traditional domestic roles, such criticism of middle-class women helped focus widespread attention on the character and value of motherhood and made it one of the central issues within what came to be known in the first decades of the century as the "woman question." As Helen Campbell observed in her popular 1910 maternal advice manual, "[motherhood] is by far the most important Woman's Question of the day, in that it must inevitably lie to a great extent at the root of those other much discussed problems of Physical Degeneracy, Social Morality, and National Welfare and Progress."[71]

Tension between certain significant changes and continuities in the actual conditions of many middle-class women's lives also contributed to making middle-class motherhood an issue of national interest. By 1900 the increasing market availability of domestic goods—from processed food to ready-to-wear clothing—plus the invention of various labor-saving devices, had indeed changed the character of household work for better-off women and had oriented their homes more toward consumption than production.[72] So too had the century-long drop in the fertility rate, a drop that was most pronounced among the white, native-born, and relatively well-off. American middle-class women were having fewer children than their mothers and grandmothers and were completing their families at an earlier age.[73] At the same time, more women than ever before were receiving formal education. By 1900 60 percent of all high school graduates were women, and by 1910 40 percent of all Americans attending college were also women.

The changes in home life and the increases in education helped contribute to what many historians have described as a profound restlessness among turn-of-the-century middle-class woman, a restlessness centered in but not limited to a clash between rising expectations and a still powerful Victorian domestic ethos that confined women to the private sphere of the home. Although most powerfully articulated by feminists such as Charlotte Perkins Gilman, that restlessness also found expression in one form or another throughout middle-class America. One form it found was in the increasing incidence of women entering the public sphere, through participating in women's organizations, pursuing careers, or becoming engaged in some other public activity. Another was in a movement by reformers and middle-class women alike to redefine maternal duties and responsibilities, make them worthy of the talents and abilities of educated women, and to invest them with social significance and national importance. As Nancy Woloch has observed, "during the Progressive era, housekeeping and child care were transformed into specialized missions that required commitment, talent, training, executive abilities and professional skills. Domestic science, home economics, household engineering and child psychology became arts and sciences that only an educated woman could master."[74]

Popular magazines, such as *Good Housekeeping* and the *Ladies Home Journal*, championed the need for educated motherhood and offered "expert" advice on every conceivable situation a mother might face. Courses in home economics and child management were offered in secondary schools and colleges. Kindergarten clubs, designed to introduce mothers to the latest theories of child psychology and development, were founded throughout America. Maternal advice manuals appeared in dizzying numbers. Writers and lecturers addressed university women and discussed the natural fit between intellectuality and maternity. And social and child welfare advocates publicly decried the ills brought about by unskilled mothers.[75] Indeed, the age-old idea that women were fit for motherhood because they were instinctively nurturing took something of a battering. While few promoting the new motherhood denied that mother love was instinctual, even fewer considered such instinct sufficient. As with other complicated activities in the modern world, successful mothering required information and skills that needed to be learned. As one writer in the *Ladies Home Journal* explained, "Ideal Motherhood, you see, is the work not of instinct, but of enlightened knowledge conscientiously acquired and carefully digested."[76]

Although the movement to educate and ennoble mothers encompassed a wide variety of concerns associated with motherhood, the care of infants and the prevention of morbidity and mortality in infancy increasingly became a central one. Before 1900, infant care was the subject of only a few, sporadic articles in women's magazines. In the decades that followed, however, it became the topic of regular features, often written by recognized or self-proclaimed experts. With every new issue of *Harper's Bazaar*, readers could turn to Marianna Wheeler for advice on such matters as how to clothe a baby, what to do when the baby begins teething, how to handle the baby's first summer, what babies should be fed, how to travel with a baby, and what were the pros and cons of pasteurized versus certified milk. Similarly, from 1903 through 1921 readers of the *Ladies Home Journal* could count on a regular feature on baby care written by Emelyn L. Coolidge, author of the popular *Mother's Manual* (1904). The *Ladies Home Journal* also published short pieces from their readers explaining how they raised their infants, or confessing to some egregious but not fatal mistake. The *Delineator* featured Leonard K. Hirshberg, author of *What You Ought to Know About Your Baby* (1910) and subsequently an advice columnist with *Home Progress* and then the *Ladies Home Journal*. The *Woman's Home Companion* offered its readers a feature written by Roger H. Dennet, a young pediatrician and author of both *The Healthy Baby* (1912) and a respected medical text on simplified infant feeding. Magazines also encouraged mothers to write in with specific questions regarding infant care and published both the questions and answers. They also competed for the services of prominent infant welfare experts and pediatricians. In 1922, after the *Delineator* signed up L. Emmett Holt to offer advice on a regular basis, the *Ladies Home Journal* responded by contracting Josephine Baker to do the same.

Some magazines also did more than just offer advice to mothers on infant care. As part of the child rescue campaign initiated by Theodore Dreiser when he took over editorship of the magazine, the *Delineator* organized an infant rescue and maternal education campaign. One part of that campaign was to be carried on in the pages of the magazine through features and advice columns on infant care. Another part was to be carried on in the field. In April of 1909, using space donated by the Children's Aid Society, the magazine established seven schools or consultations for mothers in lower Manhattan. Hiring eight nurses and six physicians to examine babies and visit homes, it cared for 442 infants that summer. The magazine also promoted the establishment of similar mothers' schools in other cities, assigning Edith Howe, an assistant editor and chair of the child hygiene committee of the National Congress of Mothers, to offer interested readers assistance and advice. By the end of the year her efforts were paying dividends, as readers formed 185 organizations in 30 states and 150 cities.[77]

In 1917 the *Delineator* also mounted what it termed a "Save the Seventh Baby Campaign" in response to published statistics showing that one American baby in seven died before the end of its first year. In addition to publishing advice columns and sponsoring classes for mothers, it hired a staff of trained nurses and offered them to communities with populations of 10,000–40,000 to work with local organizations in surveying the causes of infant mortality and making recommendations. It also made available a lab chemist to analyze milk supplies, sent in a traveling exhibit, and supplied items on infant mortality and infant care to local newspapers. Its aim was not only to save the seventh baby but also to improve all babies so they would be models of health and happiness. Such model infants the magazine labeled "*Delineator* babies."[78]

Promoting the development of perfect babies was also a task taken on by the *Woman's Home Companion*. In 1913 the magazine came up with the idea of encouraging "better baby shows" and hired Anne S. Richardson to promote it. The idea was not entirely original, however. Baby shows or contests had become rather commonplace in England since the first one was held in Manchester in 1905. Nevertheless, the idea was new to Americans and when the first such show was held in Colorado in the spring of 1913, it immediately caught the fancy of the public. By the end of the summer, hundreds of shows had been held throughout the country in town squares, summer resorts, and county fairs. Frequently organized by middle-class women's clubs or by companies that sold infant products, such shows involved the judging of infants according to criteria contained on a scorecard. The infant who scored highest was awarded a ribbon and was paraded around by its proud mother as proof of her superior maternal devotion and skill. More often than not, however, the scoring criteria were rather vague and the baby who won was usually the plumpest, fairest, and most blue-eyed. This led to objections from various quarters. The *Literary Digest* described the contests as "human cattle shows" and the *Journal of the American Medical Association* editorialized against them. Interestingly, though, the AMA did not find anything intrinsically wrong in judging infants like so much cattle on the hoof. Its objection was that the criteria for such judging were too often unscientific. It thus established a committee to devise a scientifically legitimate scorecard to be used at future contests.[79]

In an effort to improve their babies and to learn all they could about their management, middle-class mothers also began purchasing infant care manuals in sufficient numbers to make some of their authors both wealthy and famous. L. Emmett Holt's *The Care and Feeding of Children*, most of which concerned infant care, approximated during the first quarter of the century the influence and popularity that Benjamin Spock's *Baby and Child Care* achieved during the third. Indeed, in 1946 when Groliers published a list of the one hundred books it judged to have had the most impact on American life and customs since colonial times, Holt's was one of them.[80] In addition, mothers could also turn to advice manuals written by a number of other renowned pediatricians as well as to a host of works written by lay writers, nurses, and less well-known physicians.[81]

The writers of these manuals and the magazine advice columnists offered their readers something still not readily available to most American parents: informed and detailed information on infant care. Early childhood medicine still constituted only a minor part of most physicians' formal education, and while pediatrics had become a recognized specialty, the number of pediatricians practicing outside major cities was negligible at best. Even fairly prosperous non-urban parents had to turn to their general practitioners when their infant became ill or developed some problem. And they, more often than not, tended to dispense vague generalities and rely on liberal doses of purgatives and cathartics. All too typical was the experience of one obviously well-off and well-educated woman who wrote to the Children's Bureau seeking advice on an infant who since birth had been discharging loose stools covered with green mucus. "I have been to the Dr. time and again," she complained. "He gives me a pink tablet, which I think contains calomel but I can never find out from him what causes the mucus to form."[82]

Although differing on minor points, most of the advice offered tended to stress certain common themes. Whether published in women's magazine columns or in infant care manuals, it emphasized that good mothering required scientific knowledge applied with care. This emphasis created something of an anomaly, however. In keeping with the growing consensus that bottle-fed infants were much more likely to develop gastrointestinal problems, the advice writers underlined the importance of maternal nursing. Yet after having done this, they usually went on to devote more time and space to explicating various methods of artificial feeding than to discussing breastfeeding. As a consequence, the implicit message they delivered was that bottle-feeding was scientific and breastfeeding was not.[83] The advice literature also stressed the wisdom of the day that infants should receive nothing but a liquid diet until they were almost one year old and that feeding should be done on a regular schedule. Whether breast- or bottle-feeding, mothers were urged to do so by the clock. Similarly, they were encouraged to foster regular bowel habits by toilet training early (beginning at three months) and by establishing a time each day when evacuation should take place. Sleeping and excercise were also to take place on schedule. Indeed, regularity was seen as such a virtue in all aspects of infant management that one chronicler of infant care advice has described the agenda of early twentieth-century advice writers as the production of a "mechanical baby."[84]

Much of the advice was also practical. Mothers were told how to bathe a baby, how to make its bed, how to fold and pin a diaper, and what sort of clothing the baby should wear during the different seasons. Directions on how to arrange a nursery were given and usually stressed that the baby's sleeping area should be sunny, airy, and warmed by dry heat to prevent respiratory infections. Advice writers also described the symptoms of various infant diseases and complaints, explained what sort of home therapy should be applied, and counseled when to call a physician. And they described the contents of various patent medicines, usually warning mothers away from them.

The central message delivered by the advice columns and manuals, however, was that raising a baby was a complicated matter that demanded intelligence and diligence. The best babies, the healthiest babies, were those whose mothers were willing to devote the time and energy to learn and implement scientific baby care. Along with ennobling full-time and educated motherhood, this message also countered the criticism that had been leveled at middle-class mothers for their declining fertility. Beginning in the second decade of the century, the argument was increasingly heard that small families were necessary if mothers were to provide each child with the attention and care it needed to develop physically and mentally. Moreover, that argument found support in a number of studies appearing at the time showing that a child born into a large family was more likely to die in infancy than one born into a small family. In probably the most influential of these studies, Alice Hamilton examined infant loss among 1,600 Chicago families of comparable income and demonstrated a direct correlation between family size and infant death rate. The reason for that correlation, Hamilton concluded, was that the more children a mother had to look after the less likely it was that she would be able to give an infant the care and devotion it needed to survive the first year of life.[85]

Limiting the number of children one had was therefore not, as eugenicists charged, a sign of selfishness and lack of concern for the propagation of the race, but was rather a decision made in the best interests of the child and the nation. In *The Task of Social Hygiene*, Havelock Ellis dismissed eugenicist alarms over the falling birth rate as "the wild outcry of many unbalanced people," and declared that the tendency of the middle class to have smaller families evidenced an admirable concern for the physical and mental well-being of their children. Florence Kiper, writing on the "new motherhood" in the *Forum* in 1914, protested that it was quality not quantity that mattered and contended that even the most ardent opponent of race suicide had to acknowledge the superior chances and condition of a child brought forth with rejoicing and tended with knowledge, devotion, and love.[86]

It would be, however, simplistic, inaccurate, and grossly unfair to charac-terize the quest for advice on infant care among middle-class mothers in the first decades of the century as simply the product of anxiety over their status in a changing society or as merely the consequence of a need to legitimate their decision to restrict family size. These were important, no doubt. But so too was genuine concern over the fate of their offspring, coupled with the hope that, unlike their mothers and grandmothers, they might have avail-able to them the means of ensuring against the loss of an infant. This may be obvious, but it needs saying. For despite losing on an average one infant for every three lost by the poor and for every two lost by the working class, middle-class parents still saw approximately sixty of every one thousand of their babies fail to survive the first year.[87] Having an infant die was thus a very real possibility for middle-class families.

Middle-class concern with infant survival was also heightened by chang-ing attitudes toward death, and particularly toward the death of infants and children. As Nancy Schrom Dye and Daniel Blake Smith have illustrated, by the end of the nineteenth century maternal attitudes toward infant and child loss had undergone a significant revolution. No longer was such loss to be accepted passively as the will of God, but was now to be battled with science and reason. Women thus turned to doctors, advice writers, and other experts in an almost desperate attempt to arm themselves with knowl-edge and skill that might enable them successfully to battle for the survival of their children.[88] Indeed, the greatest attraction of the published advice manuals and columns may have been that the concrete knowledge and skills they taught (whether medically useful or not) provided psychological and emotional assurance and served to combat the powerlessness felt by parents facing the possibility of infant loss. Anyone who has raised a child knows that the parents of infants experience tremendous insecurity. And it must have been especially so in the early decades of the century when heightened parental expectations were too often mocked by the unavailability of sound medical advice and care and by a continuing high rate of infant morbidity and mortality.

It would also be inaccurate to characterize the quest by early twentieth-century American mothers for advice on infant care as an exclusively middle-class phenomenon. While it was certainly most visible and pro-nounced among the middle class, it was not limited to them. The Children's Bureau's *Infant Care* made its way into the hands of women of all so-cioeconomic classes and geographic regions. Between 1914 and 1921, nearly 1,500,000 copies of the pamphlet were distributed. Moreover, the pamphlet inspired thousands of women to write the bureau, explaining their concerns about the welfare of their infants and often asking for specific advice in some matter relating to illness or general infant care. Although many of those letters were from fairly well-educated women who seem to have been conversant with infant care and feeding theories, others were not. According to one historian who has closely examined the letters, a large number were from working-class women and from women who lived on farms or in small towns in rural areas.[89] While some of these letters were barely literate, they were also eloquent in their expression of concern and in their description of the hardships attending the rearing of infants by those who did not have access to good medical care and did not have the economic security to devote themselves solely to caring for their babies. As one poor Michigan farm woman wrote:

Dear Sir:

I read in one of your leaflet that there is no resin why a Mother could not nurse her baby, if she had no bad disease. There is not a thing [wrong] with me, only what I eat hurts me. I have a little Female weakness so it leaves me feeling weak. And we are poor farmers and have 4 children, so I have to over do. All my milk leakes out. I have to give [the] baby cow's milk alot, and days I wash I have no milk. And when I have to give him the bottle all together, I can hardly get his bowels [to] move at all. And my milk is get[t]ing less all the time. So if I can't get help at once I must put him all together on the bottle, then what I am to do about his bowels I don't know. I have follow what you Drs and my own Dr says as near I can. So please tell me what to do. [sic][90]

Other women wrote with similar concerns and like the above writer especially requested information on feeding and the treatment of bowel troubles. Such requests not only testified to the continued prevalence of gastrointestinal disorders among infants but also to the tendency of infant welfare experts to elevate such disorders above all other causes of infant morbidity and mortality. Indeed, Infant Care estimated that 90 percent of all infant diseases could be traced to faulty feeding. More than a few women also complained that the doctors they consulted did little more than prescribe pills and give rather vague counsel. They therefore turned to the bureau in hope that something more could be done. The bureau responded to as many letters as it could and sought to give advice that was both consistent with medical theory and suited to the actual conditions of its correspondents' lives. Convinced that fatigue dried up a nursing woman's milk yet cognizant that the demands of farm life precluded significant periods of rest, the bureau advised the Michigan farm woman to spread her washing out over several days so that its effect on her strength would not be so concentrated. In giving that type of practical advice, the bureau attempted to offset the somewhat skewed orientation of Infant Care, which, as a number of letter writers commented, was written as if all women lived in cities and enjoyed a middle-class standard of living. Moreover, the women who requested it seemed to find the advice applicable. For they continued to flood the bureau with letters. Indeed, by the 1920s the bureau was receiving more than 100,000 letters a year.

Whether such advice had any significant influence on improving infant health is another matter, however, and speaks to the question that must be asked about the entire maternal educational campaign. Did that campaign serve significantly to reduce infant mortality in America? Most of the advice sought and given was aimed at countering deaths from gastrointestinal disorders, and such deaths did indeed drop substantially after 1910. According to U.S. Census Bureau tabulations for America's registration cities from 1906 through 1910, the average annual ratio of infant deaths from that cause to 100,000 people living was 111.3. From 1911 through 1915, it was 85.0. And by 1916 through 1920 it had dropped to 65.7. For the entire registration area the pattern was the same, with the ratio declining from 96.2 in 1906 through 1910 to 55.4 in 1916 through 1920.[91] Furthermore, according to one recent demographic analysis, the period between 1910 and 1920 also witnessed a profound change in the seasonal patterns that had characterized urban infant mortality for as long as records had been kept. In 1910 summer epidemics of infant diarrhea still scourged American cities, making the hottest months the most dangerous time in an infant's life. By 1920, however, those epidemics had all but disappeared, and infant deaths during the winter months had begun to outnumber those during the summer.[92]

Yet it is one thing to show that infant diarrheal deaths dropped concurrently with the campaign to educate mothers and quite another to prove a causal link. The decade from 1910 to 1920 was also a period in which living standards were rising and in which large municipalities, especially, were making significant strides in the expansion and purification of water supplies, in the implementation of functioning sewerage and garbage disposal systems, and in the regulation and improvement of commercial milk. It is therefore difficult, perhaps impossible, to pinpoint with even a modicum of precision what effect, if any, the maternal educational campaign had on infant mortality rates. One can, it is true, point to Baker's 1908 demonstration as offering ample proof that an intensive instructional effort, involving home visiting and infant supervision, could indeed reduce infant mortality where summer diarrhea was a scourge. In addition, the dramatic plunge in the infant diarrheal death rate in New York City—from 47.6 per 1,000 live births in 1905 to 15.8 in 1919—suggests that the efforts of public health departments and private agencies to educate poor mothers were not without effect. But we must be careful not to generalize too much from the experience of New York. For in many respects that experience was somewhat anomalous. While other cities might have sought to emulate New York's commitment to infant welfare, few actually succeeded in doing so. In 1915, through the combined efforts of the Bureau of Child Hygiene and private agencies, New York had 443 nurses in the field visiting and instructing mothers. This was thirteen more than the combined total of the next nine largest American cities.[93] As with many reform activities, the effectiveness of the municipal maternal education campaign was directly tied to the amount of funding that was allocated it. And in most American cities, that amount was sadly inadequate.

One could also argue with certain justification that while some of the advice offered by manual and magazine writers, as well as by the Children's Bureau, represented an unnecessary complication of infant care in an effort to make it scientific, the information provided on safeguarding infant food held the potential for significantly reducing digestive disorders. The typical mother did not need formal training in bacteriology to grasp that milk exposed to flies and filth or left to spoil could be harmful to an infant. Nor did she have to understand the finer points of asepsis to grasp that fecal contamination of bedsheets, clothing, diapers, and even her own hands could transmit diarrheal diseases to her infant. The emphasis that infant welfare reformers placed on hygiene may have been reinforced by their middle-class preoccupation with domestic and personal cleanliness, but it also was etiologically sound.

It is similarly arguable that the maternal education campaign served to heighten awareness of infant mortality, thereby creating a demand, especially from women, for better medical services for their infants and for protective action by the government. In response to the former, early childhood medicine began to improve and become a more important part of medical education. In response to the latter, politicians, both on the local and the national level, began considering legislation and other action to protect and promote the health of the young, and began advertising their concern for infants by kissing them at election time.[94] Indeed, perhaps the major benefit of the maternal education campaign was that it mobilized American women as a potent political force behind infant welfare. Although male physicians, male social workers, and male public health officials continued to play an important role, the nation's women, along with their magazines and organizations, came to provide the leadership and support in the continuing battle to save American babies.

Yet even these two arguments need qualification. By emphasizing the promise that reforming mothers held for reducing gastroenteric related infant deaths, the maternal education campaign tended to push into the background other specific and underlying causes of infant mortality and to inhibit reform aimed at countering its socioeconomic determinants. Personal and domestic hygiene may have been of critical importance in protecting infants from diarrheal diseases, but they were often difficult to achieve in crowded, unsanitary tenements with poor plumbing. Moreover, gastroenteric disorders were not the only major pathological cause of infant death. Finally, educating mothers did not really resolve the issue of poverty and its relation to infant mortality. Rather it allowed it to be sidestepped. Although infant welfare activists invariably cited poverty, bad surroundings, and ignorance as the three principal conditions influencing the infant death rate, they frequently dismissed the first two as intractable, defined them as conse-quences of the last, or most commonly, argued that proper care and feeding could buffer the infant from their effects. Indeed, the appeal of maternal education was the relatively simple antidote it offered for what was in reality a very complex problem.

Not all infant welfare activists were oblivious to the limitations of mater-nal reform. Indeed, the consensus on the efficacy of maternal instruction in infant care had never been complete. As Robert Bruere's comments at the 1910 AASPIM meeting illustrate, a barely submerged current of doubt had long existed as to whether the promotion of infant care and feeding was sufficiently broad enough to deal adequately with all the causes of infant mortality. By 1915 that current of doubt had surfaced as critics within and without the infant welfare movement began challenging on two fronts the sufficiency of a reform program that placed so much emphasis on improving the way that mothers cared for and fed their infants. One front was econom-ic and developed after the Children's Bureau began publishing the results of the investigations it had been conducting since 1913 into the causes of infant mortality during specific years in certain American communities. Although confirming the importance of proper feeding and care and the usefulness of infant welfare activity designed to promote both, the bureau studies also presented compelling evidence that the ill effects of inadequate family in-come penetrated even the supposedly impregnable barrier offered by breast-feeding. They also showed that the type of care and feeding an infant received was dictated not only by maternal knowledge and choice, but also by economic necessity. The second front was essentially pathologic and developed as mounting statistical evidence suggested that a large and in-creasing proportion of infant deaths were taking place within the first few weeks after birth. Since the vast majority of these deaths were from pre-maturity, congenital debility, malformation, and injuries at birth—causes related to the prenatal and natal health and care of the mother—they in no way could be ascribed to improper feeding and care.

While the discovery of neonatal mortality and the rediscovery of poverty did not ultimately dislodge maternal education from its position as the centerpiece of American infant welfare, they did force those concerned with reducing the infant death rate to expand their focus to include the health and social welfare of the mother. This in turn forced them to confront a question, which though logically implicit in their definition of infant mor-tality as essentially a problem of motherhood, had to this point been largely ignored. If a mother's ability to carry, bear, and rear her infant successfully was tied to her physical and social well-being, to what extent did the reduc-tion of infant mortality demand that maternal education be complemented with medical and social assistance?

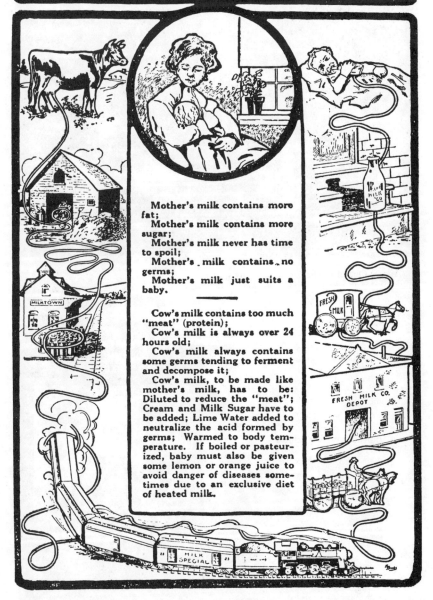

MOTHER'S MILK BEST FOR BABIES
COW'S MILK BEST FOR CALVES

Mother's milk contains more fat;
Mother's milk contains more sugar;
Mother's milk never has time to spoil;
Mother's milk contains no germs;
Mother's milk just suits a baby.

———

Cow's milk contains too much "meat" (protein);
Cow's milk is always over 24 hours old;
Cow's milk always contains some germs tending to ferment and decompose it;
Cow's milk, to be made like mother's milk, has to be: Diluted to reduce the "meat"; Cream and Milk Sugar have to be added; Lime Water added to neutralize the acid formed by germs; Warmed to body temperature. If boiled or pasteurized, baby must also be given some lemon or orange juice to avoid danger of diseases sometimes due to an exclusive diet of heated milk.

1. A widely used poster illustrating the advantages of human breast milk over commercially marketed cow's milk.

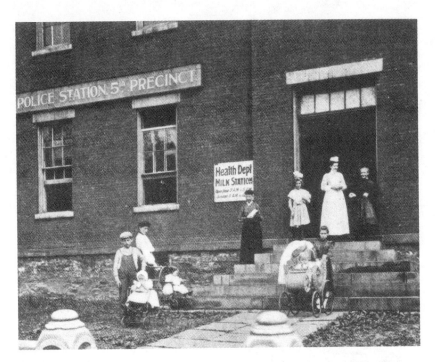

2. (*Above*) One of Rochester's pioneering municipal milk stations, shown in 1905.

3. (*Right*) A wall panel from a Children's Bureau traveling exhibit.

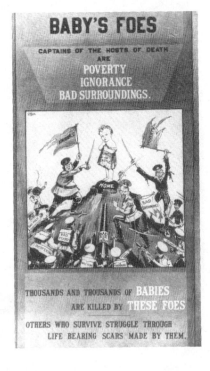

BABY'S FOES

CAPTAINS OF THE HOSTS OF DEATH
ARE
POVERTY
IGNORANCE
BAD SURROUNDINGS.

THOUSANDS AND THOUSANDS OF BABIES
ARE KILLED BY THESE FOES

OTHERS WHO SURVIVE STRUGGLE THROUGH
LIFE BEARING SCARS MADE BY THEM.

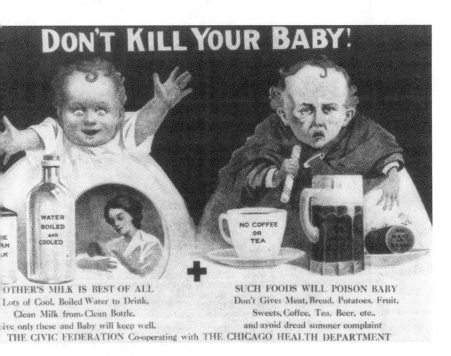

DON'T KILL YOUR BABY!

WATER
BOILED
AND
COOLED

NO COFFEE
OR
TEA

OTHER'S MILK IS BEST OF ALL
Lots of Cool, Boiled Water to Drink.
Clean Milk from Clean Bottle.
ive only these and Baby will keep well.
THE CIVIC FEDERATION Co-operating with THE CHICAGO HEALTH DEPARTMENT

SUCH FOODS WILL POISON BABY
Don't Give: Meat, Bread, Potatoes, Fruit,
Sweets, Coffee, Tea, Beer, etc.,
and avoid dread summer complaint

4. (*Above*) The English-language version of a poster pasted on walls and fences in Chicago's tenement districts.

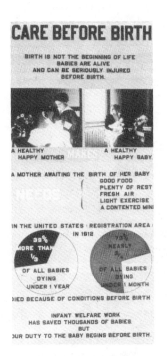

CARE BEFORE BIRTH

BIRTH IS NOT THE BEGINNING OF LIFE
BABIES ARE ALIVE
AND CAN BE SERIOUSLY INJURED
BEFORE BIRTH.

A HEALTHY
HAPPY MOTHER

A HEALTHY
HAPPY BABY

A MOTHER AWAITING THE BIRTH OF HER BABY
GOOD FOOD
PLENTY OF REST
FRESH AIR
LIGHT EXERCISE
A CONTENTED MIN

IN THE UNITED STATES (REGISTRATION AREA)
IN 1912

38%
MORE THAN
1/3

73%
NEARLY
3/4

OF ALL BABIES
DYING
UNDER 1 YEAR

OF ALL BABIES
DYING
UNDER 1 MONTH

DIED BECAUSE OF CONDITIONS BEFORE BIRTH

INFANT WELFARE WORK
HAS SAVED THOUSANDS OF BABIES.
BUT
OUR DUTY TO THE BABY BEGINS BEFORE BIRTH.

5. (*Left*) A wall panel on prenatal care from a Children's Bureau traveling exhibit.

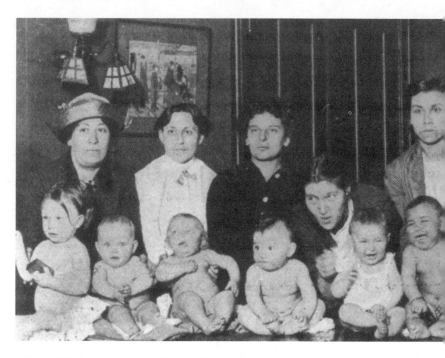

6. Some of the babies who scored high in a better baby contest sponsored by the University Settlement in New York City.

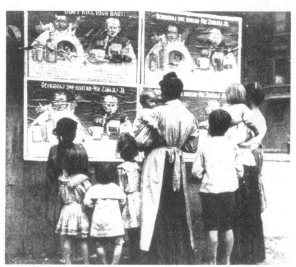

7. Chicago tenement-district women reading infant welfare posters distributed by the municipal health department.

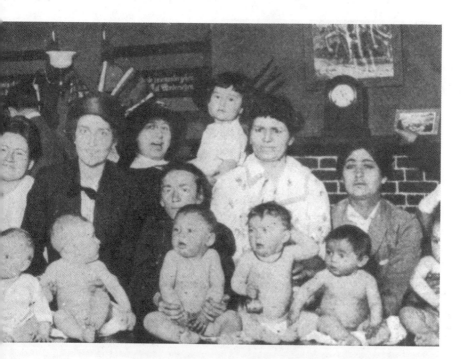

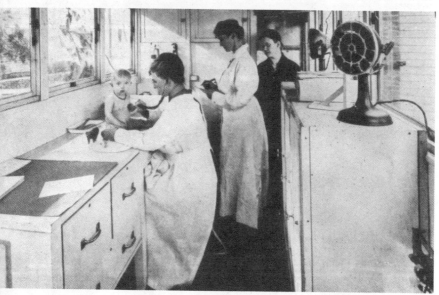

8. The interior of a mobile "child welfare special" used to reach rural women and their infants.

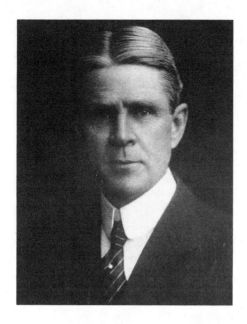

9. L. Emmett Holt

10. (*Below*) Well-baby examinations given in a schoolroom as part of a small town's celebration of National Baby Week.

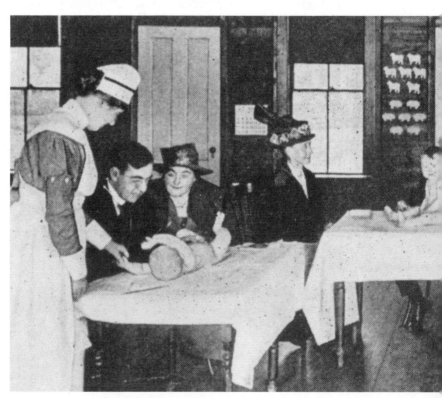

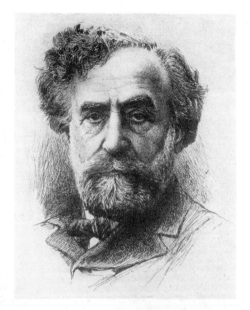

11. Abraham Jacobi

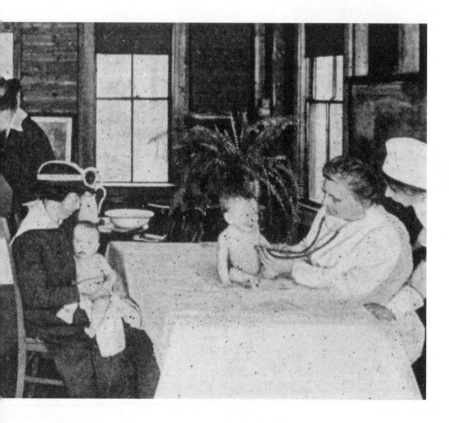

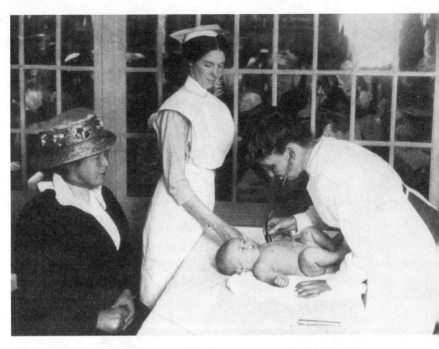

12. An infant being examined at a well-baby clinic.

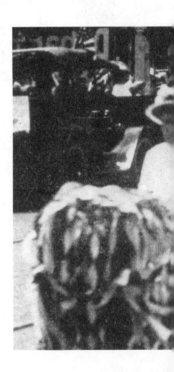

13. Julia Lathrop

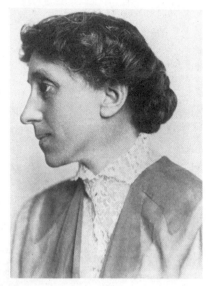

14. A section of a baby-week parade held on Staten Island in the
summer of 1915.

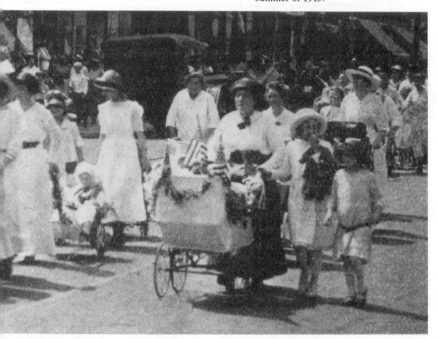

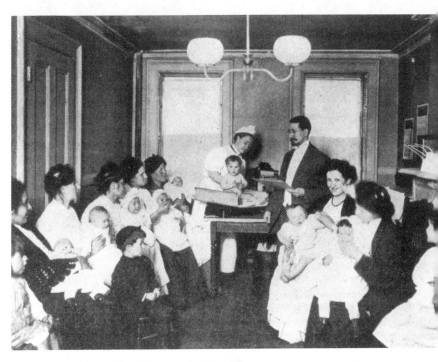

15. A volunteer doctor and a public health nurse conducting an infant hygiene class and baby-weighing demonstration for a group of immigrant mothers.

16. (*Opposite*) Often coupled with the caption, "Save the Babies," this dramatic poster illustration was used in both American and English infant welfare campaigns.

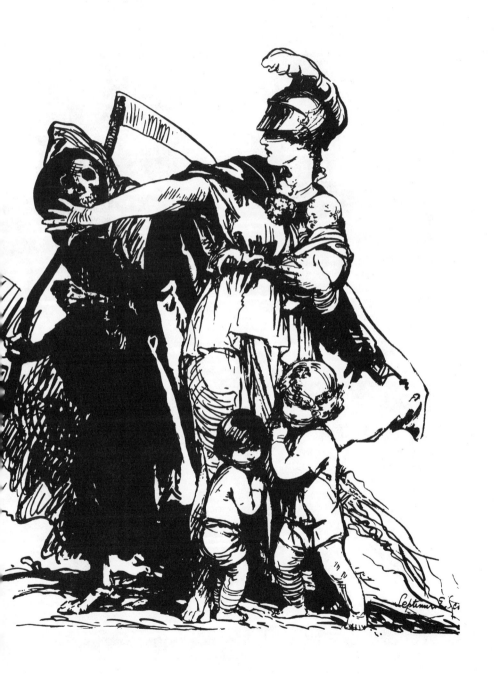

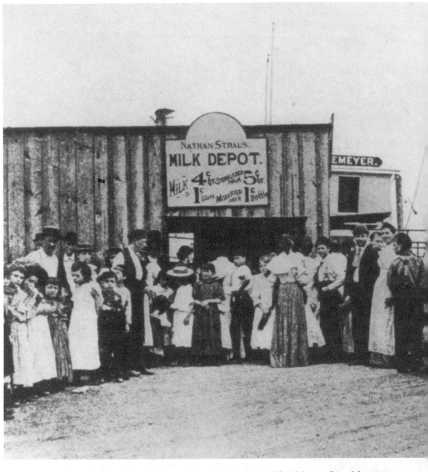

17. (*Above*) The first Nathan Straus Milk Station on the East Third Street Pier, New York City, shown in 1893.

18. (*Opposite, above*) A widely distributed poster linking the promotion of infant health with female suffrage.

19. (*Opposite, below*) A popular baby-week newspaper cartoon.

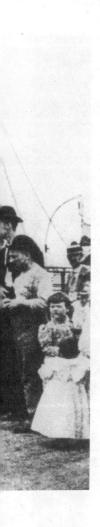

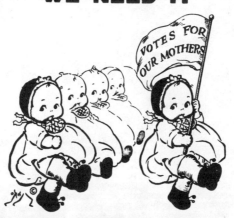

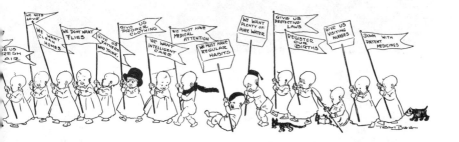

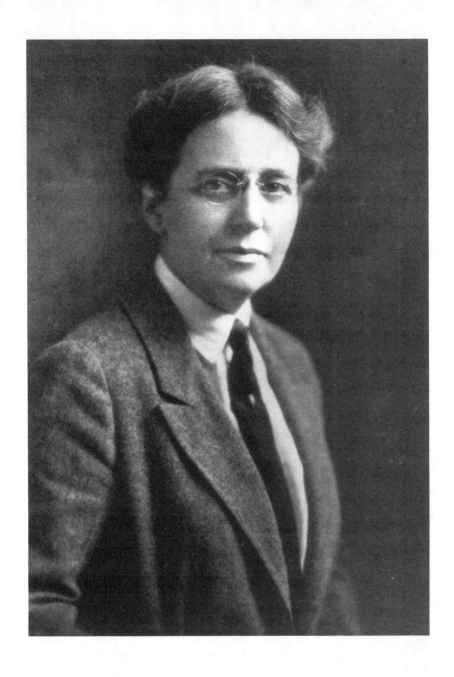

20. S. Josephine Baker

6

Before the Baby Comes:
Neonatal Mortality
and the
Promotion of Prenatal Care

Surveying the current state of the infant welfare movement in 1914, future AASPIM president Philip Van Ingen observed that many of those actively involved in saving babies had begun to doubt that weighing and examining infants, providing them with clean and wholesome milk, and instructing their mothers in the basics of infant and domestic hygiene—while of proven and critical importance— would alone be sufficient to reduce infant mortality to a level acceptable in a civilized society. In explaining the source of this doubt, the veteran infant welfare activist pointed to what was becoming painfully obvious to anyone familiar with published statistics on the causes and rates of infant death. Such statistics showed that while deaths among infants one month and older had begun to decline substantially, those among infants less than a month (neonates) remained high as ever, and, indeed, seemed to be rising. Since almost two-thirds of such deaths were attributed to premature birth and congenital debility, they could not be ascribed to improper feeding and care nor diminished by efforts to reform mothers in these areas. As a conse- quence, Van Ingen observed, he and others in American infant welfare had come to accept that neonatal mortality was "caused by conditions acting on the child through the mother and must be attacked by methods directed at pregnant women."[1]

Van Ingen was not the first to note the mounting concern with neonatal mortality and consequent interest in reaching pregnant women. Two years earlier, at the Fifteenth International Congress on Hygiene and Demogra- phy, Josephine Baker pointed to budding interest in prenatal reform as one of the most important new developments in infant welfare.[2] Similarly, in her 1912 report to association members, AASPIM's executive secretary com- mented,

159

In all quarters greater significance is being attached to the fact that the greatest reduction in infant mortality so far has been in the digestive and respiratory diseases and that little headway has been made in cutting down the appalling death rate of the first few weeks of life. This is leading to a more general recognition of the importance of prenatal care and instruction as an essential initial step in any plan of prevention.[3]

Other infant welfare activists were making similar observations. Taken together their comments pinpoint an important shift in infant welfare work. For over four decades the primary aim of such work had been to counter postnatal threats to infant life, chiefly by improving the domestic sanitary environment and the quality of infant nutriment and care. While this aim remained central to infant welfare, after 1914 or so it was increasingly joined by another, namely, improving the care and health of gestative and parturient women. As more attention was given to reducing the neonatal death rate, more importance was granted to prenatal maternal health and behavior. In short, infant welfare became maternal and infant welfare.

If neonatal mortality and the health of expectant and new mothers were somewhat belatedly discovered by infant welfare activists, it was not because there existed no prior appreciation of the connection between infant and maternal health. Recognition that infant survival and health were intimately connected to the physical condition and behavior of women during gestation was certainly not new. It had long found expression in the protective rituals and customs pertaining to pregnant women common to the cultures of both comparatively advanced and primitive societies. Nor was suspicion new that the first few weeks of life constituted a particularly hazardous period for infants and that deaths during that time were somehow connected to the prenatal condition and activity of their mothers. Aristotle had suggested that "the majority of deaths in infancy occur before the child is a week old"; and Avicenna had argued that survival of early infancy depended a great deal on in utero conditions.[4] Similarly, those eighteenth- and nineteenth-century physicians who pioneered Anglo-American pediatrics also stressed the connection between prenatal conditions and death in early infancy. In his 1781 obstetric manual, Alexander Hamilton encouraged pregnant women to maintain their health and carefully avoid any activity that would hinder fetal development and neonatal survival. William Dewees complained that too many infants were born sickly and soon died because of the failure of their mothers to follow simple rules of prenatal hygiene. And Andrew Combe declared: "The first circumstance which affects the mortality of infants, is the degree of health and comfort the mother enjoyed during pregnancy."[5] Additionally, as public health reformers in the latter half of the nineteenth century focused their attention on reducing infant mortality, they did so acknowledging that deaths during the first month after birth constituted a significant proportion of that mortality and were related to the health and activity of expectant mothers. In 1873, for instance, Edward Jarvis observed that more infants seemed to die in the first few weeks of life than in any other period, and suggested that this was traceable to "prenatal conditions which belong to or may be controlled by the parent."[6]

Despite the long recognized connection between the health and activity of a pregnant woman and the survival of her infant once born, infant welfare activists had initially decided to focus their attention almost exclusively on preventing deaths attributable to postnatal environment and care. Indeed, preventive prenatal work had all but been ignored. The decision had been a strategic one, based in part on the conviction that the prevention of such deaths could be more readily effected. Behind that conviction was the recognition that the causes of neonatal death, and indeed the physiology of gestation itself, were still shrouded in medical uncertainty. Despite a well-established tradition of offering advice to pregnant women on hygiene and life style, medicine's systematic interest in and understanding of the mechanics of fetal development were decidedly limited prior to the end of the nineteenth century. In 1842 the *Encyclopaedia Britannica* characterized what for some time continued to be the state of medical knowledge concerning gestation by observing, "the immediate agency by which one living being is rendered capable of giving rise to another similar to itself is enveloped in the most profound and most hopeless obscurity."[7] Coupled with spreading revulsion against the interventionist excesses of heroic medicine, this dearth of medical knowledge had encouraged physicians through much of the latter half of the nineteenth century to regard gestation as a somewhat mysterious but essentially natural physiological process that required patience more than direct supervision and intervention. Consequently, they tended to give pregnant women little attention and rarely if ever examined those whom they delivered before labor had actually commenced. In his highly regarded *Treatise on the Science and Practice of Midwifery* (1876), William S. Playfair, for instance, made no mention whatsoever of prenatal exams and gave fetal development only cursory attention.[8]

Admittedly, even if physicians had wished to be more involved during pregnancy, it is doubtful that they would have received much support from their patients. The dictates of Victorian modesty rendered vaginal exams out of the question and abdominal ones of questionable propriety. More importantly, the economics and patterns of medical care militated against prenatal supervision. Through the early twentieth century, people tended to engage the services of a physician only when they were seriously ill, or, as with the case of a difficult birth, some form of medical attendance was clearly required. Even among those who could afford regular medical care, visiting a physician for preventive reasons was exceptionally rare. Among those who could not, it was unheard of. Since prenatal care was essentially preventive in nature, few expectant mothers regarded it as necessary or as economically justifiable.[9]

There were, of course, a few exceptions. In the 1850s overcrowding at the Dublin Maternity Hospital forced prospective obstetric patients to present themselves months in advance, at which time they were given an examination. Thus was established what may have been the first prenatal clinic. In 1866, Dr. William Goodell opened Philadelphia's Preston Retreat, a lying-in hospital dedicated to serving the poor, and encouraged his patients to admit themselves two weeks before delivery. In the late 1870s Pierre Budin began offering prenatal supervision and instruction to pregnant women. And in the 1880s Dr. Anna Broomwell ran an obstetrical clinic at Women's Hospital in Philadelphia that included in its services the observation of expectant women. Moreover, in the late 1800s, male obstetricians, who for at least a century had been becoming increasingly involved in the birthing process of more prosperous women, developed a number of techniques for early discovery and correction of conditions that complicated delivery and demanded operative and surgical intervention. Nevertheless, formal obstetric involvement in prenatal care did not seriously begin until the turn of the century.[10]

Among those initiating that involvement was John W. Ballantyne, a lecturer in obstetrics at the University of Edinburgh who advocated preventive prenatal care as a means of reducing stillbirths and neonatal deaths from congenital problems and morbid states arising during pregnancy. In 1901 Ballantyne published a widely read and much discussed article in the *British Medical Journal* calling for the establishment of prematernity hospitals as annexes to the lying-in hospitals that had existed in many English cities since the eighteenth century. Such hospitals, he argued, would provide physicians the opportunity to observe pregnant women in a clinical setting and would do much to reduce infant mortality that had its origins in prenatal pathological complications.[11] That same theme—that prenatal clinical supervision would increase medical knowledge of the physiology of gestation and therefore contribute to the reduction of infant mortality—was also central to the massive, two-volume *Manual of Ante-Natal Pathology and Hygiene* that Ballantyne published between 1902 and 1904. By far the most comprehensive work to that point in English on the physiology, pathology, and therapeutics of gestation, it served for years as an authoritative text on the subject. Lending scientific legitimacy to prenatal supervision, it also lent it social significance. Contending that it was necessary to care for the fetus in the womb to reduce the large number of neonatal deaths that occurred each year, Ballantyne stressed that the first step "in the direction of successful treatment of the unborn infant must be successful treatment of the pregnant mother."[12]

The work of Ballantyne and other turn-of-the-century advocates of prenatal medical supervision has been described by sympathetic historians as initiating effective and beneficial prenatal care and by less sympathetic historians as advancing modern medicine's medicalization of and arrogation of control over pregnancy.[13] However described, such work advanced and was predicated on a new view of pregnancy, one which held that the process of gestation was at least potentially pathological and therefore required medical supervision and assistance. While hesitating to call pregnancy a pathological condition, Ballantyne defined it as a state of "health under strain"; that is, a state in which natural "physiology [was] working under high pressure."[14] In other words, while gestation involved physiological processes that were inherently natural, its successful completion demanded that the pregnant woman and her reproductive organs be strong, healthy, and sufficiently developed to operate without a hitch under extremely taxing conditions.

Although not as involved as their English and European counterparts in advancing medical understanding of gestation, leading American obstetricians quickly adopted the position that pregnancy was potentially pathological and also used it to promote prenatal care and supervision. J. Whitridge Williams opened a chapter on pregnancy in the 1912 edition of his famous obstetric text[15] with the following observation,

> From a biological point of view, pregnancy and labor represent the highest functions of the female reproductive system, and *a priori* should be considered a normal process. But when we recall the manifold changes which occur in the maternal organism, it is apparent that the border-line between health and disease is less distinctly marked during gestation than at other times, and derangements, so slight as to be of little consequence under ordinary circumstances, may readily give rise to pathological conditions which seriously threaten the life of the mother or child, or both.
>
> It accordingly becomes necessary to keep pregnant patients under strict supervision, and to be constantly alert for the appearance of untoward symptoms.[16]

Indeed, so convinced was Williams of the importance of prenatal care and supervision that in his own practice he provided his patients with a printed card establishing a schedule for examinations, directing them regularly to send him urine samples for analysis, and giving them detailed instructions on exercise, diet, and clothing.[17]

The view that pregnancy was potentially pathological was not, admittedly, entirely new to the end of the century and had roots in popular belief that modern life was having a deleterious effect on the health and organic functions of women, and particularly women of the uppermost and lowest classes. Through much of the latter third of the nineteenth century, medical and social commentators had complained that overcivilization among the wealthy classes and privation, degenerate behavior, disease, and hard labor among the poorer classes were having detrimental effects on the ability of many women to gestate healthy infants As early as 1874, Henry Hartshorne, in a talk before the American Public Health Association, declared that the primary cause of infant mortality traceable to prenatal conditions was re-productive deficiency. Such deficiency, he suggested, resulted "from *Alco-holism, Syphilis, Scrofulosis,* debility from *overwork and under-feeding,* in the poorer classes; in those more prosperous, excess of the *nervous temperament,* and *deficient organic development in women who become mothers*" (italics in original).[18]

What was new was medicine's conviction that it could medically counter such prenatal influences and its use of the purported organic enervation or debility of upper and lower-class women to argue the need for prenatal supervision and therapeutic, operative, and surgical intervention. Just as late nineteenth-century pediatricians advanced scientific artificial feeding as a narrow medical antidote to modern life's perversion of the natural alimentary function, so too did early twentieth-century obstetricians ad-vance scientific prenatal supervision and intervention as a similarly narrow medical antidote to supposedly perverted gestative capabilities.[19] Where Hartshorne could offer only a broad program involving "*popular education, moral reform,* and *sanitary police*" to counter the prenatal effects of modern life, his early twentieth-century successors could turn to the new obstetrics for a narrower medical approach to the problem (italics in original).[20] If pregnant women would submit to supervision and instruction and take advantage of competent medical attendance, then the consequences of ei-ther overcivilization or poverty might be countered.

Medical interest in pregnancy and prenatal care also developed as part of a larger transformation of childbirth from a social event, managed largely by women, to a medical event managed and controlled by physicians. That transformation involved an upgrading of obstetrics to a modern medical specialty, a transference of decision-making power from parturient women and their families to doctors, and, ultimately, a shift in the birthplace from the home to the hospital. It also involved the increasingly widespread use of invasive birthing techniques and the redefinition of medical attendance at birth from assistance to surgery. Begun in the last quarter of the eighteenth century, the transformation was more or less complete by the second quarter of the twentieth century.[21]

Toward the end of the first decade of the twentieth century, obstetrics' new systematic interest in pregnancy motivated a few medical and phi-lanthropic organizations to experiment in providing prenatal care to small groups of American women. By 1906 all women registered to be delivered by the outpatient department of the Boston Lying-in Hospital were receiving at least one visit from a nurse prior to confinement. Two years later the New

York Milk Committee told its nurses to instruct pregnant women when and if they came across them in their normal rounds. The following year Mrs. William Lowell Putnam of the Committee on Infant Social Services of the Boston Women's Municipal League began a program providing intensive prenatal care to obstetric patients registered at the Massachusetts Homeo-pathic Hospital and the Boston Lying-in Hospital. And in 1910, the Russell Sage Foundation sought to promote interest in prenatal care as a means of preventing birth complications and fetal and infant mortality by publishing a study of the types of instruction and supervision available to women in European countries.[22]

Not until 1911, however, did prenatal care as a means of preventing infant mortality attract any really significant publicity. In that year the New York Milk Committee began an experiment which it hoped would prove that an intensive program of prenatal care could significantly reduce stillbirths and neonatal deaths among the urban poor. Dividing the poorer sections of the city into small districts, the NYMC put each district in charge of a trained obstetrical nurse who through house-to-house canvassing and through re-ports from churches, settlements, charity organizations, and infant welfare stations sought the names of all pregnant women. Each woman was then paid an initial visit, and if she agreed to enroll in the program, was visited at ten-day intervals. During such visits her blood pressure was checked and a urine sample was taken (to detect the possible onset of pre-eclampsia), and she was examined for any other possible complications. If such complica-tions were detected, she was referred to a clinic or private physician. She was also instructed on what to eat and the types of work to avoid, urged to make arrangements for a midwife or doctor, and was apprised of the value of breastfeeding once the infant was born. Among the 2,644 women super-vised during the two years that the NYMC experiment ran, stillbirths were 8 percent lower than in the rest of Manhattan and neonatal deaths were 12 percent lower. These impressive results served to inspire other infant wel-fare activists to begin considering prenatal care a necessary part of the effort to reduce infant mortality. Citing the accomplishments of the NYMC exper-iment during its first summer, AASPIM's Section on Nursing and Social Work passed a resolution late in 1911 urging that prenatal instruction and supervision be made an integral part of infant welfare station work.[23]

By 1912 other social welfare and voluntary and municipal health organi-zations were also beginning to experiment with the provision of prenatal care. The Visiting Nurse Association of St. Louis, in conjunction with Washington University Hospital Obstetric Dispensary, began monitoring all pregnant women who applied to the dispensary for care. In Baltimore, a similar program was begun by the Maryland Association for Study and Prevention of Infant Mortality with the aid of the city's four leading hospi-tals. In Providence, the District Nurse Association began visiting pregnant women and the city health department issued a leaflet on prenatal care. Similar leaflets were distributed by Milwaukee and Portland, Oregon. In Detroit, the Babies' Milk Fund sponsored pregnancy clinics at obstetric dispensaries. In New York, the Diet Kitchen Association transformed one of its infant welfare stations into a prenatal care station, and the NYAICP expanded its Caroline Rest Program (begun in 1907 to provide convalescent care to exhausted post-parturient women) to include prenatal visitation and monitoring.[24]

The following year saw further growth in prenatal work as a means of preventing infant mortality. New York's Bureau of Child Hygiene set up a special training center for obstetric nurses and by the following year had seven such nurses in the field. In Boston, the Division of Child Hygiene established a prenatal subdivison and also began pursuing prenatal work. In Chicago, the Mary Crane Nursery began providing prenatal instruction to pregnant women of the Hull House neighborhood. And the Children's Bureau, recognizing that a program of postnatal instruction represented an incomplete approach to the reduction of infant mortality, published the first edition of its popular pamphlet, *Prenatal Care*.[25]

Despite the growing interest in prenatal care, it was still very much the stepchild of the infant welfare movement. Compared to the money and effort devoted to reducing postnatal infant mortality, that devoted to combating stillbirths and neonatal deaths remained inconsequential. Moreover, at least a few involved in infant welfare continued to question the efficacy of such work. Despite the new attention that obstetrics was giving to pregnancy, the physiology of gestation was still anything but well understood and the precise causes of prematurity and congenital malformations remained shrouded in uncertainty. Also, eugenicists were still arguing that stillbirths and neonatal deaths were a consequence of hereditary weakness and therefore not only unpreventable but also nature's way of weeding out the unfit.[26] Indeed, as Mrs. Max B. [Mary Mills] West, author of the Children's Bureau's pamphlet on prenatal care, noted in 1914: "systematic prenatal work, undertaken as a recognizable means of combating infant mortality and of improving the health of the succeeding generation is a distinctly new idea."[27]

Nevertheless, a definite shift in focus was taking place in infant welfare as concern mounted over the number of deaths occurring within a few hours and weeks of birth. Helping crystallize that concern was the publication in the summer of 1913 by the Bureau of the Census of its mortality report for 1910. The report had a major impact because it was the first to include a special table detailing the number of registration area infant deaths by age within the first year.[28] Previous reports, while enumerating deaths by cause, had lumped all infant mortality into a single age category. The 1910 report, however, not only showed what infants were dying from, but also when in the first year they were doing so. The figures confirmed what infant welfare activists had long suspected: that early infancy was a particularly deadly period of life. Of the 154,373 infants who died in the registration area during 1910, 38 percent failed to survive the first month, 24 percent expired within the first week, and 10 percent did not even last a day. (See Table 8.) The figures also confirmed opinion that diarrhea and enteritis—the targets of most reform activity thus far—were only of minor importance as causes of death among neonates. Although causing 29 percent of all deaths during the first year, they accounted for only 8 percent of those deaths that occurred in the first month and less than 2 percent of those that occurred within the first week. In contrast, prematurity, congenital debility, and malformation— causes of death presumed to be related to prenatal conditions—accounted for 61 percent of infant deaths during the first month and 74 percent during the first week. Here, then, was clear illustration that improving the quality of the milk supply and instructing mothers in the hygienic care and feeding of their babies would do little to save the some 60,000 registration area infants who were failing to survive early infancy each year.[29]

Table 8
Registration Area[a] Deaths[b] of Infants During First Day, Week, Month, and Year of Life, 1910

Cause	First Day	First Week	First Month	First Year
Contagious diseases[c]	9	57	507	6,614
Dysentery and erysipelas	—	20	248	1,442
Tuberculosis[d]	6	32	127	2,416
Syphilis	90	228	608	1,658
Meningitis	5	114	356	2,372
Convulsions	120	1,144	2,070	4,089
Respiratory diseases[e]	54	886	4,094	23,187
Diarrhea and enteritis	25	684	4,477	44,695
Premature birth	8,808	16,197	19,498	20,275
Congenital debility	2,007	5,943	10,273	15,361
Malformations	1,437	4,380	5,901	7,501
Injuries at birth	1,740	3,430	3,689	3,725
External causes	99	308	510	1,497
Ill-defined or unknown	272	742	1,056	6,900
All other causes[f]	274	2,186	4,675	12,641
Total	14,946	36,351	58,089	154,373

Source: U.S. Department of Commerce, Bureau of the Census, Mortality Statistics, 1910 (Washington, D.C.: Government Printing Office, 1913), p. 533.
[a]In 1910 the Registration Area was made up of 21 states, the District of Columbia, and 43 cities in nonregistration states.
[b]Exclusive of stillbirths.
[c]Measles, scarlet fever, whooping cough, diphtheria and croup, and influenza.
[d]Tuberculosis of the lungs, tuberculous meningitis, and other forms of tuberculosis.
[e]Acute bronchitis, bronchopneumonia, and pneumonia.
[f]Including but not limited to tetanus, organic diseases of the heart, and diseases of the stomach.

Providing a statistical breakdown of deaths during the first year, the 1910 mortality report heightened concern with neonatal mortality. Moreover, within less than six months of its publication, the Bureau of the Census issued its reports for 1911 and 1912. These successive reports confirmed what was revealed in the first. Deaths occurring within the first few weeks of life constituted a large proportion of infant mortality and would not be reduced by efforts aimed at diminishing digestive disorders. Coming on the heels of the 1910 report, they kept alive discussion of neonatal mortality and provided an opportunity for immediate computation of trends across time. The results of those computations were highly disturbing to infant welfare activists. While the proportion of infant mortality caused by diarrhea and enteritis had declined from 29 percent in 1910 to 23.5 percent in 1912, the proportion ascribed to prematurity and congenital debility and malformation had risen from 27.9 percent to 35.5 percent. Accordingly, the proportion of total infant mortality occurring during the first month had also risen during the period from 37.6 percent to 43.5 percent.[30] In actuality, however, the figures in the reports did not really prove that the incidence of neonatal deaths was rising, only that the proportion of total infant mortality they constituted was. But infant welfare activists were not inclined to make such subtle distinctions; they interpreted the data as proving that neonatal mortality was a serious and mounting problem that was not being affected by existing programs. Pointing to the evidence contained within the reports purportedly showing that neonatal mortality was on the rise, the Children's Bureau concluded that while existing "efforts to save babies through pure milk and more intelligent care have produced results," it was quite apparent that the "infant mortality problem cannot be solved adequately by any measures that leave out of their scope some attention to the care of expectant mothers."[31] Van Ingen also cited the reports as extremely influential, claiming that they precipitated a new awareness that neonatal deaths were high and rising.[32]

While this new level of awareness and the expansion of sponsored activities to include promotion of maternal as well as infant health signaled a broadening of the compass of infant welfare, it did not, initially at least, entail any significant departure from a strategy based on the assumption that maternal education represented the most effective approach to preventing infant deaths. In attempting to reduce the prenatal and natal complications that were believed to cause so many deaths in early infancy, philanthropic and government infant welfare agencies merely applied to pregnant women the educational and supervisory techniques they had developed to combat deaths from postnatal causes. Visiting obstetric nurses and prenatal clinics adopted the preventive educational and supervisory approach of visiting infant welfare nurses and well-baby stations. The only significant difference was that the education, examinations, and referrals provided were aimed at preventing gestative and birth complications among pregnant and parturient women rather than at improving the quality of infant care provided by post-parturient mothers. Moreover, as was true with postnatal infant welfare work, provision of free medical services was not part of the program, except for those whose destitution qualified them for admittance to charity hospitals and clinics.

For those involved in infant welfare, an extension to pregnant women of the type of supervisory and educational program initially adopted to improve the care and feeding of older infants, had considerable attraction. Much of the machinery was already in place, and it required only a small outlay of additional funds to extend services to pregnant women. Also, maternal education had shown itself to be effective in reducing mortality among older infants and was consistent with the emphasis that the "new public health" was putting on the promotion of personal hygiene as an antidote to public health problems. At the same time, however, it was apparent early that reducing neonatal mortality would involve different and more complex challenges than those posed by the reduction of mortality among post-neonates. For one thing, the specific causes of neonatal death were more numerous, and their precipitating or underlying causes were not so easily isolated, defined, and attacked. Nor were they necessarily within the increasingly narrow confines of the self-defined province of public health. Although there was sharp debate over the relative efficacy of specific ameliorative measures, postneonatal infant welfare had been informed by a consensus that gastroenteric disorders, the chief killer of older infants, were specifically caused by the ingestion of food, particularly milk, that was pathogenically contaminated and/or nutritionally unbalanced. There was also a consensus that the problem could be combated by improving and regulating the commercial milk supply, instructing mothers in home modification and domestic hygiene, and convincing them to breastfeed: all of which public health accepted as within its ability to do. No such consensus, however, could inform neonatal infant welfare. For no single cause, pathogenic or otherwise, could be identified as primary. It was one thing to agree that death within the first month of life was related to maternal condition during gestation, yet quite another to define the precise physiology of that relation, pinpoint the various influences that affected maternal health, and explain with any certainty why and how they did so.

Equally problematic, the relationship that pregnant women had to their social, economic, and physical environment was obviously much more complex and less circumscribed than that of infants. The initial phase of the maternal reform campaign had proceeded on the assumption that the immediate environment of the infant was largely domestic and primarily shaped and controlled by the mother. Infant welfare reformers therefore assumed that enlightened mothering, particularly in regard to domestic hygiene and proper feeding, was capable of erecting a buffer between the infant and potentially dangerous environmental conditions. Indeed, they regarded good mothering, and especially breastfeeding, both of which they felt could be effected by advice, as socioeconomic equalizers, capable of offsetting the admittedly deleterious influences of poverty conditions. It seemed less clear, however, that advice held the same promise for guaranteeing maternal health. It was one thing to assume all mothers capable of constructing an hygienic environment for their infants and of adhering to a simple program of infant care; and quite another to assume them capable of isolating themselves and of adhering to a prenatal regimen that required of them rest, freedom from worry, and good nutrition. Even those infant welfare activists who evinced greatest faith in the power of advice, had to admit that a mother's ability to carry and bear healthy infants could be seriously affected by a pre-gestative life of poor nutrition, debilitating physical activity, and exposure to infectious disease. Most physicians, for instance, were aware that childhood rickets, a common disease among the malnourished, often produced pelvic deformities that later complicated childbearing.

Obstetric science's increasing insistence that gestation and parturition were potentially pathological states also complicated the application of a simple educational strategy to the prevention of neonatal mortality. Maternal education in the care and feeding of infants was conceptualized as well-baby care and thus was aimed at keeping the healthy baby healthy by protecting it from external morbific influences. Preventive rather than therapeutic, it rested on the assumption that infant development, though sensitive to interdiction, was a natural physiological process that in most cases would proceed relatively smoothly. The provision of medical services, beyond advice and supervision, was therefore not seen as an essential part of the program. Indeed, the success of the maternal education program was gauged against the extent to which such services were unnecessary. To a certain degree this was also true of the effort to reduce neonatal mortality. It too was conceived of as preventive.[33] Yet, because gestation and parturition were regarded as potentially pathological, the type of prevention promoted placed a high premium on the availability and consumption of quality medical care. Even the healthiest and most enlightened woman could develop complications in pregnancy and have a problem labor and delivery—both of which could adversely affect the survival of her newborn. It followed, then, that medical supervision and attendance were of critical preventive importance. Indeed, central to the instruction that infant welfare aimed at expectant mothers was the message that pregnancy, labor, and delivery could be dangerous to both mother and infant and thus that the best possible medical attendance should be secured.[34]

Because of the causal complexity of infant death within the first month, the difficulty of controlling morbific influences on expectant mothers, and the assumed potential pathology of pregnancy and parturition, the discourse on neonatal mortality was considerably more divisive than that which had centered on the prevention of mortality among older infants. At issue were two questions. First, would an essentially educative campaign—designed to acquaint women with the possible dangers of carrying and bearing children and thus to convince them of the need to employ skilled medical attendants and to follow a hygienic regimen during pregnancy—be an adequate and realistic strategy for combating the causes of death during early infancy? And second, if quality medical care was of critical importance, how could its availability be ensured? Americans, of course, were not the only ones debating these questions. Indeed, they informed the discourse on neonatal mortality that was simultaneously taking place throughout the industrialized West. Yet the American response was unique and gave shape to what became its relatively singular approach to ensuring maternal and infant health.

Within the American infant welfare movement, two positions on these questions early crystallized. One was defined and promoted primarily by physicians, especially a small group of obstetricians who were beginning to exert considerable influence within the movement. Although obstetricians had from the beginning been involved in the discourse on infant mortality, they had initially taken a backseat to pediatricians in shaping the character and focus of that discourse. But as concern over neonatal mortality and its prenatal and natal causes increased, so too did the influence of those medical specialists whose province was prenatal and natal care. Signaling the new prominence of obstretrics and obstetricians within infant welfare was the 1914 election of J. Whitridge Williams to the presidency of AASPIM. Williams, who was a professor of obstetrics at Johns Hopkins and a leading figure in the reform of obstetric education and practice, chose as the topic of his presidential address prenatal and natal care as a means of preventing stillbirths and neonatal deaths. While admitting that the causes of stillbirths and deaths in early infancy were still only imperfectly understood, he was nevertheless emphatic in his belief that increasing the amount and quality of obstetric advice and care would drastically reduce both fetal death and neonatal mortality. If stillbirths and deaths in early infancy were to be prevented, Williams argued, obstetric practice would have to be reformed from within, mothers would have to be educated as to the necessity of contracting skilled medical attendants, and prenatal and obstetric clinics, similar in function and compass to well-baby stations, would have to be established to educate and supervise pregnant women.[35]

Given the state of obstetric knowledge at the time, Williams' plan made considerable sense. It was decades before physicians comprehended the role that chromosomal and genetic aberrations and defects played in producing congenital problems or had the surgical ability to rectify such problems. Similarly, even the most sophisticated physicians at the time had only a rough appreciation of the impact of maternal conditions and exogenous influences on fetal development and newborn viability. But they did have available enough clinical evidence to suspect that late-term fatigue or trauma, alcoholism, hypertension, toxemias, maternal age, birth history, general health and nutrition, and certain infectious diseases such as syphilis all seemed connected in some way to either stillbirth or neonatal death from prematurity, congenital debility, and malformations.[36] Any program that heightened maternal awareness as to potential pathological conditions, encouraged pregnant women to submit to medical supervision, and modified their behavior so that they escaped infection, ate well, received enough rest, and avoided teratogenic agents thus seemed to hold great preventive potential.

Williams' tripartite plan for reducing neonatal mortality also reflected the particular professional challenges obstetrics was facing at the time. Although long able to attract a few elite and highly trained physicians, obstetrics had historically been one of the least esteemed branches of medicine. In the nineteenth century, for instance, the Royal College of Physicians and Surgeons branded it manual labor, unworthy of pursuit by a gentleman.[37] That prejudice continued through the beginning of the twentieth century and was reflected in the cursory exposure to obstetric theory and practice that most medical students received. Indeed, in his immensely influential 1910 survey of medical curricula, Abraham Flexner reserved his harshest criticism for obstetric education, calling it "utterly worthless" and a threat to the safety and comfort of mothers and infants.[38] Similarly, Williams, who had himself charged that even those teaching obstetrics were too often sadly incompetent, lamented that the average medical student "cannot be blamed for believing that obstetrics is a pursuit unworthy of the broadly educated man, but is suitable only for midwives and physicians of mediocre intelligence."[39]

In an attempt to increase the status of obstetrics and attract better students to its practice, Williams and other leading American obstetricians embarked upon a reform program aimed at legitimizing the specialty by improving obstetric training and practice, by wresting control of pregnant and parturient women from midwives and general practitioners, and by promoting the idea that gestation, labor, and birth were potentially pathological processes and therefore justified the expense of comprehensive care from highly skilled attendants capable of detecting and successfully handling those complications that might arise.[40] Almost exclusively drawn from the profession's elite, the obstetricians involved in infant welfare shared this commitment to reforming and elevating the specialty and thus tended to emphasize a definition of neonatal infant mortality and promote a course of action to counter its causes that were consistent with the attainment of their professional objectives.

On the positive side, obstetricians' commitment to reforming and legit-imizing their specialty focused much needed attention on the inadequacy of obstetric services available to most American women and helped reveal the mortal cost that unskilled attendants were inflicting upon both infants and their mothers. At the same time, however, it tended to skew the medical discourse on the causes of neonatal mortality. While deaths from injuries at birth (resulting from unskilled obstetric intervention) constituted the small-est proportion of neonatal mortality, their prevention was the subject of most of the medical discourse.[41] More importantly, perhaps, the specialists' commitment to elevating obstetrics guaranteed their opposition to any pro-gram to improve obstetric services and reduce neonatal mortality that would not also promote their professional objectives. In particular, obstetri-cians expressed unshakable opposition to any plan to incorporate female midwifery into obstetric practice, as had been done in England, Scan-dinavia, and Europe.

What to do with female midwives became a divisive issue in American infant welfare during the second decade of the century. In part the attention it attracted was due to the growing interest in preventing congenital and birth-related problems and neonatal mortality. But it was also the conse-quence of a resurgence in female midwifery in the United States that had begun in the late nineteenth century. Although female midwives had domi-nated birth attendance during the colonial era, they had gradually been displaced by male physicians, especially among the upper and middle classes and among those living in cities.[42] After 1880, however, the influx of mil-lions of immigrants from eastern and southern Europe gave renewed life to female midwifery. Because of tradition and personal experience, the new immigrants usually turned to female midwives when they sought a birth attendant. As a consequence, the practice of midwifery by women enjoyed a comeback, especially in cities with large immigrant populations. One study conducted in 1905 revealed that 42 percent all births in New York City were being attended by midwives. Another done in 1908 showed that midwives attended 86 percent of all Italian-American births in Chicago.[43]

Immigrant women preferred female midwives for a variety of reasons. One reason was experience and familiarity. In the towns and villages from which the new immigrants came, midwives were usually well-trained and competent and were favored as birth attendants. Moreover, many midwives were immigrants themselves and spoke the language of their clients. An-other reason was custom. Especially among Italian immigrants, a strong cultural taboo existed against men in the birthing chamber. Price was also a factor. Midwives charged between $5 and $10 while physicians charged $20 and up. Midwives also offered a greater range of services. Whereas doctors rarely visited pregnant women and usually arrived only once the final stages of labor had begun, midwives spent considerable time with their clients.

Also, they often helped with the housework and with the other children.[44]

The resurgence and visibility of female midwifery among urban immigrants prompted public health officials and social analysts to take a closer look at midwifery in the United States, especially as it existed among those who continued to have little access to mainstream medicine. It soon was revealed that somewhere around 90 percent of southern black births were attended by midwives and that a sizable proportion of poor, rural white women gave birth attended only by female friends, neighbors, or relatives. Indeed, it soon became common wisdom that between 40 and 50 percent of all births in the United States were being attended by other than regular physicians.[45]

For American infant welfare activists, increasingly concerned with the prenatal and natal care received by women, the revelation that nearly half of all births in the nation were being attended by "untrained women" was shocking and precipitated an intense debate over what was termed the "midwife problem."[46] AASPIM, and particularly its session on obstetrics, became one of the major forums of that debate. Many of the papers delivered there were subsequently published in medical and public health journals. Williams initiated the AASPIM debate in 1911 when he delivered a provocative and immensely influential address entitled, "The Midwife Problem and Medical Education in the United States."[47] Basing his remarks on the response to a questionnaire he had sent to those teaching obstetrics in 120 American medical schools, Williams savaged prevailing obstetric instruction and practice and blamed them for the death or permanent injury of thousands of women and children. Convinced that few general practitioners were competent to handle any but the simplest of births, he charged that they were at least as dangerous, and in all probability more so, than the average female midwife. Yet Williams had little interest in defending midwives. They looked good in comparison, he advised his audience, only because general practitioners were so bad. He therefore argued that the remedy for the low level of obstetric care in America lay not in licensing and legitimizing female midwifery, but in improving the skills of doctors. Indeed, he was adamantly opposed to any effort to give midwifery a permanent place in American obstetrics, contending that to do so would impede improvement of available services. If female midwifery were institutionalized, Willaims warned, obstetric fees would remain inadequate and so too would the care they purchased. "Doctors who are obliged to live from their practice," he counseled, "cannot reasonably be expected to give much better service than they are paid for."[48]

Williams' arguments were reiterated in subsequent AASPIM meetings by other leading American obstetric reformers. Charles Ziegler, professor of obstetrics at the University of Pittsburgh, contended in 1912 that the only way to reduce birth-related deaths and injuries among women and infants was to "train the physician until he is capable of doing good obstetrics, then make it financially possible for him to do it, by eliminating the midwife."[49] Joseph DeLee, a prominent proponent of hospital birth, agreed. Encouraging female midwifery, he warned AASPIM, would impede efforts to reform obstetrics from within and would postpone the day when the American public would be "brought to realize that there is a high art to obstetrics and that it must pay as well for it as for surgery."[50]

As in other areas of infant welfare, race and ethnicity played an important role in the debate over female midwifery. Noting that most midwives were foreign-born or black, physicians frequently characterized midwifery as a backward and alien practice kept alive by women who were ignorant, super-stitious, and dirty. In an editorial on the midwife problem, the *Boston Medi-cal and Surgical Journal* railed against the ignorance and low character of the typical midwife and asserted that "the tolerance of such persons is an anom-aly in an enlightened civilization."[51] Opponents of midwifery also used ethnic and racial slurs to argue that the type of midwife training and educa-tion programs common in Europe could not be implemented here because the typical American midwife was incapable of benefiting from formal in-struction.

Although obstetricians had an increasingly influential voice in infant wel-fare, they did not have the only voice, and their position on female midwif-ery was generally opposed by public health officials, social workers, and a number of pediatricians. Although frequently agreeing that many American midwives were ill-trained and incompetent and posed a threat to women and infants, many infant welfare activists argued that abolishing or ignoring midwifery offered no solution to the problem. Contending that it would be years before there was a sufficient supply of adequately skilled doctors, they favored training and licensing midwives so that midwifery could be im-proved and controlled. Among those most forcibly supporting this position was Josephine Baker. Convinced that custom, preference, and economic necessity would continue to motivate many women to choose midwives, Baker was instrumental in initiating training and regulatory programs in New York City. She also lobbied for their adoption elsewhere, and as early as 1911 stood before AASPIM and praised the success of such programs in Europe. Baker was joined by the social workers attached to various charity organizations and to the Children's Bureau and by public health officials such as Julius Levy who headed Newark's Division of Child Hygiene. She also received the support of pediatricians such as Philip Van Ingen and Abraham Jacobi. Indeed, Jacobi published a long paper in the *Journal of the American Medical Association* in which he harshly criticized the members of that organization for allowing their greed and self-interest to outweigh their concern for the welfare of America's mothers and infants.[52]

Infant welfare activists with a more sociological orientation also took issue with the tendency of obstetricians and other physicians to characterize the problems faced by mothers and newborns as essentially medical ones. At the 1914 meeting of AASPIM's obstetric session, Baker complained about what she described as the purely medical focus of many of the papers. Although agreeing that improving the quality and consumption of obstetric care would contribute significantly to the reduction of mortality in early infancy, she argued that any reform program limiting itself to that would be inadequate because it ignored the social and economic dimensions of neonatal mortality. Observing that while it might be natural for physicians to regard neonatal mortality as primarily a medical problem, Baker objected to the narrowness of this view, contending that mortality in early infancy was "in a larger sense a social problem."[53] In particular, she pointed to prematurity—which accounted in 1912 for 47.5 percent of all registration area deaths that occurred in the first week of life and 37.5 percent that occurred in the first month—as a problem that had social and economic as well as medical and hygienic dimensions. Noting that prevailing medical opinion held that the possibility of premature birth was greatly increased by overwork and fatigue toward the end of the gestative period, Baker argued that it was naive to think that a program limited to advising pregnant women to rest was sufficient. Although such advice might be suitable to some classes of women, she observed, it was of little use to the many women who were compelled by economic necessity and domestic responsibilities to engage in hard work in the factory or in the home right up to confinement.

Baker delivered her comments during a discussion that followed a paper given by Mrs. West of the Children's Bureau. While concurring with the obstetricians present that much benefit would be derived from improving obstetric training and educating mothers to avail themselves of skilled attendants and follow their advice, West suggested that the problem was somewhat more complex. Even if quality obstetric service was available and its value appreciated, she observed, many women could still not afford to take advantage of it. West also spoke at length of the need for legislative and other action that would discourage gestating women from working right up to the time they gave birth and post-parturient women from returning to work immediately after confinement. Noting that virtually every European and Scandinavian country had laws prohibiting the employment of women for several weeks before and after birth, she lamented that in the United States only four states had seen fit to pass similar laws.[54] Moreover, she charged that even in those states with laws, the actual protection provided pregnant and nursing mothers was minimal at best. Not only were the laws worded so as to make enforcement all but impossible, but as strictly prohibitive measures they did little to relieve, and indeed exacerbated, the economic necessities that compelled many women to work. "One of the obstacles of protective labor legislation of this sort," she declared, "is that unless it carries with it some provision for the payment of a woman's wages during the time she is required to be away from work, the law will work hardship where it is intended to relieve."[55]

Baker concurred. "It is farcical," she observed, "to pass laws that women cannot work a month before or a month after labor, when such prohibition may mean starvation for themselves and their children; therefore unless we can provide some sort of payment during this period, I think our laws are quite useless."[56] Homer Folks made essentially the same point. In his opinion, merely advising pregnant women and new mothers not to work or passing laws that prohibited them from doing so without compensation was an absurdly inadequate response to infant mortality. He therefore advised,

> We have to face the fact that this baby-saving business means money, and means interference with the ordinary methods of earning money, and that interrupted earnings have to be made up somehow if the baby is going to be saved. In other words we must study maternity insurance, and the many economic aspects of baby-saving."[57]

The argument put forth by Baker, West, and Folks—that neonatal mortality, indeed all infant mortality, was more than a medical problem and thus required some form of protective legislation combined with social and medical welfare or maternity insurance—was one heard with increasing frequency toward the end of the second decade of the century. Prompted both by a spate of studies conducted by the Children's Bureau and by social welfare developments in Europe, American infant welfare activists rediscovered poverty and, at least briefly, contemplated adopting maternity insurance to ameliorate its effects.

7

The Steps Not Taken:
The Rediscovery of Poverty
and the
Rejection of Maternity Insurance

As the second decade of the century progressed, the Children's Bureau played an increasingly central role in shaping the discourse on infant mortality. Limited by the Congress to conducting and assisting child-related research, the bureau initially focused its energies on promoting birth registration. At the same time, however, it recognized that even if birth records were complete, they would not throw light on such hypothesized determinants of infant survival as type of care and feeding, domestic and community sanitation, size of family, and access to medical advice and care. Consequently, beginning in 1913 the bureau launched a series of comprehensive investigations into the causes and rates of infant mortality in various American communities during specified years.[1] In total, the bureau examined ten communities and published its findings between 1915 and 1923. In keeping with the still prevalent assumption that infant mortality was highest among the urban immigrant poor, seven of the targeted communities—Johnstown, Pennsylvania; Manchester, New Hampshire; Waterbury, Connecticut; Brockton and New Bedford, Massachusetts; Akron, Ohio; and Gary, Indiana—were mid-sized, industrial cities with significant immigrant populations. The other three communities, chosen for the sake of comparison, were Montclair, New Jersey, a fairly prosperous suburban town; Baltimore, Maryland, a major urban center; and Saginaw, Michigan, a diversified industrial city with a small immigrant population.[2]

In an attempt to achieve unprecedented comprehensiveness and accuracy, bureau investigators supplemented official birth and death records with information gleaned from house-to-house canvassing and sought to determine precisely the ratio of infants born in one year who died rather than relying on the approximation of that ratio provided by the standard infant mortality statistic.[3] They also gathered standardized and comparable data on the social, sanitary, civic, and economic conditions in each community,

and carefully interviewed the families of each infant born during the specified year. Bureau investigators entered the selected communities only after
the cooperation of municipal officials, civic organizations, and women's
clubs had been obtained and after the populations had been apprised of the
purpose of the study by their newspapers and clergy. Having done this, they
first attempted to determine as precisely as possible the actual number of
infants who had been born during the year being studied. They then elimi-
nated from this number all infants whose families had moved away or could
not be found.[4] Visiting the households of all the remaining infants, they
determined whether each infant had survived twelve months and verified
official records of the sex and cause and age of death of those infants who had
not. In addition, they collected detailed information on household and
neighborhood sanitary conditions, on methods of childcare and feeding, on
parental ethnicity and race, on maternal health, reproductive history and
type of birth attendance, on birth order and family size, on maternal employment and domestic responsibilities, and on paternal earnings.[5]

As the Children's Bureau had hoped, its studies proved to be more comprehensive and sophisticated than anything previously undertaken. The
combined studies provided a detailed picture of infant mortality in America
that both confirmed and challenged prevailing opinion. Proving what had
long been suspected, nearly 75 percent of all the infant deaths which took
place in the communities studied were attributable to three major categories
of pathologic causes. The first, problems specific to early infancy and traceable to the condition and care of the mother during pregnancy, accounted for
36.3 percent of all deaths during the first year and represented a rate of 40.4
deaths per 1000 live births. Within this category, 43.1 percent of such deaths
were ascribed to prematurity, 36.9 percent to congenital debility, 10.6 percent to congenital malformations, and 9.4 percent to injuries at birth.[6] The
second major causal category was gastric and intestinal diseases, accounting
for 29.1 percent of all infant deaths and a rate of 32.4 per 1000 live births. Of
these deaths, 96.6 were ascribed to diarrhea and enteritis, with the re-
mainder being attributed to so-called diseases of the stomach. Making up the
third major pathologic category were respiratory diseases, including bronchitis, bronchopneumonia, and pneumonia. These totaled 17.6 percent of all
infant deaths and represented a mortality rate of 19.6. Accounting for the
remaining 17 percent of infant deaths were "external" causes (.5 percent);
epidemic and communicable diseases, including whooping cough, tuberculosis, and syphilis (6.4 percent); other defined diseases, including meningitis, convulsions, and heart disease (7.8 percent); and ill-defined diseases
(2.3 percent).[7]

Although at 111.2 deaths per 1000 live births the overall infant mortality
rate for the investigated cities was somewhat higher than that which the
Bureau of the Census claimed obtained in the entire registration area, the

proportion of deaths ascribed to each pathologic category was quite similar.[8] The Children's Bureau's findings thus substantiated the basic accuracy of the mortality reports that the Bureau of the Census had been publishing since 1906. Children's Bureau investigators, however, were less interested in validating Bureau of the Census statistics than they were in supplementing them. The studies were designed to reveal much more than simply the pathologic causes of infant death and their respective mortality rates. Indeed, the studies aimed especially at revealing the secondary or underlying causes—medical, environmental, socioeconomic, and behavioral—and hoped to correlate those causes with the pathologic ones. This aim reflected the orientation of those who ran and staffed the Children's Bureau. But it was also a product of the battle for survival that the bureau was constantly forced to fight. Challenged from its inception to prove that it was not duplicating other agencies that gathered vital statistics, the bureau formulated its studies to collect data that were not available anywhere else.[9]

In seeking to discover and reveal the underlying or secondary causes of infant mortality, bureau investigators had two principal tools. One was a standardized schedule for recording the socioeconomic, physical, and civic environment of the various cities. The other was a similarly standardized set of questions, the answers to which were sought by visiting the individual domiciles of all infants born during the year under study. Armed with the first, bureau investigators recorded general information on each city's history, topographic and climatic characteristics, industrial profile and conditions of employment, and more specific information on population makeup, sewerage, water supplies, garbage disposal, milk distribution, and the extent to which public health and infant welfare work was being actively supported and pursued. While the findings were somewhat mixed, the information collected enabled the bureau to draw a number of general conclusions. In particular, it provided confirmation of what many public health officials and infant welfare activists had long been arguing: that in most mid-sized American cities, public health and infant welfare activity was minimal at best; and in those few where it was not, the infant mortality rate was significantly lower.[10]

More fruitful and revealing, however, was the information collected by visiting the homes of infants born in each city. Along with recording neighborhood and domestic sanitary conditions, bureau investigators interviewed parents to obtain individualized data that would enable them to correlate infant mortality and age and cause of death with ethnicity and race, family and household size, methods of infant care and feeding, maternal health and reproductive history, type of birth attendance, maternal employment and domestic duties, and paternal earnings. With those interviews the bureau studies were able to demonstrate on a large scale what previous smaller investigations had suggested were the critical factors influencing survival of older infants. All the studies, for instance, illustrated and con-firmed long-held opinion that both methods of feeding and infant hygiene and seasonal temperature correlated strongly with deaths from gastric and intestinal disorders. (See Table 9.) Such deaths, they showed, were thirteen times higher in August than in January and three to four times higher among artificially fed infants than among those who were breastfed. The studies also provided detailed information on deaths from respiratory diseases and emphasized that such deaths, while declining, still accounted for a signifi-cant proportion of existing infant mortality.

The collection of individualized data through interviews also enabled bureau investigators to verify on a large scale and among a normal popula-tion the influence on neonatal mortality of certain maternal factors which smaller studies of obstetric clinic patients had suggested were important. Among these were maternal age, multiple births, number of previous births or birth order, interval since preceding birth and before succeeding pregnan-cy, previous occurrence of prenatal complications and perinatal loss, and type or manner of delivery. For instance, the data collected by the bureau investigators showed that infant mortality peaked at 160.3 for infants born to mothers less than eighteen years of age, dropped to its lowest ebb at 101.4 among infants whose mothers were 25–29 years of age, and steadily climbed again to 131.3 for infants born to mothers 40–44 years old. Similarly, they

Table 9
Infant Mortality Rates[a] by Month and Type of Feeding in Eight Communities[b]
Studied by the Children's Bureau

Month of Life	All	Type of Feeding		
		Solely Breastfed	Partly Breastfed	Solely Artificially Fed
First	44.8	16.9	36.4	54.7
Second	9.3	5.8	14.7	24.6
Third	8.1	3.7	12.9	21.2
Fourth	8.0	3.4	9.0	19.2
Fifth	7.7	3.3	5.7	18.1
Sixth	7.4	2.1	5.9	17.7
Seventh	6.3	1.9	4.0	14.1
Eighth	5.8	2.9	3.3	11.3
Ninth	5.7	3.2	2.9	10.7
Tenth	5.3	3.8	2.3	9.3
Eleventh	3.9	2.4	2.5	6.0
Twelfth	4.5	4.4	2.7	6.4

Source: Robert Morse Woodbury, Infant Mortality and Its Causes (Baltimore: Williams and Wilkins, 1926), p. 79.
[a]Deaths per 1,000 live births among a population of 22,422 live births. Population excludes 545 live-born infants who did not live long enough to be fed.
[b]Table based on data from all the communities studied by the Children's Bureau except for Montclair, New Jersey, and Gary, Indiana.

showed that twins and triplets were much more likely to die than single issue, that family size correlated with infant survival, that infants born after a two-year interval had almost a 50 percent better chance of living than did those born after a one-year interval, that women who had previously miscarried or lost an infant were significantly more likely than other women to do so again, and that infants delivered by instruments suffered a mortality rate 20 percent higher than those who were not.[11]

The bureau's studies had their greatest impact, however, not in the revelation of these underlying medical causes but in their demonstration of and insistence on the overwhelming causal significance of family economic status. From the Johnstown study onward, the bureau had carefully collected data on father's earnings and sought to evaluate the extent to which income correlated to both the pathologic and the underlying causes of infant mortality. What that evaluation showed, bureau researchers argued, was that the amount of money a father earned during the year was one of the most accurate predictors of infant survival. (See Table 10.) As the bureau's first released study, that of Johnston, concluded: "the economic factor is of far-reaching importance in determining a baby's chance of life."[12] In demonstrating the significance of economic status, the bureau studies mounted a powerful and controversial challenge to what had been and still was the operating assumption of American infant welfare. While not denying the importance of convincing mothers to seek and follow medical advice on the care and feeding of their infants and on the hygiene of pregnancy, they questioned its efficacy in the face of inadequate family income.

The initial adoption of maternal education as the primary strategy for preventing infant deaths had been based on the conviction that intelligent maternal care provided an effective buffer against the influence of conditions attending poverty. The Johnstown study sent the shocking message that this was less true than believed. While confirming that infant mortality was indeed higher among bottle-fed than breastfed babies, bureau researchers pointed to an anomaly. Although the babies of poor, immigrant mothers were more likely to die than those born into more prosperous, native families, they were also more likely to be breastfed. Rather than explain this anomaly, as others had, by suggesting that the higher infant death rate suffered by the immigrant poor could be attributed to the astronomical mortality of those of their infants who were artificially fed, bureau researchers sought an explanation by correlating infant deaths and type of feeding with maternal nativity and paternal earnings. What they found, in the words of the Johnstown report, was that "the manner of feeding is one of the most important considerations in the life and health of a baby. But a comparison of the number of deaths among infants whose fathers earned specified sums, shows that the influence of poverty reaches even the breast fed baby. Where fathers' earnings are small, a large number of babies die despite breast feeding."[13]

Aside from illustrating that "even the care given the baby by its mother often must be offset by the evils resulting from an income insufficient for a family's needs," the bureau studies offered compelling evidence that quality of care, and particularly lack of breastfeeding, was more often dictated by economic necessity than maternal knowledge, concern, or choice.[14] Since the data collected included information on methods of care and feeding, paternal earnings, and maternal employment, bureau researchers were able to draw conclusions as to the extent to which those mothers who early curtailed breastfeeding did so to return to work to supplement meager family incomes. In one city, for instance, it was discovered that in families where fathers earned less than $450 per year, over 73 percent of the mothers were gainfully employed either inside or outside the home during the year imme- diately following their confinement. As paternal income rose, however, the proportion of gainful maternal employment dropped, as did the infant mor- tality rate: in part because the death rate of babies whose mothers worked was over 80 percent higher than those whose mothers did not.[15]

Bureau investigators acknowledged that the relationship between mater- nal employment and infant mortality was a complex one because the effects of gainful employment were different for mothers working inside and out- side the home, and because in both cases the income brought in had a mitigating influence. But they felt the character of the relationship was clear enough to support at least two conclusions. The first was that contrary to popular opinion, mothers who worked did so primarily out of economic necessity. As the authors of the Manchester study observed,

It has often been alleged that in industrial communities such as Manchester, which offer ready employment for women, the reason married women and moth- ers seek employment is either because of the temptation to earn pin money or money for some special purpose such as buying a home or because women learn economic independence before marriage and prefer the factory to housework. Individual instances of this sort were encountered in Manchester, but insufficient or low earnings on the part of the father appear to be the most potent reason for a mother's going to work.[16]

The second conclusion was that no matter what benefits maternal employ- ment outside the home might bring to sustaining the family, it robbed infants of mothers' care, required artificial feeding, and thus contributed substan- tially to infant mortality. "Mothers who are obliged to work," concluded the authors of the Waterbury study, "must perforce substitute artificial feeding for nursing and intrust to others the care of their infants. The result is a high mortality rate for infants of working mothers."[17]

Along with implicating inadequate family income and maternal employ-ment as causes in all infant mortality, the bureau studies showed them to be important factors in neonatal mortality. For eight of the cities studied, neonatal mortality was 56 percent higher for infants whose mothers worked away from home during pregnancy than for those whose mothers were not gainfully employed.[18] Moreover, bureau researchers argued that even when poor women were not gainfully employed outside the home, they more often than not were engaged in hard labor right up to confinement. While few married women in the steel and factory towns of Pennsylvania and the Great Lakes region actually left home to work, many took in boarders or wash and thus had rigorous and fatiguing "domestic" duties. And even those who did not engage in income-producing work in the home could not afford to hire domestic help or interrupt their household chores and child care duties for more than a few days. Bureau researchers also contended that meager family income prevented many women from availing themselves of adequate medical supervision and care during pregnancy. The Baltimore study, for instance, showed that even in a city that was a leader in promoting prenatal care, less than 45 percent of women whose husbands earned under $850 per year had any form of prenatal medical attendance while over 87 percent of women whose husbands yearly earned over $1,850 did.[19] (See Table 10.)

Table 10

Infant and Neonatal Mortality Rates by Earnings of Fathers in Seven Communities[a] Studied by the Children's Bureau

Earnings of Father for Year	Live Births	Deaths	IM Rate[b]	NM Rate[c]
No earnings	313	66	210.9	60.7
Under $450	3,085	515	166.9	55.8
$450 to $549	2,827	355	125.6	46.0
$550 to $649	2,908	339	116.6	43.3
$650 to $849	5,050	543	107.5	46.5
$850 to $1,049	3,345	277	82.8	38.0
$1,050 to $1,249	1,391	89	64.0	33.1
$1,250 and over	2,252	133	59.1	38.2
Unknown	365	51	139.7	41.1
Total	21,536	2,368	110.0	44.4

Source: Robert Morse Woodbury, Infant Mortality and Its Causes (Baltimore: Williams and Wilkins, 1926), p. 131
[a]The commuinities not included are Johnstown, Pennsylvania, Montclair, New Jersey, and Gary, Indiana.
[b]Infant mortality (IM) rate computed as: deaths of infants < one year old/live births in specified year × 1000.
[c]Neonatal mortality (NM) rate computed as: deaths of infants < one month old/live births in specified year × 1000.

While the bureau studies did not deny that ignorance among immigrant and poor expectant mothers significantly contributed to those prenatal and natal complications that increased neonatal mortality, they did question whether a reform program limited to promoting personal hygiene and the consumption of medical services was alone an adequate response to the problem. Such a program assumed that only obduracy would prevent gestating women from following a medically acceptable regimen once they were apprised of its importance. According to bureau researchers, however, this was not the case. As Robert Morse Woodbury, the bureau's director of statistical research, observed in an analysis of neonatal mortality differentials by income,

> Though ignorance in poorer families of the rules of health doubtless played some part in producing these differences, the obvious relation between lack of means and inability to purchase medical and nursing services and competent advice and to follow that advice suggests that lack of means or economic pressure must have borne a heavy responsibility. The health program recommended by the best medical authorities for pregnant women includes wholesome and nourishing food, spending at least two hours a day in the open air, and freedom from worry and overwork. This program is obviously one which can be more easily and faithfully observed by women in comfortable circumstances than by those who have to struggle daily to make ends meet.[20]

With their consistent reiteration of the influence of family income, the Children's Bureau studies helped reinvest the American discourse on infant mortality with a substantive economic dimension and put forth a powerful argument that the causes of infant mortality would not be sufficiently countered simply by eradicating maternal ignorance in regard to prenatal and infant hygiene. Nor were they alone in doing so. Other American sociomedical analysts were beginning to advance the same argument. Among these was Louis Dublin. Head of the Metropolitan Life Insurance Company's statistical bureau, Dublin was then earning recognition as one of America's most sophisticated and informed experts on the relation of morbidity and mortality to public health and socioeconomic conditions. In 1915 he published an influential essay in which he took issue with a 1912 U.S. Bureau of Labor Statistics Study of infant mortality and maternal employment in Fall River. Part of a massive, congressionally mandated investigation of women and children in industry, the earlier study had concluded that whatever influence maternal employment and other economic conditions had on infant mortality in Fall River, it paled before the overriding influence of improper care and feeding devolving from maternal ignorance and ethnic custom. As Charles H. Verrill, the study's chief investigator, contended: "The causes of excessive infant mortality in Fall River may be summed up in a sentence as the mother's ignorance of proper feeding and proper care and of the simplest requirements of hygiene."[21]

Dublin disagreed. Basing his analysis on data collected in the summer of 1913 by the Fall River District Nursing Association, he contended that it was economic status as much as ignorance or ethnic custom that explained why immigrant mothers lost babies more frequently than native-born mothers and why certain immigrant groups suffered higher rates of infant death than others. Demonstrating that those immigrant groups who had the highest neonatal and infant mortality also had the lowest family incomes and the largest percentage of mothers working outside the home, Dublin argued the importance of economic status. "It is the factor of income," he contended, "which determines the number of rooms occupied, their location in the city, the amount and character of food, the need for supplementary work by the mother outside the home, and other considerations which bear directly on infant mortality."[22] Dublin's analysis was soon supported by other sociomedical investigators such as Henry Hibbs, whose *Infant Mortality: Its Relation to Social and Industrial Conditions* (1916) was a carefully documented plea for recognition of the socioeconomic causes of infant death. In conjunction with the Children's Bureau, these analysts advanced a powerful argument for the expansion of infant welfare beyond maternal educational reform and toward the inclusion of some form of social and medical welfare for mothers. And, as Mrs. West predicted in 1914, they raised the issue of maternity benefits or insurance, some type of which had already been adopted by most of the other industrialized Western nations.

Although maternity insurance varied from country to country, in general it aimed at providing two types of assistance. First, whether through the direct provision of medical services, sick benefits, or cash grants, maternity insurance sought to ensure that pregnant and parturient women had available to them adequate medical attendance. Second, through some combination of lost wage compensation, nursing premiums, and domestic assistance, it sought to encourage mothers to breastfeed their infants and to guarantee them the economic security required to avoid fatiguing work before and after confinement.[23] Whatever form it took, maternity insurance was designed to complement rather than replace existing instructional services organized around well-baby and prenatal clinics, mothers' classes, home visitation, and the general dissemination of information. Indeed, even in countries that established maternity insurance systems, infant welfare continued to operate on the assumption that infant mortality would be substantially reduced if mothers would follow offered advice on the care of themselves and their infants. Rather than challenging that assumption, maternity insurance represented an extension of it, an extension based on the recognition that many mothers needed material assistance if they were to follow the regimen infant welfare experts promoted as necessary for the successful

carrying, bearing, and rearing of infants. Maternity insurance thus represented an attempt to meet a need at least implicitly recognized ever since
infant welfare reconceptualized infant mortality as essentially a problem of
motherhood.

Although there had been some discussion of material assistance to mothers throughout the nineteenth century, maternity insurance and the benefits
it provided became a significant social and political issue only after the 1870s
when a number of industrialized nations began passing laws prohibiting the
employment of women during the weeks surrounding confinement.[24] Since
such laws made no provision for lost wages, it soon became apparent that
what good they did was frequently offset by the economic hardship they
imposed on families where the mother's income was critical for survival in
normal times and was doubly so when the burden of confinement expenses
was added. Maternity insurance was thus conceived and promoted not only
as a means of combating infant mortality, but also as a type of social insurance designed to stabilize income and prevent the impoverishment of the
working poor from the loss of wages and the expenses of childbirth. Indeed,
except in Australia, where all new mothers were granted a lump sum payment regardless of income, and in Italy, where a separate and independent
maternity benefit system was created, maternity insurance was incorporated into compulsory sickness insurance.[25] Compulsory sickness insurance
was one of the several types of social insurance created and put into effect by
the governments of most Western industrial nations at the end of the nineteenth and the beginning of the twentieth centuries to protect the working
poor from being thrust into dependent poverty by loss of income and catastrophic expense due to industrial accidents, temporary unemployment, old
age, sickness, debility, or death. In order to understand the evolution of
maternity insurance and to explain its fate in the United States, then, it is
necessary to consider it not simply as part of the infant welfare movement
but also as part of the development of state-initiated compulsory sickness
insurance.

The first compulsory sickness insurance system was established in Germany in 1883 when the Reichstag approved a law mandating coverage for
low-income workers in certain industries. Both a reform measure designed
to protect the working poor from income disruption and catastrophic expense due to sickness, disability, and death and a defensive action intended
to quell mounting political and labor unrest, the system was the brainchild
of Chancellor Otto von Bismark who later commented that his purpose had
been "to bribe the working classes, or if you like, to win them over to regard
the State as a social institution existing for their sake and interested in their
welfare."[26] Amended several times during the following decades and
codified in 1911, German sickness insurance offered essentially four types of
benefits: a cash benefit which compensated sick workers for lost wages; a

medical benefit that covered physician and nursing care; a maternity benefit that provided wage compensation, midwife, or physician attendance, and a nursing premium; and a funeral benefit that helped cover the cost of burial.[27]

Confronted with similar economic and political conditions, other nations eventually followed Germany's lead: Austria in 1888, Hungary in 1891, Luxembourg in 1901, Norway in 1909, Serbia in 1910, Great Britain in 1911, Russia and Rumania in 1912, and the Netherlands in 1913. In addition, Sweden, Denmark, Switzerland, and to a lesser extent France and Italy began subsidizing existing private sickness insurance funds.[28] Although specific coverage, funding, and administration varied from country to country, by the second decade of the twentieth century most sickness insurance systems had at least four common characteristics. First, they were aimed at the working poor, extending coverage only to workers, usually industrial workers, whose incomes were below a set amount. In short, eligibility involved a means test. Second, they were compulsory, requiring from covered workers and their employers a specified contribution that was frequently, though not always, subsidized by the state. Third, they were usually administered by existing private sickness funds under government supervision. And fourth, the benefits they provided generally included both cash payments to compensate for lost wages and free or subsidized treatment by sickness-fund doctors and nurses.

From the beginning, maternity benefits were part of the benefit package offered in most sickness insurance systems. However, because maternity benefits were in large part designed to counter economic hardship caused by factory laws restricting female employment in the weeks surrounding confinement, most, initially at least, restricted coverage to women workers, although provision was made in some countries to allow for the voluntary purchase of insurance by other women. One of the major exceptions to this rule was the British system, whose chief architect and promoter, Lloyd George, considered a broadly inclusive maternity benefit critical to achieving necessary popular support for his compulsory insurance plan. In addition to covering eligible women workers, British maternity insurance also covered the wives of insured men. Yet what the British system gave with one hand, it took away with the other. While the 1911 law establishing maternity benefits as part of national sickness insurance provided a lump cash payment of 30s. (approximately $7.20 in 1911 dollars), it expressly prohibited the use of the medical benefit to cover obstetric and midwife services during pregnancy and confinement. Although clearly inadequate to do so, the cash payment was expected to cover both lost wages and the medical expenses of birth.[29] While this inadequacy characterized the British system until World War II, it was, to some extent at least, compensated for by assistance programs established by Parliament in 1914 and by the Maternal and Child Welfare Act of 1918. The former gave grants-in-aid to voluntary associations

working in infant and maternal welfare and the latter provided local authorities with matching funds that they could use to furnish needy women
with the services of midwives or pay the expense of physician attendance
and hospital confinement when complications arose.[30]

Although various American medical and social science journals reported
upon their adoption and development in Germany and elsewhere, little
discussion of or agitation for either maternity or sickness insurance took
place in the United States until 1911 when Parliament passed the National
Insurance Act. Inspired by Lloyd George's success in Britain and encouraged that several states had recently enacted workmen's compensation laws,
American Progressives began a push for the creation of systems of compulsory sickness insurance to protect the working poor from the consequences of
sickness, debility, and death. Spearheading that push was the American
Association for Labor Legislation (AALL), a small but influential group of
"Social Progressives," who in 1913 decided to focus their energies on securing enactment of sickness insurance laws within the various states. By 1915
they had drawn up a model bill which would require that most manual
workers earning less than $1,200 a year have available to them sickness
insurance that included a medical benefit, lost wage compensation, maternity benefits, and a death benefit.[31] In addition, the bill stipulated that some
medical assistance and maternity benefits be provided to wives and depen-
dents, guaranteed the right of beneficiaries to choose among participating
doctors, and allowed other workers and self-employed persons with incomes
of less than $100 a month to buy into the system on a voluntary basis.
Funding was to come from equal compulsory contributions from employees
and employers, as well as from a 20 percent subsidy from the individual
states.[32]

Although acknowledging that considerable debate existed over whether
maternity should be classified as a temporary disability in the same way
sickness was, the AALL justified the inclusion of maternity benefits within
their plan for compulsory sickness insurance by arguing that for many of the
working poor, carrying and bearing children frequently posed the risk of
bankrupting meager family resources. "In the life of the working-class,"
contended Isaac Rubinow, the AALL's most articulate and passionate proponent of compulsory sickness insurance, "maternity has proved a fruitful
source of destitution."[33] Advocates of the maternity benefit also pointed to
the accumulating evidence showing that labor outside the home, and especially industrial labor, had a serious negative impact on women's ability to
gestate, bear, and rear healthy infants and therefore not only contributed to
the unnecessary death of many newborns but also condemned a large number of those who survived to a life of unproductive physical debility. To its
proponents, then, maternity benefits, estimated at less than .9 percent of the
total annual wages paid to working women, seemed a small price to pay for a

good that both compassion and social efficiency demanded.[34] The maternity benefit included in the model bill assumed that employed women should refrain from work for at least two weeks before and six weeks after confine' ment. During that time they would be supplied with medical supervision and attendance and would receive wage compensation equal to that of sick pay. The unemployed wives of insured men would receive only the medical benefit.[35]

In January 1916, modified versions of the AALL model bill were placed before the state legislatures of New York and Massachusetts. Although neither passed, the AALL and its allies remained optimistic. Aware that a number of other states had appointed commissions to study the appropriate' ness of considering similar bills and heartened by the positive response of many state legislators, proponents of sickness insurance expressed the belief that it was only a matter of time before their state'by'state campaign was crowned with success. That belief, however, proved to be illusory. Al' though between 1915 and 1920 eleven state sickness insurance commissions were formed and bills were considered by the legislatures of sixteen states, not one state enacted a compulsory sickness insurance law. Indeed, only in New York, where in 1919 a much modified version of the original 1916 bill passed the Senate before it died in the House, did enactment seem a real possibility. Moreover, in California, the only state where it was put to a popular vote, compulsory sickness insurance was soundly defeated. By 1921, then, compulsory sickness insurance had become a dead issue in the United States.[36]

Why did sickness insurance fail in the United States and with it any hope of maternity benefits or insurance? In answering that question historians have often pointed to the withering opposition it faced from special interest groups with solid functional reasons for considering it a threat to their welfare. Compulsory sickness insurance was strongly opposed by commer' cial insurance companies, who faced the loss of a lucrative business in death benefits, and by employer associations, who feared that employer costs would far outweigh any gains in worker productivity. It also met intense opposition from organized medicine, which after initially reacting with luke' warm support tinged by apathy, mounted an increasingly vociferous, hos' tile, and effective campaign to block the enactment of sickness insurance laws.[37]

The almost complete absence in the United States of already existing private and public bureaucratic structures to facilitate and administer sick' ness insurance also contributed to the failure of the proposed bills. Unlike in Europe, no established network of voluntary sickness insurance funds ex' isted to incorporate into a government'sponsored system. Nor was there a professional civil service bureaucracy sufficiently competent to oversee and regulate the system. The lack of private and public bureaucratic structures made the mechanics of sickness insurance a much more problematic issue in the United States. It also shaped organized medicine's response to sickness insurance. In Europe, the question for physicians was whether they wished to have their fees and actions controlled by voluntary funds in which they had little input or by a government bureaucracy which they could conceiv-ably influence. In the United States, however, the question for physicians was not what type of control they would be willing to submit to, but whether they would be willing to submit to any control at all.[38]

Historians have also noted that, unlike much of the rest of the indus-trialized West, early twentieth-century America did not have a political challenge from the left that was clear and powerful enough to force a signifi-cant modification in the classically liberal orientation of American govern-ment and to counter a strong ideological tradition that fostered suspicion of government's ability to solve social problems. Indeed, in Europe, social in-surance in general and sickness insurance in particular developed and were adopted as a compromise between a tradition of laissez-faire government subscribed to by the right and an emergent tendency toward the welfare state championed by an increasingly powerful left. In the United States, however, no such compromise was necessary, for the left was too weak and too fragmented to force it. Socialism, though at the peak of its American influence, was politically inconsequential, and organized labor contained within it a powerful element opposed to anything that smacked of govern-ment paternalism.[39] In a political spectrum that ranged from center to right, sickness insurance appeared not as a moderate alternative to more radical schemes, but as a radical alternative to the status quo.

American government was also highly decentralized and at the national level had no commitment to or experience in providing welfare services. In contrast to Europe where sickness insurance was debated and implemented as a national reform—and not insignificantly pushed from within national governments by political figures wielding immense power—in the United States, it was considered and debated at the state level and promoted pri-marily by advocacy groups with little or no formal political power. As a consequence, the American battle for sickness insurance was never truly a national one. Like the contemporaneous fight for improved infant welfare services, it was, with a few notable exceptions, confined largely to the industrial Northeast and Midwest. Moreover, the fight took shape not as one between government and opposing special interests, but between those interests and reform advocates. The role of government was thus not one of advocacy, but at most one of mediation, evaluating the relative merits of each group's case.[40]

Timing also worked against the adoption of maternity and sickness insur-ance in America. In England, they had been debated and adopted at a time when Anglo-progressivism was at the peak of its influence, when concern with social reform had not yet been eclipsed by the exigencies of fighting a world war, and before the initiation of what was an international postwar trend toward political conservatism. In the United States the story was quite different. Not only were sickness insurance and its included maternity benefit introduced after progressivism and the reformist impulse had begun to wane, but they were also victimized by the war, having the misfortune of being caught up in the feverish anti-German hysteria that attended America's 1917 entry into the fighting. War-provoked antipathy toward all things German was certainly not the origin of opposition in the United States to sickness insurance. But it did significantly add to that opposition, and more importantly, gave special interest opponents a vocabulary with which to arouse popular sentiment. Pointing to the origin of sickness insurance in Germany, while conveniently neglecting its adoption by most of our allies, opponents of sickness insurance painted it as a German-inspired plot to bring about the Prussianization of America. "What is Compulsory Social Health Insurance?" rhetorically asked one organized opponent in 1918. "It is a dangerous device, invented in Germany, announced by the German Emperor from the throne the same year he started plotting and preparing to conquer the world."[41] The war, then, served to poison the atmosphere in which sickness insurance was debated and to ensure that its consideration would be attended by rhetorical hysteria. Moreover, that hysteria did not abate with the armistice in 1918. During the Red Scare of the postwar era, opponents of sickness insurance merely switched from an anti-German vocabulary to an equally resonant anti-Bolshevik one.

Finally, maternity benefits were not adopted in the United States in part because they received only somewhat ambivalent support from the infant welfare community. As could be expected, physicans and especially obstetricians involved in infant welfare were less than wholeheartedly convinced of the absolute necessity of sickness insurance and maternity benefits. Although some, like Arthur B. Emmons and George Kosmak, initially endorsed the AALL proposal, they did so with hesitation. Moreover, as opposition to sickness insurance mounted within the entire profession, it also increased among the ranks of infant welfare physicians. Obstetricians in particular echoed the AMA's condemnation of sickness insurance as dangerous to medical standards and expressed the fear that maternity insurance, by controlling fees and restricting freedom of practice, would seriously impede their efforts to attract better students to the specialty and thus improve the quality of available obstetric care.[42]

Although more supportive, public health officials active in infant welfare were also somewhat ambivalent toward maternity insurance. While many of them joined Josephine Baker in calling for the adoption of such insurance, they were markedly reluctant to endorse the AALL model bill. The source of that reluctance was twofold. Conceiving of both sickness and maternity insurance as public health measures, they were disappointed that the AALL bill did not place administrative authority within health departments. In short, they were willing to support such insurance but only if they could administer it.[43] Secondly, the underlying argument for maternity benefits— that meager income swelled the infant death roles—ran counter to the emphasis that public health had come to place on hygienic instruction as a panacea for community health problems. In a 1919 talk before the National Conference on Social Work, Julius Levy, the director of Newark, New Jersey's Division of Child Hygiene, spoke for many of his colleagues when he declared, "I cannot believe that low income bears any very constant causal relation to infant mortality." The primary cause, he continued, was maternal ignorance or obduracy in regard to proper prenatal and postnatal hygienic regimens.[44] Thus, even when sickness insurance bills placed administration of maternity benefits within health departments—as did a 1920 bill before the Massachusetts legislature—opposition was still voiced by some public health officials. Appointed to investigate the need for that bill, a commission headed by Merrill Champion, director of the Massachusetts Department of Health's Division of Child Hygiene, took issue with the economic interpretation of infant mortality, reporting that up to 50 percent of the state's infant deaths seemed to have occurred in families where mothers were not compelled to work and where income was sufficient to afford adequate medical attendance for both mother and offspring. The commission concluded that "infants die in Massachusetts largely because of lack of hygiene," and went on to suggest that "this conclusion justifies us in continuing the plan we have always followed of directing our efforts towards the education of our citizens in matters of personal hygiene."[45]

Ambivalence even characterized the response that maternity insurance evoked among social workers and social scientists, that contingent of the infant welfare community who were most committed to the idea that economic conditions exerted a powerful influence on infant death rates. Despite the Children's Bureau studies, a strong suspicion remained that both the tendency of mothers to work and the underutilization of skilled medical attendance were rooted in ethnic custom as much as poverty. Moreover, accepting the necessity of maternity insurance meant accepting the necessity of married women working. And this—challenging deep-seated American convictions regarding the responsibility of the father for providing his family with sufficient economic support so that the mother could remain home caring for the children—was something that even those who embraced an economic analysis of infant mortality had difficulty doing. Committed to an ideal vision of the family as small and nurturing, most middle-class social workers and social scientists saw employment of any family member but the father as deviant. Writing in the *Survey* in 1916, S. Adolphus Knoph summed up that view, proclaiming the superiority of "the social and moral life of the smaller family where the father earns enough to support his wife and children, and where the mother can devote her time to the care of them, and where neither she nor the children go out and help in the support of the family."[46] Similar sentiments were expressed even by Lee K. Frankel, co-author of an authoritative work on social insurance in Europe and a leading advocate of its adoption in the United States. Contending that the "need for sickness insurance can no longer be denied," Frankel admitted to fellow AASPIM members that he nevertheless had mixed feelings about including maternity benefits within it. While observing that the number of women in industry was growing, he declared that he and other American social scientists considered this neither normal nor desirable. "For the present, at least," he informed his listeners, "we have not accepted the European principle that the wife's earnings must be an element in the family budget," and argued that the real solution to the problems caused for infants by their mothers working was "not insurance but a better wage" for fathers. While ultimately suggesting that the association support maternity insurance, he advised that it do so only as a stopgap and temporary measure.[47]

Other social workers and social scientists were even more ambivalent than Frankel. Although somewhat moderated, the legacy of nineteenth-century antipathy to direct relief was still strong in the American welfare community and prompted concern that the cash benefit part of maternity insurance might work to the detriment rather than to the benefit of women. Florence Kelley voiced the opinion that providing wage compensation grants to married women posed the danger that husbands, and especially immigrant husbands, might force their wives into the factory in anticipation of a future benefit. Indeed, on those grounds she successfully lobbied to have the cash payment part of the maternity benefit removed from the 1916 New York sickness insurance bill.[48] And Kelley was not alone. Concern over providing cash payments to families that included an able-bodied husband was widespread throughout the social service community and is attested to by the much more avid support given to mothers' pensions—a type of economic assistance for widowed and deserted mothers which had built into it strict rules requiring the absence of adult males in the household.[49]

Even the Children's Bureau, whose infant mortality studies provided some of the most compelling evidence for the proposition that compensation was necessary if mothers were to be convinced not to work before and after confinement, tended to back away from actively supporting that proposition. Despite being on record as in favor of its consideration, neither Lathrop nor any of the other major figures within the bureau played a particularly prominent role in the battle for maternity insurance. When pressed as to whether their economic interpretation of infant mortality meant that they were in favor of cash subsidies to families with able-bodied fathers, they defensively responded that such was not the position of the bureau, that what the bureau was in favor of was raising paternal wages so that mothers' incomes would not be needed.[50] As Lathrop frequently argued: "The power to maintain a decent family living standard is the primary essential of child welfare. This means a living wage and wholesome working life for the man, a good and skillful mother at home to keep the house and comfort all within it."[51] Lathrop and others in the bureau also apparently entertained serious reservations about the overall efficacy of cash payments, noting their alleged frequent misuse in Britain and arguing that existing evidence from Australia and New Zealand seemed to question the impact they had on infant death rates.[52]

The bureau's decision not to actively promote sickness insurance and maternity benefits may also have been prompted by politics. Although committed to the idea that many impoverished women needed material assistance to protect the health of themselves and their infants, Lathrop was a political pragmatist and all too aware that the continued existence of her bureau was dependent on funding from a Congress that contained many members who already were grumbling that she was in the forefront of a socialist attack on the family.[53] Taking the lead in promoting a measure that was increasingly being characterized as of foreign and socialist origin would do little to still that grumbling. The bureau also seemed reluctant to alienate its traditional allies in the medical profession. As organized medicine's opposition to the compulsory character of sickness insurance grew more vocal and intense, the Bureau began modifying its original position and by 1920 was contending that whatever system was adopted, "it must not be compulsory."[54]

Of equal importance, however, was the serious doubt that Lathrop and others in the bureau shared that an essentially urban industrial social insurance could adequately deal with the reality of infant mortality in America. The thousands of letters that American women sent to the bureau convinced Lathrop and her co-workers that infant welfare's traditional urban/industrial emphasis was far too narrow. Pushed by its own Frances Sage Bradley and by other pioneers of rural health reform, the bureau by 1917 was exhibiting an acute awareness that most Americans lived outside large cities and industrial centers and therefore had no access to the maternal and infant health programs thus far established. In her annual reports to Congress and elsewhere, Lathrop had begun emphasizing that lack of prenatal maternal care and postnatal infant supervision was a problem most serious in rural areas and small towns. It thus seemed to her that, while helpful, an insurance system that protected working women and the wives of industrial workers was fundamentally inadequate to deal with actual American conditions.

Indeed, Lathrop seemed more inspired by the infant welfare work of New Zealand, than that of the industrial nations of Europe. Not only did New

Zealand have the lowest infant mortality rate in the world but also, according to Lathrop, it was like the United States, "a young and vigorous country with a scattered population."[55] From 1914, when the bureau issued a report on New Zealand baby-saving work in rural areas and small towns, until her retirement in 1921, Lathrop continually held up that nation's approach to infant welfare as a model which the United States might emulate. That approach centered on the establishment of state maternity hospitals for treating problem cases and for training maternity nurses, state registration of and training for midwives, compulsory birth registration, and a nation-wide system of "educational" prenatal centers, well-baby clinics, and visiting nurse services, available to all women regardless of economic status. What that approach did not include—at least prior to the late 1930s—was free medical service (other than examinations and advice) or any type of cash maternity benefit.[56]

Ambivalence toward maternity insurance was not unique to American infant welfare activists.[57] Yet it was particularly strong among them. Combined with the other sociopolitical and ideological conditions unfavorable to the adoption of maternity insurance and rooted in a discourse on public health problems that was historically more constrained and narrow than its European counterpart, it assured maternity insurance's defeat and helped end the brief and uneasy flirtation that American infant welfare had with maternal reform encompassing social and medical welfare as well as supervision and education. Having belatedly, unsteadily, and with historic reluctance followed most of the rest of the industrialized West near to the threshold of providing mothers with economic assistance and medical services, the United States faltered and withdrew, refusing to take the final steps.

The defeat of maternity insurance was certainly not the only turning point in the evolution of contemporary American infant and maternal health policy.[58] Developments during the Roosevelt and Truman administrations as well as health policy decisions made during the Kennedy and Johnson years are arguably as important and perhaps more important. Moreover, just as the adoption of such insurance by the rest of the industrialized West did not immediately give birth to comprehensive and state-provided maternal and infant health care services (it took a world-wide depression and another world war to do that), so too its rejection by the United States did not abort all effort to have such services provided here. Like state-sponsored health insurance, maternity insurance and other forms of state-provided maternal and infant health assistance remained on the American reform agenda and continued to be the object of heated and divisive political discourse. Yet as the first major battle over such assistance, the Progressive fight for maternity insurance was formatively important for, to a significant degree, it shaped the contours of subsequent battles and helped determine their outcomes.

In rejecting maternity insurance, the United States in large part rejected the conception of infant mortality as a multifaceted problem demanding a comprehensive response involving social and medical assistance measures. In the decades that followed infant mortality was increasingly medicalized. Strategies for reducing the death rate of American babies came to focus almost exclusively on improving the availability and quality of medical care and convincing mothers to use it. The medicalization of infant mortality was not, admittedly, unique to the United States. The rest of the industrialized West also increasingly turned to improved medical care as a primary weapon in the fight for infant survival. Yet they also complemented such care with social programs designed to aid mothers in carrying, bearing, and rearing their infants. For the most part, the United States did not.

Along with ensuring that the United States would take a comparatively narrow medical approach to combating infant mortality, the defeat of maternity insurance also ensured that such an approach would be fraught with problems and inequities. It did so by helping to precipitate four interrelated developments in the organization and provision of American health care. The first development was the ideological and political marginalization of government-provided health care services—including maternal and infant health care—as radically leftist and un-American. Admittedly, this marginalization was not solely the product of the early twentieth-century battle over sickness and maternity insurance, and can be seen as devolving more from America's historic veneration of private enterprise than from any single event. Moreover, the comparative narrowness of the American discourse on the prevention of infant mortality had from the beginning located on the fringe in the United States what were advanced as centrist and compromise programs elsewhere in the industrialized West. Yet, as Paul Starr has convincingly argued, the American Progressive-era fight over maternity and sickness insurance was intensely ideological and political—perhaps even more so than in Europe.[59] As such, it ideologically and politically concretized that marginalization and provided subsequent adversaries of government health care for mothers and infants with a powerful opposing rhetoric and strategy.

Secondly, while not solely responsible, the defeat of maternity and sickness insurance was instrumental in firmly establishing a pattern of private control over the dispensation of medical services to nonindigent Americans outside the military, a pattern that continues to be the defining characteristic of America's health care system. In rejecting maternity and sickness insurance, the United States rejected direct state involvement in and control over the provision of medical care to all private citizens except the needy. In the process, it sharply demarcated the boundaries of public health, granting it responsiblity for only those services that private practitioners could not or would not provide. It thus helped relegate public health to its present secondary status of aiding private practitioners with diagnostic and laboratory services while taking infinite care not to intrude on their well-guarded domain. And in so doing, it, implicitly at least, granted to private medicine the right to determine what was and was not in its domain. Indeed, as private practitioners expanded the services they provided to include preventive medicine, they came to regard public health's traditional activity within that sphere as state intrusion into private medicine. In the 1920s, then, as well-baby and prenatal supervision were increasingly incorporated into the services that doctors offered their patients, private medicine began vociferously and effectively objecting to the state's involvement in what it had previously conceded to it.

The defeat of state-sponsored maternity insurance also necessitated the eventual development of private health insurance to cover childbirth medical costs. While ultimately guaranteeing medical attendance to the majority of American women and their babies, the development of such insurance served to make maternal and infant care a minority issue and to rob it of its historic constituency. As private health insurance increasingly covered wealthy, middle-class, and upper working-class women, government-sponsored programs of maternal and infant health protection lost the broad political support among women that they had previously enjoyed.

The idea of state medicine did not, of course, die in America with the defeat of maternity and sickness insurance. Nor was the privatized nature of the American health care system never again challenged. It was and continues to be. Yet those challenges have proven decidedly ineffective, in large part because of the fourth major development accompanying and precipitated by the Progressive sickness insurance debate. That development involved a change in the political orientation and representation of the American medical profession and was rooted in two phenomena that were of major consequence to the subsequent course of American infant and maternal welfare. One was the resurgence, after a brief flirtation with Progressive social reform, of the medical profession's traditional political conservatism and self-protectionism; the other was the emergence of the American Medical Association as the recognized and profoundly influential leader of American medicine.

Although historically conservative as a whole, the American medical profession had always contained an articulate element among its well-educated elite who actively promoted social reform. This was especially true in the Progressive era, when socially minded elite physicians embraced the promise of state medicine, joined Progressive medical organizations like the American Academy of Medicine, and actively called for more government involvement in protecting and promoting the health of the nation's citizenry. By 1920, however, as progressivism began to wane, so too did the reformist impulse in medicine.[60] The reform elite of the profession did not, of course, abandon en masse their commitment to social medicine. Although suffering defections from their ranks, they and their disciples continued to fight for state medicine into the 1930s and beyond.[61]

But the influence and privileged position these socially minded elites had previously held as both the conscience and voice of medicine were increasingly undercut by the prominence and power that the American Medical Association came to enjoy as the politically dominant representative of the profession.[62] Although founded in 1847, the AMA at the turn of the century was still only one of a number of American medical organizations and had fewer than 6 percent of the country's physicians as members. By 1920, however, it was the premier American medical organization, with over 50 percent of the nation's doctors enrolled as members.[63] Although the AMA's ascendancy began before the battle over sickness insurance, the part it ultimately played in that battle and the position it took not only assured it unchallenged authority in articulating the medical profession's views on social and medical issues but also greatly determined what those views would be. During the American debate on sickness insurance, the AMA established itself as the best-financed and most politically influential voice of American medicine, and devoted itself to challenging any legislation that might provide an "entering wedge" for government encroachment on private practice.[64]

Combined with the defeat of maternity insurance, these four developments served to guarantee that as the United States continued to pursue the preservation of infant lives after 1920, it did so along a path that was not only comparatively narrow but also studded with obstacles. Indeed, the ultimate historical significance of the failure of maternity insurance may be that not only did it prevent the expansion of governmental responsibility for infant welfare beyond its traditional role as provider of information and advice, but that it also made even that role problematic. Nowhere was this more dramatically illustrated than in the controversy that surrounded the enactment and subsequent repeal of the Sheppard-Towner Act. A relatively conservative medical welfare measure, the Sheppard-Towner Act funded maternal and infant health education programs between 1921 and 1929 and established the formula that largely continues today to govern American infant and maternal health care policy.

8

Defeat in Victory,
Victory in Defeat:
The Sheppard-Towner Act

Although the nationalistic senti-
ments released by the entry of the United States into World War I helped
defeat maternity insurance, the overall effect of the war on American infant
welfare was not entirely negative. For as was true on the other side of the
Atlantic, the war served further to heighten American concern with the
conservation of its young. As Josephine Baker recalled near the end of her
life: "the World War was a backhanded break for children," in that the
nation "began to see that new lives, which grow up to replace brutally
extinguished lives, were extremely valuable national assets."[1] Wartime concern over the conservation of infant lives was not sufficient to overcome the
ideological, economic, and political opposition to maternity insurance. But
it did provide impetus for expanded government involvement in those infant
and maternal welfare activities that remained confined to education and
supervision. In short, while helping to ensure that the nation would pursue
infant welfare only along a narrow path, the war also served to accelerate
the speed of that pursuit.

On the principle that the "protection of its children is a primary essential
to a nation at war," the Children's Bureau and the Women's Committee of
the Council on National Defense designated 1918 "Children's Year" and
launched a campaign to improve child welfare services throughout the country. Scheduled officially to begin on April 16, the anniversary of America's
entry into the war, and characterized by its sponsors as "a definite war
measure," Children's Year aimed at improving the health and welfare of
children of all ages. Central to it, however, was a major drive to effect a
further reduction in infant mortality by lobbying states to improve birth
registration, increase private physician and hospital services, create divisions of child hygiene, expand health department programs of maternal
education, enlarge their corps of visiting nurses, and both increase the number of prenatal and well-baby clinics in urban areas and establish them in

rural areas.[2] Children's Year thus sought to continue and enlarge the type of infant welfare activities first promoted nationally during the baby week campaigns.

Yet, if Children's Year signaled a renewal of national interest in conserving the lives and health of the young, it also signaled a refocusing of that interest, a refocusing that expanded early childhood health reform beyond infant welfare. This too was a product of the war. Prior to World War I, child health reform in America had been pursued along two related but essentially separate tracks. One track had as its destination improving the health of the older child and involved the promotion and implementation of school medical exams and other school health services. The other track was directed at reducing infant mortality, and involved a wide array of infant welfare activities. Almost completely ignored was the preschool child; that is, the child roughly between the ages of two and six.[3] Indeed, when late nineteenth- and early twentieth-century health reformers spoke of conserving the health and lives of the very young, they almost invariably meant promoting infant welfare.[4]

During the war years, however, the lack of interest traditionally shown the preschool child by American child health reformers was rapidly replaced by profound concern. Essentially, two developments, both war related, prompted this new concern. The displacement of thousands of people in war-torn Europe created a large population of refugee children, whose plight was given much attention in the American press. As a consequence, many American infant welfare activists volunteered for duty in the Red Cross, the Commission for Relief in Belgium, and later in the Relief Administration Children's Fund headed by Herbert Hoover. Moreover, the Children's Bureau sent over staff and volunteer doctors and nurses.[5] Although some of the work of the volunteers was directed at infant welfare, more involved combating the effects of malnutrition among very young children and battling the epidemics of early childhood disease that continuously swept through the refugee populations. When they returned home, the American volunteers brought with them a heightened awareness of the health problems and needs of the preschool child.

Probably more important, though, in directing reformer and public attention toward the young child were the shocking results of the physical and medical examinations given to American draftees. Altogether, 29.1 percent, or 730,000 young American men were judged physically unfit for military service. Revelation of this revived earlier concern with national degeneration and prompted calls for remedial measures. Since most of the defects in the draftees appeared to be the result of early childhood diseases (for example, heart murmurs due to scarlet fever, and physical deformities due to rickets), it was argued that such measures would have to focus on improving the health of the preschooler. In the immediate postwar years, infant welfare was thus expanded to include the early detection of disease in young children. Signaling that expansion, AASPIM in 1919 changed its name to the American Child Hygiene Association and declared itself devoted not only to infants but also to young children.[6]

In addition to heightening interest in preschool children, the war also cast into bold relief another health problem that had been gradually moving from the periphery to the center of infant welfare. This problem was maternal mortality resulting from pregnancy and childbirth. That bearing children carried with it the danger of death was certainly not startling news to Americans and especially not to American women. Its historical prominence in popular and religious literature and the considerable attention devoted to it in women's diaries from the colonial era onward testify to that.[7] But with the exception of the attention that danger was given by obstetric reformers in their late nineteenth- and early twentieth-century battles against both puerperal fever and midwives, it did not become a significant public health issue until the war years, when both its extent and its relation to infant welfare were realized and publicized.

In 1916, not long after Arthur Newsholme and Britain's Local Government Board issued the war-inspired "Report on Maternal Mortality in Connection to Childbearing and Its Relation to Infant Mortality," the Children's Bureau conducted a study of American maternal mortality and transmitted a similar report to Congress. The Children's Bureau report used the English study as both a model and source of information, and was authored by Grace L. Meigs, a physician and director of the Bureau's Division of Child Hygiene. Aware that her report seemed to move the bureau into a new area of public health, Meigs took pains to assure federal lawmakers that in looking into maternal mortality the bureau was not exceeding its mandate. "In the progress of work for the prevention of infant mortality," she observed, "it has become ever clearer that all such work is useful only in so far as it helps the mother to care better for her baby. It must be plain, then, to what a degree the sickness and death of the mother lessens the chances of the baby for life and health."[8] Such sickness and death, Meigs suggested, was far more prevalent than was commonly imagined. She estimated that in 1913 alone 15,376 American women had died from causes related to pregnancy and childbirth, thus ranking motherhood second only to tuberculosis as a killer of women aged 15 to 44. She also noted that in contrast to the experience of many other countries, there seemed to have been no appreciable decline in American maternal mortality since 1890; and that as a consequence, mothers in the United States faced a significantly greater risk of dying in childbirth than did mothers in virtually all the European countries as well as in New Zealand, Australia, and Japan.[9] (See Appendix B.)

In revealing the high level of mortality in pregnancy and childbirth suffered by American women, the bureau's report further accelerated a trend begun with the discovery of neonatal mortality, the trend toward linking maternal and infant welfare. Indeed, by the end of the second decade of the century, the two were seldom spoken of separately. That which had begun as an effort to save infant lives was now one also dedicated to saving the lives of their mothers. One consequence of this trend was to focus increasing attention on medical services independent of socioeconomic conditions. In its initial studies of infant mortality, the bureau had stressed that inadequate family income frequently forced women to ruin their health through strenuous industrial labor and denied them proper nutrition and sanitary living environments. But in its studies of maternal mortality, the bureau tended to downplay the importance of such socioeconomic factors. While conceding that "overcrowding, overwork [and] low incomes" all contributed to maternal mortality, it emphasized that the danger of dying from problems related to gestation and parturition cut across all classes and had as its chief determinants the quality and availability of obstetric services and the willingess of women to use them. Beneath the high level of maternal mortality in America, the bureau asserted, "lie two chief causes: First general ignorance of the dangers connected with childbirth and the need of skilled care and proper hygiene in order to prevent them; second, such difficulties related to the provision of proper obstetrical care as are characteristic of conditions in this country."[10]

Behind the bureau's assertion that the limited availability and underconsumption of quality obstetric services were responsible for America's high rate of maternal mortality was its conviction that the two chief killers of mothers—puerperal septicemia and eclampsia—were largely preventable with proper medical and hygienic care.[11] By 1917, for instance, it was widely believed that eclampsia, which accounted for 27.2 percent of recorded puerperal deaths that year, was related to diet and could early be detected through urinalysis and blood pressure monitoring. Similarly, it was commonly assumed that puerperal septicemia, which in 1917 accounted for 41.6 percent of recorded puerperal deaths, was essentially a wound infection, primarily caused by birth attendants and preventable by the application of "the same measures of cleanliness and asepsis which are used so universally in modern surgery to prevent infection."[12]

In defining the chief causes of maternal mortality as medically preventable, the bureau advocated a solution very similar to that promoted by J. Whitridge Williams and other obstetric reformers.[13] Echoing the arguments of those physicians, the bureau suggested that a critical first step in reducing maternal mortality involved increasing the demand for quality obstetrics by convincing the public that gestation and parturition were potentially pathological processes that required skilled supervision and attendance.[14] "By most people," it observed, "childbirth is regarded as an entirely normal process, and, happily, in the great majority of cases this is true. But the figures given in this report show that it is not true of all. . . . Knowledge of the need for good care at childbirth is essential; the lack of such knowledge and the demand for such care has been, probably, the chief factor in producing the present indifference to this phase of preventive medicine."[15] In promoting increased demand as a solution, the bureau report did not, however, spell out how such demand would actually increase the availability of quality obstetric services. Rather, it contented itself with vaguely concluding: "As women, their husbands, physicians, and communities realize the absolute need of skilled care for the prevention of needless deaths from childbirth, methods for providing such care will be developed."[16]

No such vagueness characterized the recommendations for "minimum standards for the protection of the health of mothers" adopted by the regional and national conferences on child welfare that were held in 1919 as the final part of Children's Year. Although deferring to the privileged domain of private medicine by declaring that their recommendations applied only to women not under the care of private physicians, the conferees resolved that public funds should be appropriated to establish maternity centers offering comprehensive obstetric care. Women who were accepted by such centers would receive complete and frequent prenatal exams and would be instructed in the hygiene of maternity and supervised throughout pregnancy. They would also be visited at home by public health nurses, would have the attendance of a physician at confinement, and would receive follow-up care by both physicians and nurses for several weeks after giving birth.[17]

Another consequence of the inclusion of maternal mortality within the infant welfare movement was to further reorient the movement's focus away from urban areas. In 1913, when the bureau formulated a plan for studying infant mortality, it proceeded on the assumption that the problem was essentially an urban one and therefore targeted a number of cities as the focus of its investigation. After becoming concerned with maternal mortality, however, it switched that focus and in 1917 began publishing a series of studies on rural maternal and infant welfare.[18] The bureau and other infant and maternal welfare activists readily acknowledged that urban mothers died more frequently in childbed and from pregnancy complications than rural mothers. But they argued that the causes of maternal mortality were more intractable in those areas of the country where the population was scattered, doctors were few and far between, and public health programs virtually nonexistent. Indeed, the bureau's 1917 report paid special attention to the problem of rural maternal mortality, noting that in sparsely populated regions "the question is not one of good or bad obstetrical care but of the inaccessibility of any care at all."[19]

Seizing upon heightened wartime awareness of infant and maternal mortality and reflecting the growing concern with rural health, Julia Lathrop in her 1917 *Annual Report* recommended to Congress that it abandon its traditional reluctance to involve the federal government in the direct provision of public health and social welfare services and adopt legislation providing matching grants to states so that they could set up infant and maternal health centers and expand visiting nurse services, especially in rural areas where none existed. Aware that her recommendation challenged strong sentiment in Congress that such matters were state responsibility, Lathrop pointed to the historic inability of states to provide for the public health needs of their nonurban residents. She also suggested that precedent for the proposed legislation existed in the Smith-Lever Act (1914), which provided states with matching funds to set up county programs to teach farmers new agricultural methods. As foreign examples of what she envisioned, Lathrop cited New Zealand's state-assisted infant and maternal welfare program and the matching grant program established by the British Parliament in 1914 through which the Local Government Board provided funds to local authorities and private agencies to operate well-baby and prenatal clinics and to hire visiting nurses.[20]

Although Lathrop's proposal was novel in its suggestion that federal funds be used, it hardly represented a significant departure from existing infant and maternal welfare policy or practice and was considerably more conservative than the call for publicly funded, comprehensive maternity centers subsequently issued by the Children's Year conferences. The health program it envisioned did not include the provision of free or subsidized medical services, other than examinations at which problems might be pointed out. Its purpose was limited to increasing public awareness of the need to follow certain hygienic rules and to demand quality private medical services. As Lathrop later explained, the typical maternity and infancy health center her proposed legislation would fund "is not a clinic for sick children nor an obstetric clinic, but an opportunity for the mother to have explained to her how to keep her baby and herself well by using intelligently the available medical service and also by improving the home care she gives herself and her children."[21] Moreover, unlike maternity insurance, Lathrop's proposed health program offered no material assistance so that mothers might follow the recommended prenatal and postnatal regimens. Indeed, it was almost a carbon copy of the type of educational and supervisory program developed by Josephine Baker and her Bureau of Child Hygiene and already in operation in New York and a number of other cities. Designed primarily to educate mothers in the care of their infants and themselves, that program fell well within the boundaries of established and accepted maternal reform. Lathrop's purpose in advancing her proposal, then, was not to expand such reform beyond the educational and supervisory services already offered by visiting nurses and by well-baby and prenatal centers, but to make those services available in areas where they had previously been lacking.

In July 1918, Representative Jeanette Rankin placed a bill before the 65th Congress that contained the fundamentals of Lathrop's proposal and likewise targeted the non-urban mother and infant. Testifying at committee hearings, infant and maternal welfare activists argued the need for the bill by emphasizing that although it had been clearly proven that the instruction and supervision of pregnant and new mothers was effective in reducing both infant and maternal mortality, outside of a few major cities neither private physicians nor public health officials were providing such. Estimating that 80 percent of American women were without adequate prenatal care, they contended that as a consequence the United States had higher rates of neonatal and maternal mortality than virtually all of the industrialized Western nations.[22] Opponents, on the other hand, raised the issue of states' rights, characterized the bill as a socialistic plot to undermine parental authority and destroy the family, and expressed concerns about the constitutionality of federal involvement in welfare matters. Although fewer in number than proponents, their arguments apparently were more in tune with the views of the majority of representatives. For although the House Committee on Labor reported favorably on the bill, Congress refused to take any action on it.[23]

The following year, at the next session of Congress, the bill was again introduced, this time jointly by Morris Sheppard, Democratic senator from Texas, and Horace Towner, Republican congressman from Iowa. Like the Rankin bill, that proposed by Sheppard and Towner was designed to fund educational and supervisory services to women and infants, especially in non-urban areas. But it also targeted preschoolers, and proposed that some of the funding be used to provide medical examinations for young children. The sponsors of the bill asked for a yearly appropriation of $4,000,000 in matching grants for states plus an additional one-time appropriation of $10,000 for each state to assist it in setting up programs. Again infant and maternal welfare activists like Josephine Baker and Philip Van Ingen trooped to Washington to testify in support of the bill at congressional hearings. The bill also became an issue in the 1920 Presidential campaign, endorsed by the Democratic, Socialist, Prohibition, and Farm Labor parties. Warren Harding, the Republican candidate, also endorsed it, though his party did not. Nevertheless, the bill languished in committee from May through December; and although passed by the Senate on December 18, it died in the House Rules Committee.[24]

Undeterred by House inaction, Sheppard and Towner again introduced their bill when Congress reconvened in January 1921. And again supporters and opponents journeyed to Washington to testify for and against it. By now the respective lines of argument were familiar. One opposition contention was that coming on the heels of a war that had cost the national treasury $42 billion, Sheppard-Towner represented fiscal irresponsibility. Another was that its program of matching grants involved the federal government in activities that traditionally had been the responsibility of the states and therefore violated the constitutional separation of state and federal authority. A third—chiefly advanced by the AMA, the American Gynecological Society, and various state and county medical organizations—was that, like proposals for sickness insurance, Sheppard-Towner would impose lay control over medical matters, impede the progress of medical reform, and create an opening wedge for the imposition of socialized medicine.[25] Supporters, on the other hand, countered that spending a mere $4 million to protect the nation's nearly five million citizens who each year were born or gave birth hardly represented fiscal irresponsibility, especially when the government was spending almost twenty times that much to protect and improve livestock. They also argued that states had already acquiesced to federal involvement in their affairs by accepting funds for a wide variety of internal improvments; and that, in any case, the general welfare clause of the Constitution empowered the federal government to allocate funds for preventive health activities. Finally, they sought to allay organized medicine's fears by pointing out that the bill respected the domain of the private practitioner, was supportive of medical authority in health matters, and offered services that were voluntary and strictly preventive in nature.[26]

Although debate on Sheppard-Towner centered on the specific issues of fiscal responsibility, states' rights, and government intrusion into private medicine, it resonated with concern over the social definition of gender roles and the relation of government to the family and to the individual. Intensified by the final push for woman suffrage, by the recent Red Scare, and by the continuing battle over child labor, strong currents of opposition to feminism, socialism and the intrusion of government into family matters were running through Congress in 1921. Not surprisingly, Sheppard-Towner got caught up in these currents, as did its administrative agency, the Children's Bureau. Some of the most vocal opposition to Sheppard-Towner came from an alliance of anti-suffrage groups, right-wing political organizations, and conservative congressmen and senators: all of whom characterized the bill as an imported radical scheme, promoted by socialists, feminists, and their allies in the Children's Bureau. The primary purpose of the scheme, they argued, was to subvert the family and destroy individual freedom by taking authority over children from parents and giving it to the state. Testifying at committee hearings, Mrs. Albert Leatherbel of the Massachusetts Anti-Suffrage Association warned that the bill would bring about "bureaucratic control of family life." Mary Kilbreth, president of the National Association Opposed to Woman Suffrage, agreed, arguing that "it is not brought forward by the combined wisdom of all Americans, but by the propaganda of a self-interested bureau associated with the feminist bloc." Kilbreth also asserted that "there are many loyal American men and women who believe this bill, inspired by foreign experiments in Communism, and backed by the radical forces in the country, strikes at the heart of our American civilization."27

Similar arguments were advanced by a powerful group of conservative congressmen and senators who tended to view feminism, suffrage, and government involvement in child welfare all as parts of a dangerous socialist assault on American institutions, an assault that was inspired from abroad but abetted at home by Progressive "do-gooders." Long suspicious of and hostile to the Children's Bureau, they interpreted Sheppard-Towner as a transparent bid by Lathrop and her allies to empower the bureau to coerce Americans to raise their children according to government dictate. Among the most influential of these congressional conservatives was Samuel Winslow, chair of the House committee holding hearings on Sheppard-Towner. An ardent anti-socialist and anti-suffragist, Winslow was also a prominent critic of the Children's Bureau and had a deep personal antipathy for Julia Lathrop. Having successfully blocked House action on the bill in 1920, Winslow acceded to it coming to a vote in 1921 only after it was amended to limit the Children's Bureau's role and after Lathrop promised to resign as USCB Chief.

Another prominent congressional critic was James Reed, Democratic senator from Missouri. In a long, rambling diatribe against the bill, Reed charged that "the fundamental doctrines on which this bill is founded were drawn chiefly from the radical, socialistic, and bolshevistic philosophy of Germany and Russia." If passed, he warned, it would bring about forced registration of pregnant women, coerced prenatal examinations, interference with the right of individuals to choose among birth attendants, and intrusion into family life by government agents.28 Reed also articulated an argument that the AMA soon took up: that Sheppard-Towner was a disguised form of maternity insurance, equally radical and un-American.

> It is allied with . . . various radical schemes inaugurated in different European countries, notably Germany, where socialistic doctrinaires have long insisted upon the establishment of maternity benefit systems. . . . All of such plans involves the assumption by the State of the authority to interfere in the family relations. They imply the right of State visitation and espionage. Such doctrines are not tolerated in a free country.29

Finally, Reed railed against the Children's Bureau and played to popular prejudice by characterizing it as staffed by childless childrearing experts. "It seems to be the established doctrine of this bureau that the only people capable of caring for babies and the mothers of babies are ladies who never had babies." Indeed, he went so far as to slander bureau staffers, calling them a "band of devoted spinsters" and arguing that it was the height of irony "to employ female celibates to instruct mothers how to raise babies."[30]

Opposition arguments that Sheppard-Towner was fiscally irresponsible, violated states' rights, endangered private medicine, was essentially socialistic, and represented a power bid by an agency staffed by spinster feminists and "do-gooders" struck a resonant chord in Congress and might have again succeeded in waylaying the bill had they not been countered by a powerful lobbying effort from supporters and by the profound influence of a unique political development. Throughout 1920, as the bill remained lodged in committee, a groundswell of support for its passage began to build. Predictably, infant welfare organizations and agencies were vocal proponents. AASPIM (now the American Child Hygiene Association) passed a resolution strongly supporting the bill and called on its members to lobby their congressmen and senators. So too did the Child Health Organization, an umbrella group of New York infant and child health agencies that was formed during the war and headed by L. Emmett Holt. Child welfare advocates also mobilized support for the bill, arguing that its passage was necessary if the nation was even to approach meeting the minimum standards for the protection of maternity and infancy adopted by the regional and national conferences on child welfare the year before. Public health officials also lined up to support the bill. With its intention of assisting infant, child and maternal health work in non-urban areas, its program of matching grants, and its assurance of state administrative control, Sheppard-Towner seemed to promise the beginning of an end to America's historic pattern of gross underfunding for public health activities outside major cities. When it met for its annual meeting in 1920, the State and Provincial Health Officers Association gave the bill its overwhelming approval. Finally, organized labor, which was split over maternity insurance, showed no such division in regard to Sheppard-Towner. Indeed, when congressional hearings on the bill convened again the following year, Samuel Gompers sent Edward S. McGrady, the national legislative representative of the American Federation of Labor, to testify in its favor.[31]

Undoubtedly, however, the most vocal and widespread support came from American women and especially from women's organizations and publications. Increasingly a "women's campaign," the infant welfare movement became especially so as it came to include the prevention of maternal death in childbirth. Targeting a historic, fundamental, and universal danger at the center of women's social and biological existence, the effort to make maternity safer had an appeal that cut across class, ethnic, and regional divisions. More than a matter of philanthropy or reform, it was one of survival; and as such was a fundamental and universal "women's issue." Indeed, with the exception of suffrage, no other political issue seemed to galvanize American women in the postwar era as did Sheppard-Towner. On their own and at the urging of various organizations and national magazines, thousands of women wrote their congressmen and senators urging passage of the bill. "I think every woman in my state has written to the Senator," reported one senatorial aide.[32] Other women joined in an organized lobbying effort that was described by many in Washington as the most intensive campaign to influence the vote on a single bill they had ever seen.[33]

Spearheading that lobbying effort was a coalition of fourteen national women's organizations, including the National Congress of Mothers and Parents Teachers Association, the Women's Christian Temperance Union, the League of Women Voters, the National Women's Trade Union League, The Young Women's Christian Association, the National Consumer's League, the General Federation of Business and Professional Women, and the National Council of Jewish Women. Joining together in a special subcommittee of the newly formed Women's Joint Congressional Committee, the coalition's chief spokeswoman was Florence Kelley. A veteran Progressive reformer, Kelley was a skilled, articulate, and effective lobbyist, capable both of working behind the scenes and of delivering highly charged testimony. Moreover, she considered her effort to gain passage of the bill to be the most important endeavor of her long career. "Of all the activities in which I have shared during forty years of striving," she declared at the time, "none is, I am convinced, of such fundamental importance as the Sheppard-Towner Act."[34] Joining Kelley and her coalition were other women's organizations, including the National Women's Association of Commerce, the Women's Press Club, the National Organization of Public Health Nurses, and the Service Star Legion. Also lending influential support was the Medical Women's National Association, its various state affiliates, and its official publication, the *Woman's Medical Journal*.[35]

An intense lobbying effort on behalf of the bill was also begun in 1920 by a number of national women's magazines. *Good Housekeeping*, *Woman's Home Companion*, *McCall's*, and *Ladies Home Journal* published numerous supporting articles and editorials and urged their readers to deluge Congress with letters. Indeed, as the bill continued to languish in committee, the magazines and their writers could barely hide their mounting frustration and bitterness. Proclaiming that "Herod is not Dead," an editorialist for *Good Housekeeping* asserted that Congress was proving itself unconcerned with the wholesale slaughter of mothers and infants. Other writers concluded that the wartime rhetoric about the national importance of mothers had apparently been empty words, since although as many American women died in childbed during the war as did soldiers at the front, the nation seemed only concerned about the latter. Writers also noted angrily that while the federal government was willing to spend $47 million to protect the nation's livestock, it was caviling at spending a mere $4 million to protect its mothers and infants.[36]

Accompanying as it did the support from child welfare advocates, public health officials, and labor spokesmen, American women's outpouring of enthusiasm for Sheppard-Towner could not be dismissed by Congress. For 1920 also witnessed the ratification of the Nineteenth Amendment to the Constitution, which granted women the right to vote. For years suffragists had been predicting that women would use that right to vote in blocs and expel from Congress those who opposed "women's issues." Not yet knowing whether this prediction would prove accurate, the vast majority of Congress chose to be prudent and to register publicly their approval when the bill finally came up for a vote. Indeed, fear of being punished at the polls by American women, not conviction of the bill's necessity, seems to have motivated Congress to vote for it. As one senator admitted to a reporter from the *Ladies Home Journal*, "if the members of Congress could have voted on the measure in their cloak rooms, it would have been killed as emphatically as it was finally passed in the open."[37] Thus, on November 19, 1921, the House passed the Sheppard-Towner Act by a vote of 279 to 39, with 113 abstentions. Two days later, after the Senate approved the House-amended bill, Harding signed it into law.[38]

Although opponents were unable to block the bill from passing, they were able to imprint their stamp on it by exacting a number of compromises from its sponsors and by adding amendments during congressional consideration. When finally passed, the bill contained language making the programs it funded voluntary and prohibiting any federal or state agent from entering a home or taking charge of a child over parents' objections.[39] It also contained language expressly prohibiting the use of granted or matching funds "for the payment of any maternity or infancy pension, stipend or gratuity."[40] The annual appropriation was cut from $4,000,000 to $1,240,000 and state control over those funds was made absolute. The power of the Children's Bureau was also diminished by an amendment investing final authority for approving state plans in an oversight board on which the USCB chief was joined by the surgeon general and the commissioner of education. Lastly, and perhaps most critically, the final version of Sheppard-Towner provided funding for five years only and thus required that the act be evaluated and approved again in 1927.[41]

Sheppard-Towner stipulated that in order to receive funds, states had to pass "enabling legislation" indicating acceptance of the act's provisions, designating or creating a state agency (usually a child hygiene division of the state health department) to administer the funds and oversee the funded programs, and appropriating state monies to be matched by the federal government. The states were also required to submit to the Children's Bureau a detailed plan of action and to make regular reports on program expenditures and activities.[42] With a few notable exceptions, the state response to these stipulations was generally quite positive. Despite the contentions of states' rights advocates, most state authorities found little of threat in the act and quickly moved to qualify their states for funds. By the end of 1922, forty-one states had passed enabling legislation and ultimately only three states refused to do so. Two of those states, Illinois and Connecticut, established their own maternal and infant health programs. The third, Massachusetts, did not and indeed filed suit (*Massachusetts v. Mellon*) with the U.S. Supreme Court challenging the constitutionality of Sheppard-Towner. The Supreme Court, however, dismissed the suit on jurisdictional grounds, as it did another (*Frothingham v. Mellon*) filed by the Women Patriots, a Massachusetts archconservative organization.[43]

Along with being quick to pass enabling legislation, most states were also quick to set up programs. In 1925 alone, 561 permanent child health and prenatal centers were established, a total of 21,935 child health and prenatal conferences held, 299,100 instructional home visits by nurses made, and 2,195,000 educational leaflets distributed. Such activity was particularly noteworthy in southern and western states. Prior to Sheppard-Towner, maternal, infant, and early childhood health programs in those states had been all but nonexistent. By 1925, however, many of these states had appropriated sufficient funds to allow them to receive near or all of the federal matching grants available to them. As a consequence Alabama was yearly examining over 12,000 infants and young children and 3,000 pregnant women and was making over 45,000 home visits. Georgia was yearly examining a total of 15,000 infants, children and pregnant women; Arkansas, 6,000; Kentucky, 13,000; Louisiana, 11,000; Montana 15,000; Nevada 2,000; and other states similar numbers. Moreover, at least some of this work was reaching nonwhites, who had been virtually ignored up to this time. Minnesota and Nebraska targeted their Native American populations for special attention. New Mexico, Arizona, and Texas employed Spanish-speaking nurses to give lecture-demonstrations and make home visits within the Hispanic community. And the South, although keeping its programs segregated, for the first time made an effort to extend public health services to blacks.[44]

Carrying out these health activities was a corps of paid and volunteer physicians, nurses, and lay people. By 1926 there were 50 full-time physicians and 812 nurses being paid by Sheppard-Towner funds. There were also over 2,200 physicians, over 300 nurses, and over 3,500 lay volunteers involved in Sheppard-Towner work. Frequently, a paid physician and a staff of nurses would enter a community, organize volunteers and set up prenatal and child health clinics. After examining and counseling many of the area's women and children, they would move on to another community, sometimes leaving behind a permanent health clinic. In those areas where neither itinerant nor permanent health clinics could be established, nurses visited households and provided examinations and consultations. Sheppard-Towner workers also traveled their states in specially designed trucks, giving clinics, and registering new mothers (to receive instructional literature) at county fairs, farmers' markets, and other large public gatherings. Using Sheppard-Towner funds, states also trained midwives, initiated correspondent courses for pregnant women and new mothers, and sent out thousands of pamphlets and letters with simple instructions on maternal and infant hygiene.[45]

According to those involved in the work, public response was enthusiastic. The Children's Bureau reported that many families traveled "long distances" so that mothers and children could be examined. Indeed, for many mothers and children such examinations were the first they had ever received.[46] Moreover, hundreds of women wrote to the Children's Bureau, to the sponsors of the act, and to the various state agencies expressing their gratitude and urging that the programs be continued. After receiving mailed literature on prenatal hygiene, one Arizona mother wrote the state's director of child hygiene: "Your letters have been such an aid to me, where I had no knowledge of how to take care of myself. My time is rapidly drawing close and I have followed your sound advice in every instance possible." An Atlanta, Georgia, woman wrote Morris Sheppard proclaiming that the local prenatal clinic saved her life and urging that such clinics be continued for "there are other poor mothers just like me who are not even able to have a doctor." Mothers also wrote that the literature and clinics gave them a sense of confidence and relieved the isolation and powerlessness they often experienced in raising infants. An Idaho mother wrote that getting the information in the mail was like "receiving advice and sympathy from a dear friend," and noted that she and her friends with small children "felt too often alone." Similarly a Kentucky woman wrote: "We live so far out in the country that without the instructions that you sent me, I do not see how it would have been possible for me to care for my baby properly."[47]

Sheppard-Towner's supporters used the letters from mothers to demonstrate the popularity of the programs made possible by the act. They also repeatedly stressed that the activities carried out under Sheppard-Towner involved education and supervision and were thus well within the mainstream of American reform tradition. "The maternity and infancy act," the Children's Bureau declared in its annual reports, "makes possible a type of work which is thoroughly in agreement with the fundamental American principle of providing education to the people—in this instance education in the hygiene of maternity and infancy. The types of work undertaken by the states are quite uniformly educational."[48] The bureau also took pains to assure organized medicine that Sheppard-Towner workers were not intruding upon the domain of the private physician. "No treatment is given nor any remedial work done in the child-health conferences. If defects or pathological conditions are found in the child examined, the parents are referred for corrections to the family physician, or, in the event of indigent cases, to community or county agencies or to treatment clinics."[49]

Convinced that the act was a popular success, its backers moved in 1926 to seek renewal. They did so, however, somewhat tentatively, requesting only a two-year extension beyond the original July 30, 1927, termination date. The modest extension request reflected a pragmatic political assess-ment on the part of the act's supporters. With President Coolidge and the Republicans promoting a reduction in government at the federal level, with the Child Labor Amendment[50] apparently stalled in the states, and with the 1926 enactment of a federal tax-cutting measure, it did not seem a particular-ly propitious moment to push for a long-term funding commitment to a social welfare measure. Supporters also knew that this time they would not be assisted by congressional fear that women would vote opponents of the act out of office. The results of the 1922 and 1924 elections suggested that women did not vote in blocs according to issues, but rather, like men, split along party lines. Sensitive to the conservative mood of Congress and the nation and aware that they no longer could rely on congressional fear of the "woman's vote," Sheppard-Towner's advocates sought the brief extension hoping that by 1929 their case would be stronger and the political environ-ment better.

When Congress began hearings on the extension proposal, it was clear that many of the opposition arguments of 1921 would be raised again. Fol-lowing the Republican victory of 1924, Congress had in its ranks even more fiscal conservatives than it had when Sheppard-Towner was originally passed. Having just pushed through the Revenue Act (1926) and thus won a major battle in their post-war fight to promote economy and reduce govern-ment at the federal level, many of those fiscal conservatives seemed primed to battle against renewed funding for any temporary programs.[51] Similarly, although the postwar Red Scare had long since abated, the forces of ideologi-cal and political archconservatism could still make their presence felt. In-deed, strengthened and encouraged by their successful fight to block ratifica-tion of the Child Labor Amendment, right-wing groups rallied in opposition to the funding renewal proposal. Moreover, this time they had a number of powerful allies they did not have before.

One such ally was the Daughters of the American Revolution (DAR). Having supported the original bill, the DAR switched sides in 1926 and mounted a virulent attack on the renewal proposal. Another ally was the American Catholic Church. Although historically somewhat hostile to child welfare reform and certainly not supportive of government interven-tion into families, the church had previously remained relatively neutral in regard to infant welfare legislation and activities. Perhaps because it was primarily health-related and did not involve the type of religious proselytism historically associated with welfare work among older children, infant wel-fare had to this point provoked no opposition from the church. Indeed, rather than establish an alternative welfare system, as it did for the care of dependent children, the church had seemed content to leave baby-saving in the hands of public health departments and nonsectarian infant welfare associations.[52] In 1924, however, Boston's Cardinal O'Connell, concerned by the broad inclusiveness of the Child Labor Amendment and apparently alarmed by an increasingly vocal birth control movement, began publicly expressing his opposition to any state involvement in what were traditionally private family matters. Other influential Catholic clerics soon followed suit, with the result that in 1926 many Catholic organizations went on record as being opposed to the funding renewal proposal.[53]

Organized medicine was also still opposed to Sheppard-Towner. Indeed, its 1926 campaign against renewal was far more intense than the one it had mounted in 1921. When the measure was initially considered and passed, the AMA had been preoccupied with defeating sickness insurance and had only belatedly joined the debate over the proposed federal legislation. While some of the more conservative state chapters had early declared themselves opposed to the bill, the national organization refrained from negative comment until February 5, 1921, when the *Journal of the American Medical Association* began an editorial campaign attacking Sheppard-Towner as another attempt to usurp medical authority and place it in the hands of government bureaucrats.[54] Additionally, during the original consideration of Sheppard-Towner, there seems to have existed within organized medicine and the profession as a whole considerable division over the bill's merits. Since the bill did not essentially challenge the fee-for-service principle of private medicine and funded programs that were consistent with the type of preventive education already conceded to public health, it did not evoke the concern and hostility that sickness insurance did. As late as December 28, 1920, the AMA's own Committee on Health and Public Instruction went on record as clearly favoring the bill. Moreover, virtually all women physicians, most prominent pediatricians, and a few leading obstetricians also favored the bill. And, at least according to one historian, the rank and file was largely apathetic.[55]

Between 1922 and 1926, however, the opposition to Sheppard-Towner within organized medicine increased and solidified, while the views of women physicians were increasingly ignored, the support of specialists squelched, and the apathy of the rank and file changed to hostility. At the 1921 annual meeting of the AMA, the medical societies of New York, Massachusetts, and Michigan—having successfully blocked sickness insurance within their individual states—introduced a resolution to the House of Delegates that would extend the national organization's stated opposition to maternity benefits to include the type of maternal and infant health programs funded under Sheppard-Towner. Although the resolution received considerable support, it was blocked by the delegates from the scientific sections, who succeeded in introducing and winning approval for a substitute resolution which declared that the AMA "approves and endorses all proper activities and policies of the state and federal governments directed to the prevention of disease and the preservation of the public health."[56]

For Sheppard-Towner's opponents in the AMA, the 1921 defeat was only a temporary setback. When the association met again the following year, they succeeded in getting the House of Delegates to condemn Sheppard-Towner as an "imported socialistic scheme" and as an example of the type of legislation to which the association was unequivocally opposed. More importantly, they pushed through a resolution on "state medicine" that guided the AMA for a long time afterward. That resolution read:

> The American Medical Association hereby declares itself in opposition to all forms of "state medicine," because of the ultimate harm that would come thereby to the public weal through such form of medical practice.
>
> State medicine is hereby defined for the purpose of this resolution to be any form of medical treatment, provided, conducted, controlled or subsidized by the federal or any state government, or municipality, excepting such service as is provided by the Army, Navy or Public Health Service, and that which is necessary for the control of communicable diseases, the treatment of mental disease, the treatment of the indigent sick, and such other services as may be approved by and administered under the direction of or by a local county medical society, and are not disapproved by the state medical society of which it is a component part.[57]

The 1922 meeting also witnessed the House of Delegates reining in the traditionally independent and more liberal scientific sections. On the same day that body condemned Sheppard-Towner and passed the resolution opposing state medicine, the Section on the Diseases of Children declared its support for the act and released the text of its declaration to the press. That action so enraged the House of Delegates that it not only formally reprimanded the pediatricians, but also soon afterward adopted a rule prohibiting sections of the AMA from independently passing resolutions or taking stances on social matters or issues.[58]

It was not, however, only the growing conservatism of the AMA and the increasing hegemony within the association of the House of Delegates that contributed to the intensive campaign mounted by the nation's physicians in 1926 against renewal of funding for Sheppard-Towner. Changes in the profession as a whole—particularly the way that doctors were being educated and the types of services they were routinely offering—also played an important role. When well-baby and prenatal stations were first established, whatever opposition they provoked from community doctors was largely offset by the support they received from the profession's elites, who regarded them as critical to the clinical training of university-educated physicians. By the mid-1920s, however, elite clinical education had moved into hospitals. As a consequence, public clinics and dispensaries lost their importance to medical education and thus lost the support they had enjoyed from the medical establishment. Where once they had served as a training ground for those young physicians who subsequently wielded considerable influence in state and local medical societies, they now served primarily as places of employment for physicians who held marginal status within the profession. Thus, by 1926, women physicians constituted the vast majority of doctors hired with Sheppard-Towner funds to run well-baby and prenatal confer-ences and to staff infant and maternal health centers.[59]

At the same time that changes in medical education were undercutting medical-profession support for well-baby and prenatal clinics, changes in the character and scope of private practice were also ensuring that the old charge of unfair competition would increase in force and substance. Infant and maternal welfare advocates had always answered that charge by main-taining that the preventive, educational, and supervisory services their pro-grams offered were unavailable from private practitioners, who largely lim-ited their activities to treating the sick. During the 1920s, however, Ameri-can doctors shifted the locus of their practice from the sickroom to the office, began scheduling advance appointments, and giving routine examinations, and for the first time made preventive health care and instruction in personal hygiene an important part of services they offered their patients. Since such supervision and education was inexpensive to provide, routinized doctors' relationships to their patients, and encouraged the consumption of other medical services, their value was quickly appreciated by private practi-tioners. By 1926 there thus existed within the rank and file of the profession considerable sentiment that the services being funded by Sheppard-Towner were not only no longer necessary, but also an intrusion by the state into private practice.[60]

In the expansion of private practice to include preventive care, the AMA played a critical role. Beginning in 1922, the AMA and its local and state medical societies embarked on a campaign urging their members to restruc-ture their practices to include supervisory and instructional services. The *Journal of the American Medical Association* and state medical journals published instructions on how to conduct well-baby, well-child, and well-adult examinations as well as on the techniques of prenatal preventive care. Local and state medical societies held training sessions for their members and provided them with standardized forms that could be used in carrying out periodic health exams. Medical schools also began offering classes in preventive care. The timing of this campaign has led at least one historian to claim that it was prompted by the passage of Sheppard-Towner and that its success enabled the AMA to persuade Congress during the renewal debate (as it had not been able to do in 1921) that the funded programs duplicated and competed with services sufficiently available from private practitioners.[61]

Yet it was not just the AMA campaign that was instrumental in trans forming the character and scope of private practice. Perhaps equally impor tant was Sheppard-Towner itself. Reflecting the conviction of its sponsors that infant mortality and especially maternal mortality would be signifi cantly reduced if women and their physicians realized the need for preven tive health care, Sheppard-Towner was designed to convince patients to demand such care and physicians to provide it. Along with producing and disseminating information to mothers on what sort of medical care was appropriate for themselves and their infants, state program officials spon sored classes and demonstrations aimed at local doctors. They also dis tributed to physicians booklets (written by committees of medical special ists) containing instructions on how to conduct well-baby, well-child, and prenatal examinations. Moreover, especially in small towns, Sheppard-Towner clinics and conferences required the volunteer assistance of local doctors, many of whom then incorporated preventive health work into their own practices.[62] In short, seeking to transform rather than challenge the private delivery of health care services, Sheppard-Towner was in some respects the victim of its own success. Having encouraged the adoption of preventive health care by private practitioners and thus the expansion of private medicine's domain, it now faced the increasingly accurate charge that it was intruding on that domain.

Despite the opposition from fiscal conservatives, from right-wing political organizations and their allies and from a transformed and vocally hostile medical profession, the renewal bill seemed at first destined to be passed. Perhaps because it was popular with their constituents and with the various county and municipal officials in their districts, the members of the House discounted opposition arguments and overwhelmingly approved the exten sion by a vote of 218 to 44. Not so the Senate. Although a majority of senators seem to have favored extension, the renewal bill was effectively blocked in the Senate by a small but powerful group of archconservative senators whom the *Survey* described as "surviving anti-suffragists."[63] Among these was Lawrence Phipps of Colorado, chair of the Senate com mittee considering the bill. After attempting to block the bill from coming to the floor, Phipps tried to force its supporters to accept a one-year rather than a two-year extension. When they refused, he led his allies in a filibuster that blocked action on the bill for over eight months. Without the votes to break the filibuster, sponsors of the bill agreed to an amendment that automatically repealed the Sheppard-Towner Act after the two-year extension was over.[64]

Supporters of Sheppard-Towner accepted the amendment repealing the bill for the same reason they chose to request only a two-year extension of funding: they calculated that the 1928 election would bring about a more hospitable political climate. It was a major miscalculation. As the unprecedented prosperity of the New Era continued, the problems of the poor and deprived increasingly received less media attention than the supposed emotional and moral consequences of abundance. Moreover, many in Congress who had supported renewal were less inclined to favor reviving a welfare program that was scheduled to end. Finally, President Hoover, whose election infant welfare activists had hoped would give them an ally in the White House, made it quite clear that he was unwilling to disregard what he took to be wishes of a previous Congress.[65] Thus, despite some last minute legislative attempts to keep Sheppard-Towner alive, funding stopped on June 30, 1929.[66]

The repeal of Sheppard-Towner crushed the hopes of American infant welfare activists. They had viewed the enactment of the legislation and the implementation of its funded programs as among their most important achievements in the eighty-year campaign to reduce infant mortality. For them, Sheppard-Towner represented a major victory for the nation's mothers and infants. But if it was a victory, it was something of a Pyrrhic one. In pushing Sheppard-Towner through Congress, infant welfare activists finally won federal commitment to funding a national maternal and infant health program. But they did so at the cost of acceding to a program based on a preventive formula that was narrowly reformist rather than comprehensive. The program established under Sheppard-Towner was one that limited government responsibility for the prevention of infant mortality to educating mothers in medically approved regimens of infant and prenatal hygiene and to convincing them of the necessity of consuming private medical services. It also, though to a lesser extent, allowed the government to help improve the quality of those private medical services and to promote their more even geographic distribution. It was thus half a program, one that left largely unaddressed the recognized reality that inequalities of social and economic status made it more difficult for some mothers than others to follow the prescribed regimens and to consume the recommended services. While it allowed for (though did not fund) medical and economic assistance to the certifiably indigent, Sheppard-Towner eschewed government responsibility for providing such assistance to anyone else. In short, it defined a maternal and infant protection policy in which the government would point out the road to health, would help improve it, and extend it to all areas of the country, but would not guarantee equal access.

Epilogue

Progress along a Narrow and Bumpy Path:
Infant and Maternal Welfare
after
Sheppard-Towner

The demise of Sheppard-Towner effectively brought to a close the American campaign to reduce infant mortality that had begun in the mid-nineteenth century and had peaked during the Progressive era. Never again would the attention of the nation be so focused on saving its babies. And never again would such a high percentage of infants fail to survive their first year. But the legacy of the infant welfare movement was more than a sharply reduced rate of infant mortality. It was also a particular way of approaching the protection of infants and the women who bore them. With the mid-nineteenth century discovery and definition of infant mortality as a social problem demanding amelioration came the recognition that conditions attending poverty were a major determinant of infant death rates. After unsuccessfully pursuing a broad program of environmental reform to combat those conditions, public health reformers narrowed the focus of their efforts and sought to save babies by improving the quality of milk available to them. When milk reform also proved an inadequate strategy, infant mortality was redefined and reconceptualized as a problem of motherhood, on the principle that good mothering could counter the many morbific, social, and environmental conditions influencing infant survival.

Implicit in this international redefinition of infant mortality as a problem of motherhood was a recognition that maternal reform would require a campaign waged on at least two fronts. The first was educational and involved instructing new and prospective mothers in the principles of hygienic infant care and feeding. It also came to include convincing them to follow a prescribed regimen during pregnancy and to make use of quality medical services. The second front was socioeconomic and involved establishing social and medical assistance programs and passing legislation to protect the working mother. In the United States, however, a powerful middle-class family ideal, a tradition of safeguarding private enterprise, an antipathy toward government involvement in correcting social ills, an increasingly hostile and powerful medical profession, a comparatively narrow range of political discourse, and a tendency to elevate racial and ethnic patterns of behavior over economic status: all combined to push infant welfare toward massing its forces primarily on the first front.

The legacy that the American infant welfare movement left was thus an established pattern of combating infant mortality in a comparatively narrow and noncomprehensive way. It was also one bequeathing to future generations of policy makers and reformers a definition of infant mortality that was primarily medical. One of the casualties of the fight over Sheppard-Towner renewal was the Progressive era consensus that infant mortality was a multifaceted problem that demanded the equal participation of public health officials, social workers, and medical professionals. By the end of the decade, even those physicians who had supported Sheppard-Towner were questioning the appropriateness of having nonmedical personnel involved in shaping and directing health programs. Indeed, at the 1930 White House Conference on Child Health and Protection, infant welfare physicians spearheaded a move to shift responsibility for promoting maternal and infant health from the Children's Bureau to the Public Health Service.[1] And although the move was unsuccessful, it marked the beginning of a running battle in which medical professionals steadily assumed an ever larger role in shaping infant and maternal health policies.

The United States, of course, was not alone in medicalizing infant mortality. All of the other nations involved in the infant welfare movement also increasingly embraced a medical definition of infant mortality. Like the United States, they sought to increase medical consumption and to improve the quality of medical care for infants and mothers by training physicians, funding research, and constructing hospitals and other medical care facilities. As in other areas of infant welfare, the uniqueness of the approach adopted by the United States was less one of kind than of degree. While the other industrialized nations came to emphasize the medical dimension of infant mortality, they never lost sight of the social dimension to the extent that the United States did. Moreover, much more than did the United States, they came to recognize that promoting medical care as an antidote to infant mortality carried with it the responsibility of ensuring equal access to that care.

That the formula for approaching infant mortality developed during the infant welfare movement would live on and shape future policy became apparent during the Great Depression of the 1930s when widespread impoverishment once again raised the issue of social and medical welfare. After initially considering government-sponsored health insurance—which would include a maternity benefit—Franklin Roosevelt's Committee on Economic Security dropped it from the Social Security bill it was designing, largely out of fear that opposition from organized medicine would condemn the entire bill to failure.[2] Instead, at the urging of the Children's Bureau, it put in provisions that effectively revived Sheppard-Towner.

As signed into law by Roosevelt on August 14, 1935 and as amended by Congress in 1939, the Social Security Act contained two sections or "titles" devoted to maternal, child, and infant welfare. Both provided matching grants to states and were aimed at strengthening local services rather than replacing them. Title IV sought to assist state authorities in aiding families with dependent children. Title V, which was divided into three parts, authorized federal funds to help states improve their maternal and infant health services, establish special services for crippled children, and expand existing general child health programs.[3] In authorizing matching grants to the states to improve maternal and infant health services, Part 1 of Title V almost exactly duplicated the formula defined in Sheppard-Towner. Indeed, those who were responsible for its design and implementation, as well as its congressional supporters and critics, all spoke of it as reviving the repealed Maternity and Infancy Act.[4]

As was true under the earlier measure, before states could receive grants, they were required to pass enabling legislation, submit a detailed plan to the Children's Bureau, and provide for the administration of the funded programs by establishing a special health department agency or bureau of child hygiene if such did not already exist. The rural emphasis also was retained, as was its underlying purpose of encouraging more even geographic distribution of infant and maternal health services. The formula also stipulated that funds were to be used for demonstrations, conferences, and examinations. Like Sheppard-Towner, the Social Security Act provided no provision for children and mothers needing treatment, recommending instead that they be referred to private physicians, or if indigent, to state or charitable agencies.

Yet some critical differences reflected the desire of the title's sponsors to avoid provoking the opposition that had scuttled the earlier measure. In contrast to Sheppard-Towner, which had aimed its programs at infants and mothers of all classes and thus had prompted the charge of unfair competition from the medical profession, the Social Security Act mandated that special attention be given women and infants in economically depressed areas—thus moving its programs in the direction of temporary medical relief. It also consciously granted to the medical profession authority to determine that which was best for promoting the health of mothers and infants. Seeking to defuse the issue of lay involvement in health matters, the Children's Bureau courted specialists to design and approve programs and placed administration within a Maternal and Child Health Division with an obstetrician as director and a pediatrician as assistant director. The bureau also granted local and state medical societies the right to approve or disapprove plans.[5] Such conscious deference to medical authority did not entirely mollify organized medicine, but it did prevent outright opposition.[6]

A subtle though significant shift had also taken place in the way that critics conceptualized and defined the limitations of the implemented programs. For Progressive infant welfare activists, the inability to afford medical care represented only one of a number of economic factors affecting infant and maternal mortality levels. For Depression-era infant welfare activists, it represented the major one. As a result, when the latter discussed the need to make the maternal and infant health programs more comprehensive, they focused primary attention on the need to make medical services available to those who could not afford them. To a certain extent this shift was the inevitable consequence of a long-term trend toward medicalizing the problem of infant mortality. But it was also the result of mounting concern with sharply rising medical costs. Surfacing in the late 1920s, that concern turned to alarm in the 1930s as plummeting personal income pushed medical care beyond the reach of increasing numbers of American families.[7] Offsetting the high cost of medical care thus steadily moved toward the top of the health reform agenda during the Depression.

One consequence of this new concern with medical costs was the proposal of several schemes for making medical care more readily affordable, including the establishment of cooperative, nonprofit, community health centers. Another was the reconceptualizing of health insurance as a method of health care financing rather than as a guarantee against impoverishment due to sickness. A third was the mounting of a major effort by infant health reformers to position the medical care and treatment of mothers and infants within reach of all American families.[8] All these were brought together in the various proposals for a national health program that surfaced after 1935 and remained on the political agenda through the early 1950s.

Beginning with its 1937 review of its maternity and infancy programs, the Children's Bureau began recommending that Congress dramatically increase the funding available through Title V of the Social Security Act so that states could establish community-based maternity and infancy plans that would ensure prenatal, natal, and postnatal physician and nursing care to all mothers and would make available hospitalization and treatment to those mothers and infants who needed it. The bureau's recommendation was echoed by those attending the National Conference on Better Care for Mothers and Babies, held in Washington, D.C. in January, 1938.[9] It was also included in *The Need for a National Health Program*, the report on national health care presented to Roosevelt in February 1938 by his Interdepartmental Committee to Coordinate Health and Welfare Activities.[10] And it was one of the recommendations made by the National Health Conference that met the following July.[11]

In February 1938, Senator Robert F. Wagner of New York introduced a

National Health Bill based on the recommendations that had been placed before the National Health Conference. Proposed as an amendment to the Social Security Act, the bill sought authorization of federal funding to assist states and communities in constructing hospitals and health centers, in improving general programs of medical care and public health services, and in making available temporary sickness and disability insurance. In addition, by amending Part 1 of Title V, it sought to expand "services, supplies and facilities for promoting the health of mothers and children, and medical care during maternity and infancy, including medical, surgical, and other related services, and care in the home or institutions, and facilities for diagnosis, hospitalization, and aftercare."[12]

Not surprisingly, the Wagner bill provoked intense opposition from the AMA. Following a meeting in May 1939, at which its House of Delegates condemned the bill in no uncertain terms, the association mounted a well-financed lobbying campaign against it. Prompting Roosevelt to withdraw his initial support of the measure and coupled with a conservative resurgence in Congress following the 1938 elections, that campaign succeeded in killing the bill before it ever reached the floor.[13] Thus, when the Social Security Act was amended in 1939, its maternity and infancy provisions retained their narrow scope. All that was changed was that federal funding for state programs was increased from the original $3.8 million to $5.82 million.

Although the failure of the Wagner bill provided yet another illustration that the narrow formula devised during the Progressive era would continue to shape maternal and infant health policy, proponents of a comprehensive national program did not abandon all hope of seeing state-supported medical care for mothers and their newborns. Indeed, within a few years they were mounting another push, encouraged by the new international concern over social and medical welfare resulting from the disruptions of World War II. In 1943, a year after the Beveridge Committee issued the report that led to England's postwar adoption of comprehensive "cradle to grave" social insurance and the establishment of a National Health Service, Wagner reintroduced his Social Security Act amendment, this time jointly with Senator James Murray of Montana and Representative John Dingell of Michigan.[14] Also in 1943, Congress approved special funding for an Emergency Maternity and Infant Care program (EMIC), the purpose of which was to provide obstetric and pediatric care for the wives and infants of enlisted men in the four lowest pay grades of the armed forces. Three years later, Senator Claude Pepper of Florida introduced a Maternal and Child Welfare bill that would authorize a federal appropriation of up to $100 million a year to be granted to states to enable them to provide, among other things, obstetric and pediatric care to mothers and their infants. At the same time, Wagner-Murray-Dingell was again placed before Congress and President Truman began calling for a national health program that would equal-ize access to medical care and would promote maternal and infant welfare. Yet the fate of the Truman proposal and of the Wagner-Murray-Dingell and Pepper bills could have been predicted. Strongly opposed and labeled com-munistic by the AMA and by Republicans and conservative southern Dem-ocrats in Congress, they went nowhere. Moreover, despite the protests of the Children's Bureau, Congress terminated the EMIC program on June 30, 1949.[15] Thus, as the first half of the century came to a close and as much of the rest of the industrial West was putting in place national health services, the United States was no closer to adopting a comprehensive maternal and infant health program than it had been for several decades.

Indeed, in some respects the nation was farther away than ever from doing so. For public support for such a program was waning. There were several reasons for this. But chief among them was the increasing avail-ability of quality private obstetric and pediatric services due to the steady growth of government assistance in the areas of hospital construction and medical research and education and to the development of voluntary health insurance. While at loggerheads over most issues, organized medicine and the proponents of a comprehensive national infant and maternal health plan did agree that at least one problem demanded government assistance. This was the geographic maldistribution of adequate facilities and of trained obstetric and pediatric personnel. Providing assistance to rectify this prob-lem thus represented a relatively safe way for elected officials to grant some-thing to both sides in the stormy debate over national health. Roosevelt, for instance, while refusing in 1939 to support the Wagner bill, did throw his support behind federal funding for hospital construction and medical train-ing. Similarly, although Congress refused in 1946 to consider the Wagner-Murray-Dingell and Pepper bills, it passed the Hospital Survey and Con-struction Act. By 1973 that act had channeled close to $4 billion into the construction of medical facilities in areas where such facilities had been lacking.[16]

As federal funding was increasing the quantity and quality of in-patient obstetric and neonatal care and treatment, private or voluntary health insur-ance was making that care and treatment affordable for a majority of Ameri-can families. In the 1950s private medical insurance became an expected employment benefit for a large and growing segment of the American middle and working classes. By 1958, nearly two-thirds of the American people had some coverage for hospital costs, and fully 55 percent of the families who had a child born that year had insurance benefits for maternity care.[17] Combined with two decades of government-assisted community hospital construction and several decades of improvement in obstetric and pediatric science, prac-tice, and training, the expansion of private health insurance coverage meant that a majority of American mothers and infants finally had available to them comparatively skilled, safe, and effective care.[18] By the 1950s, then, the availability and affordability of maternal and newborn care was fast being transformed from a majority problem to a minority one.

One major consequence of this transformation was a significant decline in the broad-based support that proposals for a national maternity and infancy program had historically enjoyed among American women and organized women's groups. From Sheppard-Towner through the Social Security Act and its proposed amendments, American women had constituted a large, vocal, and interested constituency upon whose support infant and maternal welfare proponents could always count. By the late 1950s, however, this was no longer true. Although women remained concerned with infant and maternal health issues, that concern was being channeled in a number of new directions. Women's labor groups, for instance, while continuing to voice their support for a national maternal and infant health program, devoted most of their energies to securing better employer-provided health benefits. At the same time, middle-class and professional women began focusing their sights on the orientation rather than on the availability of maternity services. Indeed, by the 1960s, the traditional complaint of lack of access was fast being replaced by the charge that scientific obstetrics had transformed birth into an experience characterized by subjugation, alienation, and indignity.

As popular support for a national maternal and infant health program was eroding, so too was the political influence of its promoters within the federal government. No government agency had done more to further maternal and infant welfare in the first half of the twentieth century than the Children's Bureau. In 1946, however, as part of Truman's vast reorganization of the federal bureaucracy, the Children's Bureau was transferred from the Labor Department to the Federal Security Administration. As one historian has characterized it, this represented a "double demotion," because it transformed the bureau from an agency reporting directly to a Cabinet Secretary to one of a number of administrative units under a non–Cabinet level official.[19] The enfeebling of the Children's Bureau continued in 1953 when it became a minor unit in the newly created Department of Health, Education, and Welfare; went one step farther in 1963 when it was switched to the Welfare Administration and divested of its responsibility for researching child health issues; and culminated in 1969 when President Nixon took away its responsibility for administering maternal and child health programs.[20]

With its popular support waning and its chief government promoter weakened, broadly inclusive infant and maternal health reform died a quiet death in the 1950s. Its demise was neither sudden nor surprising; its fate had been sealed three decades earlier when Americans had refused to establish economic and medical support systems for mothers and their babies and to impose government control on the provision of medical care. In so doing they established the basis for the development of private and unequally distributed systems of social and medical insurance and assured that the state's relationship to private medicine would be complementary rather than competitive. By the end of the 1950s that relationship had produced a maternal and infant medical care system that was scientifically advanced, relatively well-distributed geographically, and accessible to a majority of American families. Yet it had also produced a system that was controlled by a monopoly wielding immense political and economic power, that empha-sized technology and was geared toward corrective rather than preventive medicine, and that excluded from its benefits a significant though politically powerless segment of American society. In the 1960s, when infant mortality was yet again discovered and defined as a social problem, these three charac-teristics of the system set the agenda for reform.

Along with witnessing the demise of the reform dream of a national comprehensive maternal and infant health program, the 1950s also wit-nessed a leveling off of the downward trend in American infant death rates that had commenced around the turn of the century. Between 1900 and 1935, infant mortality declined at an average annual rate of approximately 3 percent. Between 1935 and 1950 the rate of decline was 4.7 percent. But between 1950 and 1964, the rate of decline slowed to under 1 percent per year. This decrease in the rate at which infant mortality had fallen through the first half of the century was particularly alarming because it did not occur in other developed nations. The United States thus began to look increasingly bad in international comparison. In 1950 the United States had the sixth lowest infant mortality rate among a group of eleven advanced industrial nations.[21] By 1960, however, it had next to the highest, and by 1964 the highest. Moreover, the gap between the world leaders and America was growing larger. In 1950, Sweden's infant mortality rate was 28 percent lower than that of the United States. By 1960 it was 36 percent lower.[22]

By the early 1960s sociomedical analysts were publishing studies illustrat-ing and analyzing the stasis of American infant death rates and calling for remedial action.[23] Soon after the popular press discovered the problem.[24] Following closely upon the election of an activist Democratic president who had promised to get the country moving again and to make the United States a model for the rest of the world, the revelation that the nation was lagging behind its international counterparts in the preservation of infant lives soon prompted yet another round of federal tinkering with the infant and mater-nal welfare formula defined by Sheppard-Towner and put in place by the Social Security Act. Expressing his deep concern that "since 1950 our coun-try has slipped from 6th to 10th place among the advanced nations of the world in saving infant lives," President Kennedy informed Congress in February 1961 that he intended to ask for a dramatic increase in federal funding for basic research into child health problems and for the expansion of the preventive maternity and infancy programs being administered by the Children's Bureau.[25]

Early in 1963 Representative Wilbur Mills of Arkansas and Senator Abraham Ribicoff of Connecticut placed before Congress a bill that would implement Kennedy's intent. Passed by Congress on October 24 of that year, the Maternal and Child Health and Mental Retardation Planning Amendments to the Social Security Act increased funding for Title V programs and added grants for mental retardation projects, research and planning. At the same time, the surgeon general, empowered by congressional legislation of the year before, established within the National Institutes of Health a National Institute of Child Health and Human Development to promote and conduct research into maternal and child health problems and into the special requirements of mothers.[26] Within a few years Congress had also passed legislation assisting medical education and providing grants for the establishment of neonatal intensive care units, first in a few teaching hospitals and then in regionally distributed centers.[27]

In many respects the federal response to the early 1960s rediscovery of infant mortality represented more of the same; that is, an expansion upon but not a departure from the infant and maternal health formula established almost a half-century before. By increasing funds to the state maternity and infancy programs and by providing more for research, education, and medical facilities, the federal government continued to battle infant mortality by improving private medical care and promoting its consumption. Yet in at least one major respect, the response went beyond that, and demonstrated a recognition that, given the organization of American medical care, more of the same would not be enough.

The leveling off of infant mortality rates during the 1950s and early 1960s presented American health analysts with a paradox. In a period when per capita income was rising sharply, when medical science and practice continued to improve, when the medical sophistication of the average American increased significantly, and when there was a mass migration from rural areas with poor health facilities to urban areas with excellent ones, infant mortality should have declined dramatically rather than leveled off. For the liberal analysts who helped shape national health policy during the Kennedy and Johnson administrations, there could be only one answer: a significant proportion of the population had been excluded from the benefits of economic and medical advance.[28] Providing these "other Americans" with access to those benefits thus became a central part of the 1960s federal program to renew the downward trend of infant mortality.

For the 1960s infant and maternal health reformers, improving access meant overcoming the fundamental failure of the American infant and maternal health care system: that it helped least those who needed help

most. That infants from families situated on the lowest rungs of the economic ladder faced the highest risk of death remained as true in the sixth decade
of the century as it had in the first. So too was it still true that the infants of
racial minorities, and particularly those of inner city blacks, had significantly less chance of surviving than did their white counterparts. Indeed, in
some respects both were more true, since nearly three-fourths of all infant
deaths now occurred in the neonatal period and were causally related to
differentials in maternal circumstances and health care, both of which correlated strongly to socioeconomic and racial status.[29] Yet it was precisely such
infants—and their mothers—who had least access to the nation's advanced
but private system of maternal and infant health care. For those whose
families were near poor but not indigent and who did not have private
health insurance coverage, the cost of services in that system prevented
them from taking more than minimal advantage of it.[30] For those who were
indigent, the care available was from a welfare medical system that was
overcrowded, underfinanced, understaffed, and, compared to the private
system, thoroughly second-rate.[31] Increasing the access of the near poor to
the private maternal and infant health care system and bringing the benefits
of that system to the indigent thus constituted two major challenges for
1960s infant and maternal health reformers.

The first step toward meeting those challenges was taken when policy-
makers in the Kennedy administration placed within the 1963 Maternal and
Child Health and Mental Retardation Planning Amendment a provision
that authorized the use of special project or "Fund B" grants (initially authorized in 1935 under Title V as direct grants to states to finance demonstration projects in economically depressed sections) to establish Maternity and
Infant Care Projects that would provide prenatal, delivery, and postpartum
care to high-risk women in low-income rural and urban areas. A second and
much larger step was taken in 1965 when Congress established the Medicaid
Program as part of a Medicare Act amending the Social Security Act.

In authorizing funding of special Maternity and Infant Care Projects,
Congress acceded to the long-standing infant welfare demand that the
federal maternity and infancy program be made comprehensive enough to
include medical services. Yet it was a relatively small accession. It was, for
instance, not until the Child Health Act of 1967 that such projects extended
care to neonates. Moreover, despite legislated increases in subsequent years,
funding was kept at a very conservative level—indeed far below what
proponents of such care in 1938 had estimated would be necessary. Only 56
projects had been set up by 1972 and most of these were limited in facilities
and personnel. By the early 1970s, then, even their strongest supporters had
to admit that the programs were assisting less than 20 percent of those
American families who could not afford the increasingly high price of private maternal and neonatal care or were dependent on welfare medicine.[32]

Reaching that remaining 80 percent was thus one of the goals of Medi-caid, the stated purpose of which was to grant the near poor and those on public assistance rolls access to private medical services. And in some re-spects that goal was achieved. Between 1968 and 1979 the number of Medi-caid recipients grew from 11.5 million to 21.5 million and the payment per recipient increased (in constant dollars) from $304 to $402. As a result the consumption of private medical services by the needy and by minorities significantly increased. Combined with the introduction of food stamps and other new public assistance programs such as the Special Supplemental Food Program for Women and Infants (WIC), and in no small measure abetted by a concurrent revolution in the surgical and medical treatment of high-risk neonates, this increased consumption probably goes a long way toward explaining why the American infant mortality rate dropped from 21.8 in 1968 to 12.6 in 1980.[33] Yet while Medicaid has probably done more to equalize access to maternal and infant care than any social welfare measure in the twentieth century, it has proven a problematic and far from perfect antidote to the problem of American infant mortality.

Although the problems besetting Medicaid as a means of combating in-fant mortality are numerous and complex, they all more or less derive from two features of the measure. First, Medicaid is basically a financer of private health care and not a comprehensive maternal and infant aid program. As such, it is limited to providing services consistent with the orientation of existing private medical care. Since, in the United States, that orientation has been toward correcting rather than preventing maternal and infant health problems, the majority of Medicaid funds expended on mothers and infants has gone to finance corrective rather than preventive care. Second, as a public assistance program, Medicaid shares the complexities, ine-qualities, and political vulnerability of the welfare system. Indeed, the effec-tiveness of Medicaid in reducing infant mortality has in many ways been undercut by it being available only to those mothers and infants who qualify for assistance under the Aid to Dependent Families with Children (AFDC) program or other categorical assistance programs.

Although liberal policy-shapers conceptualized Medicaid as a vehicle for giving the poor access to mainstream medicine, it was fashioned and pre-sented primarily as a means of reorganizing and rationalizing the system by which the federal government, since 1950, had been assisting states in reim-bursing medical vendors providing services to those in the various federal categorical assistance programs.[34] As a consequence, eligibility for Medicaid was tied to eligibility for public assistance, and the program retained the joint federal-state structure of the welfare system—and the inequalities attending that structure. The bill reserved for the federal government the right to require that certain services be funded, to set the categories of persons eligible, and to determine the percentage of each state's program it would fund. But it granted to the states the right to administer their programs, to define eligibility requirements for each assistance category, to determine the amount or level of each service included, to make eligible for services the near poor or "medically needy,"[35] to set reimbursement rates, and to decide how much money they would devote to their programs.[36] The result was the development of fifty unique programs that vary considerably in inclusiveness and amount of services offered. As a consequence, the infant and maternal medical services provided under Medicaid have proven to be anything but uniform.[37]

If Medicaid shares the welfare system's complexities and inequalities it also shares its lack of a powerful constituency and therefore its vulnerability to changes in the political and economic climate. As with other social welfare measures adopted or expanded upon during the economically robust and politically liberal 1960s, Medicaid was soon facing an environment in which stagnation and inflation and dramatically rising state and federal welfare expenditures eroded liberal faith that the nation could afford to equalize access to the benefits of a prosperous society. Indeed, Medicaid elicited an unusual amount of concern, largely because its cost proved so unexpectedly high. Although the designers of the program suspected that their original estimate of a $1.5 billion combined federal-state expenditure might be low, they did not in their wildest dreams imagine that such expenditure would exceed $20 billion by 1979.[38]

Although concern over escalating Medicaid costs began surfacing before the end of the 1960s, it was not until the 1974–75 recession that both the states and the federal government became preoccupied with the "Medicaid crisis" (and a welfare crisis in general). With the economy souring, tax revenues falling, and increasing numbers of families falling below the poverty line, states were caught in a vise between rising Medicaid expenditures and declining government income. As a consequence, they seriously began attempting to cap costs. Initially, this was done by a kind of neglect, by failing to raise income limits for AFDC or medically needy eligibility so that they matched inflation. Soon, however, eligibility requirements were being tightened and restrictions were being placed on physician fees.[39]

Despite these efforts, Medicaid expenditures continued to rise, in large part because of a dramatic increase in hospital costs. Thus, the Medicaid crisis continued into the 1980s and prompted a second round of cost-cutting, this time initiated primarily at the federal level. In 1981, the Reagan administration, convinced that it possessed a mandate to shrink federal expenditures and trim the welfare rolls, pushed through Congress an Omnibus Budget Reconciliation Act, which severely tightened AFDC eligibility requirements and prohibited states from making cash assistance payments to first-time pregnant women until their sixth month. It also reduced funding for Title V maternity and infancy programs (including a 16.5 percent cut in

Fund B grants and a 22 percent cut in family planning grants), and froze funding for WIC at existing levels. One result was that states had to trim their infant and maternal health programs. Another was that at a time when unemployment was rising and when the number of families living below the poverty line was increasing, thousands of women and infants were excluded from public assistance and therefore made ineligible for Medicaid. Thus, where in 1975, 63 percent of all poor or near poor families were receiving Medicaid benefits, by 1983 the proportion had dropped to 46 percent.[40]

The cuts, however, were not made without protests by some legislators, sociomedical investigators, and public advocacy groups, many of whom predicted that the decline in infant mortality during the previous decade and a half would be slowed or even reversed.[41] Early in 1984, when infant mortality statistics for 1983 were released, those predictions seemed to be borne out. After declining between 1965 and 1982 at an annual rate of 4.4 percent, infant mortality dropped only 2.6 percent in 1983. The Food Research and Action Center and the Children's Defense Fund—two public advocacy groups who had taken the lead in protesting the new restrictions on medical and social welfare—immediately charged that the rate slowdown offered direct evidence that the Reagan administration's budget tightening was being paid for with the lives of the nation's babies. Not surprisingly, administration officials and their defenders rejected this charge, arguing that the cuts were not seriously affecting maternal and infant care and that the slowdown was either temporary or the result of infant mortality having reached a plateau where many of the remaining major causes of infant death—teenage pregnancy and smoking, drinking and drug-taking by pregnant women—were primarily cultural and behavioral and therefore beyond the reach of social and medical welfare programs. They also contended that their liberal opponents were politicizing infant mortality and using it to block much needed reform of an overbloated welfare system.[42]

Following the initial salvos, the debate over the causes and implications of the slowdown in the decline of infant mortality grew increasingly complex and inconclusive. Because the mortality statistics employed in the debate were necessarily short-term and frequently local, their statistical validity was open to question and their meaning open to differing interpretation. As a consequence, it was difficult to prove with any degree of conclusiveness that administration policies were having a negative impact on the infant death rate. Nevertheless, since 1985 opponents of the cuts to Medicaid and maternal and infant assistance programs have won a number of victories and have been able to reverse the trend toward restriction. That they have testifies to the extent to which infant mortality remains an emotionally powerful issue, as useful today as it was one hundred years ago in prying loose government funding for public health. More importantly, it testifies to the success that infant and maternal welfare advocates have had in taking the fiscal concerns of the budget cutters, adapting them to their own use, and advancing an argument that in its mating of cost-efficiency and humanitarianism would have won the approval of their Progressive forebears.

Critics of the Reagan administration contended that both the cuts in funding for maternal and infant assistance programs and the new restrictions for Medicaid and AFDC eligibility were "penny wise and pound foolish." While reducing outlays for comparatively low-cost prenatal health and nutritional assistance, they did little to control—and indeed, may have fueled—what many believed to be the major catalyst behind rising government expenditures on maternal and infant health care: skyrocketing hospital costs. The reasons that hospital costs increased so dramatically during the 1970s are numerous and complex, as are the reasons why state and federal governments found themselves paying a large proportion of that increase. In regard to infant and maternal care, however, one reason stands out above the rest. This is that the decade witnessed the development of costly technological procedures to improve the survivability of high-risk neonates.

The 1960s rediscovery of infant mortality eventually highlighted three characteristics of American infant deaths. The first was that a large and increasing proportion of such deaths was among high-risk neonates, particularly low birthweight (LBW) or premature babies,[43] primarily because such babies are prone to life-threatening problems such as hemorrhages, infections, and respiratory ailments. The second was that LBW babies were much more likely to be born to those socioeconomic and racial groups who suffered the highest rates of infant mortality. Blacks, and particularly inner-city blacks, gave birth to a much higher percentage of LBW babies than any other group.[44] The third and final characteristic of American infant mortality highlighted was that the percentage of LBW babies was higher in the United States than in most of the advanced industrial nations of the world.[45] Recognition of these characteristics led to a new emphasis on prenatal care, to some changes in the type of advice given to pregnant women, and to the development of a number of labor-inhibiting drugs. But more importantly, it led to at least an implicit policy decision to marshal national resources behind an intense effort to improve hospital capability for keeping LBW and other high-risk neonates alive. That effort produced the neonatal intensive care unit, a high-technology and labor-intensive addition to hospital nurseries which provided such babies with careful regulation of their environment, constant supervision, and an ever-increasing array of surgical, pharmaceutical, and technological intervention.

The success of these units in reducing mortality among high-risk neonates has been truly phenomenal. For instance, after an NICU was set up at New York's Mount Zion Hospital in 1970, the mortality rate among its LBW neonates dropped from 21.8 percent to 6.6 percent.[46] But that success has come at a tremendous financial cost, both to hospitals and to those who pay their expenses. By the end of the 1970s the average cost per baby admitted to an NICU was almost $14,000 and could individually run well over $100,000. By the mid-1980s the upper range of cost was pushing $200,000 and total national expenditure on intensive neonatal care was approaching $2 billion. Because those who qualify for welfare are more likely to bear LBW babies and other high-risk neonates than those in more prosperous economic strata, Medicaid has borne a significant share of the rising cost of neonatal intensive care. Moreover, because the cost of such care is so high, Medicaid frequently ends up paying the bills of "medically needy" near-poor infants whose mothers do not qualify for prenatal care coverage. Finally, because hospitals do not generally deny such care to those without government or private health care financing, they recover the cost of such care by increasing their average charges. Society as a whole thus continues to pay for neonatal intensive care, even when eligibility requirements are tightened.

It did not take a great deal of financial or sociomedical acumen to realize that spiraling public expenditures on neonatal intensive care would not be controlled unless the incidence of LBW births was also controlled. The ratio of such births to all births had declined somewhat since hitting a postwar peak in the mid-1960s, but had not done so evenly across racial and economic categories or at a rate even remotely comparable to the concurrent decline in overall neonatal mortality. Indeed, it was the common consensus of sociomedical researchers that the reduction of infant deaths in the first month had not been achieved through any significant reduction in the underlying causes, but rather through the increased application of high-cost intensive care technologies and procedures.[47] Advocates of more government involvement in maternal and infant protection were therefore able to present a powerful case that increased government spending on programs designed to accomplish a reduction in LBW births would ultimately be cost-efficient. In particular, by citing studies showing that access to prenatal care was a major deterrent of prematurity and by using estimates as to the comparative costs of preventive and corrective care, they were able argue that if government would provide prenatal care to all low-income women it would not only effect a reduction in infant mortality but also save several hundred million dollars.[48]

Advanced against a backdrop of mounting national concern over the large and burgeoning proportion of the gross national product being swallowed each year by the country's technologically advanced but high-cost medical care system,[49] the cost-efficiency argument was a powerful one, and provided state and federal legislators with both a humanitarian and a fiscally sound rationale for increasing spending on maternal and infant health care programs. On the assumption that it would save both money and infant lives, Massachusetts in 1985 established a Healthy Start Program. With an allocation of $6.1 million in state funds for the first year and $15 million for the second, the program funded comprehensive prenatal and maternity care for all women with no other health insurance and incomes at or below 185 percent of the federal poverty level. At the same time California set up a state-financed prenatal and natal care program that was projected to save the state $26 million a year on intensive neonatal care costs. Maryland allocated $1.5 million to provide maternity care for all women under 21 with incomes below the federal poverty level. And in January 1988, Rhode Island began a Rite Start Program guaranteeing prenatal, natal, and postnatal care to mothers and infants in families with incomes up to 185 percent of the poverty level. Other states, such as South Carolina, Florida, and Texas loosened eligibility requirements for welfare and expanded state-financed programs for pregnant women.[50]

In 1985 Congress also began a piecemeal reversal of the 1981 Medicaid restrictions, usually by attaching expanded coverage provisions to bills that had nothing directly to do with welfare. One such provision, attached to a bill passed in 1986, allowed states to provide Medicaid services to all pregnant women with incomes below the federal poverty level, regardless of whether they qualified for welfare. Another, attached to a bill passed in late 1987, allowed states to extend Medicaid coverage to pregnant women and infants in families with incomes up to 185 percent of the federal poverty level.[51]

Although it is too early to tell conclusively, these state and federal initiatives promise positive results. The experience of a few municipalities where prenatal care is widely available, even to the economically disadvantaged, suggests that the increased provision of such care will help reduce the incidence of LBW births and thus help diminish both neonatal mortality and the need for costly neonatal intensive care.[52] Indeed, like all the other relatively narrow health measures adopted since 1850, the provision of prenatal care to expectant women will undoubtedly further reduce infant mortality. At the same time, however, the measures taken so far to expand publicly financed prenatal care programs fall far short of providing the long sought-after solution to the problem of American infant mortality. Indeed, the new programs seem highly vulnerable. Designed to meet an immediate "crisis" and limited to the poor and medically needy (and thus without a large and politically influential constituency), they could easily be cut when the crisis is perceived to have passed, when tax revenues fall, or when it is concluded that they are not as cost-efficient or as effective as predicted.

More importantly, prenatal care is no magic bullet and never will be. Infant mortality remains, in the broadest sense of the term, a social problem; and as such demands today, just as it did at the turn of the century, a comprehensive program for combating all the conditions of economic privation and for improving maternal ability to carry and bear healthy infants. Counseling pregnant women on the risk of certain behaviors and on the

benefits of others, monitoring the health of the fetus and mother, and providing treatment when necessary constitute an important part of such a program. But it is only one part, and as Progressive infant welfare advocates
recognized, needs to be complemented with more wide-ranging social reform
and assistance programs.

Scientific medicine has come a long way in its ability to identify infant and
maternal risk factors and to correct both their prenatal and postnatal consequences. But it has not succeeded in making infant mortality solely a medical problem. The further reduction of LBW births and neonatal and postneonatal mortality thus requires that the nation reconceptualize its responsibility to its infants and to those who give birth to them and finally adopt
and implement a comprehensive and nationally uniform maternal and infant
welfare program. In addition to guaranteeing universal access to quality
prenatal, delivery, and neonatal services, such a program would also have to
ensure that pregnant and post-parturient women have the means to follow
risk-lowering regimens. This means more than simply providing bare-bones
economic support and nutritional supplements to those prospective and
new mothers who meet the eligibility requirements for public assistance. It
also means the design and implementation of systematic maternity leave and
wage compensation policies for working pregnant and new mothers and a
national investment in day care. And it means detaching maternal and
infant welfare from public assistance; making the program, like Medicare, a
uniform federal one, rather than a hodgepodge of federally assisted state
programs; and guaranteeing access to the program as a benefit of motherhood
rather than as compensation for poverty. But most of all, such a program
would require a national willingness to expand government responsibility
for the amelioration of social problems, particularly in the nation's inner
cities, and to accept as legitimate government intervention in the provision
of health care, even to those who are not indigent. If over a century of
battling infant mortality should have taught any lesson, it is that no narrow
panacea exists. One hundred and fifty years after the nation first embarked
on a systematic effort to reduce mortality among its youngest citizens, it
might be time to learn that lesson and to broaden the discourse to include
more comprehensive options.

Appendix A

Abbreviations

AAM	American Academy of Medicine
AASPIM	American Association for Study and Prevention of Infant Mortality
AFDC	Aid to Families with Dependent Children
AFL	American Federation of Labor
AMA	American Medical Association
GFWC	General Federation of Women's Clubs
GRO	General Register Office (Great Britain)
LBW	Low Birthweight
LGB	Local Government Board (Great Britain)
MOH	Medical Officer of Health (Great Britain)
NASPT	National Association for Study and Prevention of Tuberculosis
NCCC	National Conference of Charities and Corrections
NICU	Neonatal Intensive Care Unit
NYAICP	New York Association for Improving the Condition of the Poor
NYMC	New York Milk Committee
USCB	United States Children's Bureau

Appendix B

Infant[a] and Neonatal[b] Mortality Rates, by Race, United States,[c] 1915–1985

Year	Infant Mortality Rates			Neonatal Mortality Rates		
	All Races	White	All Other	All Races	White	All Other
1915–19	95.7	92.8	149.7	43.4	42.3	58.1
1920–24	76.7	73.3	115.3	39.7	38.7	51.1
1925–29	69.0	65.0	105.4	37.2	36.0	47.9
1930–34	60.4	55.2	98.6	34.4	32.5	48.2
1935–39	53.2	49.2	81.3	31.0	29.5	41.4
1940	47.0	43.2	73.8	28.8	27.2	39.7
1941	45.3	41.2	74.8	27.7	26.1	39.0
1942	40.4	37.3	64.6	25.7	24.5	34.6
1943	40.4	37.5	62.5	24.7	23.7	32.9
1944	39.8	36.9	60.3	24.7	23.6	32.5
1945	38.3	35.6	67.0	24.3	23.3	32.0
1946	33.8	31.8	49.5	24.0	23.1	31.5
1947	32.2	30.1	48.5	22.8	21.7	31.0
1948	32.0	29.9	46.5	22.2	21.2	29.1
1949	31.3	28.9	47.3	21.4	20.3	28.6
1950	29.2	26.8	44.5	20.5	19.4	27.5
1951	28.4	25.8	44.8	20.0	18.9	27.3
1952	28.4	25.8	47.0	19.8	18.5	27.3
1953	27.8	25.0	44.7	19.6	18.3	27.3
1954	26.6	23.9	42.9	19.1	17.8	27.0
1955	26.4	23.6	42.8	19.1	17.7	27.2
1956	26.0	23.2	42.1	18.9	17.5	27.0
1957	26.3	23.3	43.7	19.1	17.5	27.8

	Infant Mortality Rates			Neonatal Mortality Rates		
Year	All Races	White	All Other	All Races	White	All Other
1958	27.1	23.8	45.7	19.5	17.8	29.0
1959	26.4	23.2	44.0	19.0	17.5	27.7
1960	26.0	22.9	43.2	18.7	17.2	26.9
1961	25.3	22.4	40.7	18.4	16.9	26.1
1962ᵈ	25.3	22.3	41.5	18.3	16.9	26.1
1963ᵈ	25.2	22.2	41.5	18.2	16.7	26.1
1964	24.8	21.6	41.1	17.9	16.2	26.5
1965	24.7	21.5	40.3	17.7	16.1	25.4
1966	23.7	20.6	38.8	17.2	15.6	24.8
1967	22.4	19.7	35.9	16.5	15.0	23.8
1968	21.8	19.2	34.5	16.1	14.7	23.0
1969	20.9	18.4	32.9	15.6	14.2	22.5
1970	20.0	17.8	30.9	15.1	13.8	21.4
1971	19.1	17.1	28.5	14.2	13.0	19.6
1972ᵉ	18.5	16.4	27.7	13.6	12.4	19.2
1973	17.7	15.8	26.2	13.0	11.8	17.9
1974	16.7	14.8	24.9	12.3	11.1	17.2
1975	16.1	14.2	24.2	11.6	10.4	16.8
1976	15.2	13.3	23.5	10.9	9.7	16.3
1977	14.1	12.3	21.7	9.9	8.7	14.7
1978	13.8	12.0	21.1	9.5	8.4	14.0
1979	13.1	11.4	19.8	8.9	7.9	12.9
1980	12.6	11.0	19.1	8.5	7.5	12.5
1981	11.9	10.5	17.8	8.0	7.1	11.8
1982	11.5	10.1	17.3	7.7	6.8	11.3
1983	11.2	9.7	16.8	7.3	6.4	10.8
1984	10.8	9.4	16.1	7.0	6.2	10.2
1985	10.6	9.3	15.8	7.0	6.1	10.3

Source: National Center for Health Statistics, *Vital Statistics of the United States, 1985*, vol. 2, *Mortality* (Washington, D.C.: Government Printing Office, 1988), part A, sect. 2, p. 1.

[a]Infant Mortality Rate = Deaths within first year per 1,000 live births.
[b]Neonatal Mortality Rate = Deaths within first 28 days per 1,000 live births.
[c]Prior to 1933 data are for birth registration states only.
[d]Figures by race exclude data for residents of New Jersey.
[e]Deaths based on a 50 percent sample.

Appendix C

Maternal Mortality Rates[a] by Race, United States,[b] 1915–1985

Year	All Races	White	All Other
1915–19	727.9	700.3	1,253.5
1920–24	689.5	649.2	1,134.3
1925–29	668.6	615.0	1,163.7
1930–34	636.0	575.4	1,080.7
1935–39	493.9	439.9	875.5
1940	376.0	319.8	773.5
1941	316.5	266.0	678.1
1942	258.7	221.8	544.0
1943	245.2	210.5	509.9
1944	227.9	189.4	506.0
1945	207.2	172.1	454.8
1946	156.7	130.7	358.9
1947	134.5	108.6	334.6
1948	111.6	89.4	301.0
1949	90.3	68.1	234.8
1950	83.3	61.1	221.6
1951	75.0	54.9	201.3
1952	67.8	48.9	188.1
1953	61.1	44.1	166.1
1954	52.4	37.2	143.8
1955	47.0	32.8	130.3
1956	40.9	28.7	110.7
1957	41.0	27.5	118.3

Year	All Races	White	All Other
1958	37.6	26.3	101.8
1959	37.4	25.8	102.1
1960	37.1	26.0	97.9
1961	36.9	24.9	101.3
1962c	35.2	23.8	95.9
1963c	35.8	24.0	96.9
1964	33.1	22.3	89.9
1965	31.6	21.0	83.7
1966	29.1	20.2	72.4
1967	28.0	19.5	69.5
1968	24.5	16.6	63.6
1969	22.2	15.5	55.7
1970	21.5	14.4	55.9
1971	18.8	13.0	45.3
1972d	18.8	14.3	38.5
1973	15.2	10.7	34.6
1974	14.6	10.0	35.1
1975	12.8	9.1	29.0
1976	12.3	9.0	26.5
1977	11.2	7.7	26.0
1978	9.6	6.4	23.0
1979	9.6	6.4	22.7
1980	9.2	6.7	19.8
1981	8.5	6.3	17.3
1982	7.9	5.8	16.4
1983	8.0	5.9	16.3
1984	7.8	5.4	16.9
1985	7.8	5.2	18.1

Source: National Center for Health Statistics, *Vital Statistics of the United States, 1987,* vol. 2, *Mortality* (Washington, D.C.: Government Printing Office, 1988), part A, sect. 1, p. 65.

[a]Maternal deaths related to pregnancy and childbirth per 100,000 live births.

[b]Prior to 1933, data are for birth registration states only.

[c]Figures by race exclude data for residents of New Jersey.

[d]Deaths based on a 50 percent sample.

Notes

Introduction

1. Given the paucity of surviving records, demographers have been reluctant to specify precise rates of infant mortality for nineteenth-century America. Nevertheless, a number of estimates have been made of mortality for infants, young children, and older children in specified populations. Many of these estimates can be found in Michael R. Haines, "Mortality in Nineteenth Century America: Estimates from New York and Pennsylvania Census Data," *Demography* 14 (1977): 325. More recently a few scholars have creatively employed federal census manuscript schedules to estimate survival rates for infants and young children during the mid-nineteenth century. See especially Richard H. Steckel, "The Health and Mortality of Women and Children," *Journal of Economic History* 45 (1988):333–45; and Eric Leif Davin, "The Era of the Common Child: Infant and Child Mortality in Mid-Nineteenth-Century Pittsburgh" (unpublished paper, 1989).

2. Again, the data do not allow for precise calculations. But informed estimates have placed infant mortality in Philadelphia in 1870 at 174; in New York in 1885 at 248; and in Boston in 1880–84 at 192. Moreover, the 1900 census estimates mortality in Savannah, Georgia; Mobile, Alabama; Fall River, Massachusetts; and Richmond, Virginia; as 300, 271, 260, and 250, respectively. Here as elsewhere infant mortality is defined as the number of infant deaths per 1,000 live births in a given year. See Gretchen A. Condrun, Henry A. Williams, and Rose A. Cheney, "The Decline of Mortality in Philadelphia from 1870 to 1930: The Role of Municipal Services," *Pennsylvania Magazine of History and Biography* 108 (1984): 156; Ernst C. Meyer, *Infant Mortality in New York City: A Study of the Results Accomplished by Infant Life-Saving Agencies, 1885–1920* (New York: Rockefeller Foundation International Health Board, 1921), table v, p. 130f; Richard A. Meckel, "The Awful Responsibility of Motherhood: American Health Reform and the Prevention of Infant and Child Mortality before 1913," (Ph.D diss., University of Michigan, 1980), p. 367; U.S. Department of Interior, Census Office, *Twelfth Census of the United States,* vol. 3: *Vital Statistics* (Washington, D.C.: Government Printing Office, 1902), pp. 292, 322, 360, 544.

3. The 1 percent figure is based on the infant death rate of 1.0 (per 1,000 live births) obtaining in the United States between July 1, 1987, and June 30, 1988. It is a provisional rate and is based on registration records indicating that there were 38,300 infant deaths and 3,855,000 live births during that twelve-month period. See National Center for Health Statistics, "Births, Marriages, Divorces, and Deaths for July 1988," *Monthly Vital Statistics Report* 37 (Oct. 19, 1988): 1.

4. For the U.S. figures for 1987–88, see ibid. The rates and figures for Massachusetts and New York City in 1985 are contained in National Center for Health Statistics, *Vital Statistics of the United States, 1985*, vol. 1, *Natality*, sect. 1, pp. 76, 83; and ibid., vol. 2, *Mortality*, sect. 2, pp. 11, 34. The figures and rates for Massachusetts in 1885 are based on there having been 48,790 births and 7,626 infant deaths that year and are contained in Secretary of the Commonwealth of Massachusetts, *Forty-ninth Annual Registration Report, 1890* (Boston, 1891), p. 293. The figures and rates for New York City in 1885 are based on there having been 9,303 recorded deaths and an estimated 37,543 births. This computes to an infant mortality rate of 247.79. The birth estimate is based on a New York City Bureau of Records assessment that recorded births in 1885 were 20 percent lower than actual births. For New York City, see Meyer, *Infant Mortality in New York City*, table v, p. 130 (facing).

5. A caveat is necessary here. The reduction of infant mortality and the reduction of mortality from specific diseases are not, strictly speaking, comparable, since infant mortality is an age-specific death rate, not a cause-specific one, and since the reduction of certain specific diseases contributed to the reduction of infant mortality. Nevertheless, the reduction of infant mortality still stands out as the premier mortality reduction of the modern era. In 1900, for instance, 55,504 people (of which 1,918 were infants) in the registration area (then ten states plus the District of Columbia) died from lumbular tuberculosis, 5,721 died from tuberculosis-related diseases, and 6,766 died from venereal disease. In the same year, however, 111,687 infants died in their first year of life while another 26,722 died in their second year. U.S. Department of Commerce and Labor, Bureau of the Census, *Mortality Statistics, 1900–1904* (Washington, D.C.: Government Printing Office, 1906), p. 82.

6. For the most often cited and influential argument that mortality dropped primarily because of improved living standards and nutrition, see Thomas McKeown, *The Modern Rise of Population* (New York: Academic Press, 1976); idem., *The Role of Medicine: Dream, Mirage or Nemesis?* (Princeton: Princeton University Press, 1979). For analyses of other factors behind the reduction of infant mortality, see W. R. Aykroyd and J. P. Kevany, "Mortality in Infancy and Early Childhood in Ireland, Scotland, and England and Wales, 1871–1970," *Ecology of Food and Nutrition* 2 (1973): 11–19; M. W. Beaver, "Population, Infant Mortality, and Milk," *Population Studies* 27 (1973): 243–54; Rose A. Cheney, "Seasonal Aspects of Infant and Childhood Mortality: Philadelphia, 1865–1920," *Journal of Interdisciplinary History* 14 (1984): 561–85; Gretchen A. Condrun and Rose A. Cheney, "Mortality Trends in Philadelphia, Age- and Cause-Specific Rates, 1870–1930," *Demography* 19 (1982): 97–123; Condrun, Williams, and Cheney, "The Decline of Mortality in Philadelphia from 1870 to 1930," pp. 153–77; Hallie J. Kitner, "The Determinants of Infant Mortality in Germany from 1871 to 1933," (Ph.D. diss., University of Michigan, 1982); Richard A. Meckel, "Immigration, Mortality, and Population Growth in Boston, 1840–1880," *Journal of Interdisciplinary History* 15 (1985): 393–417; Randall Reves, "Declining Fertility in England and Wales as a Major Cause of the Twentieth Century Decline in Mortality: The Role of Changing Family Size and Age Structure in Infectious Disease Mortality in Infancy," *American Journal of Epidemiology* 122 (1985): 112–26; P. A. Watterson, "The Role of Environment in the Decline of Infant Mortality: An Analysis of the 1911 Census of England and Wales," *Journal of Biological Science* 18 (1986): 457–70; Robert Fogel, "Nutrition and the Decline in Mortality Since 1700," in *Long-Term Factors in American Economic Growth*, ed. Stanley L. Engerman and Robert E. Gallman (Chicago: University of Chicago Press, 1986), 439–555.

7. Although there has been a recent withdrawal of unqualified support, most demographers continue to agree with McKeown's contention that curative medicine had little impact on mortality levels prior to the last half century. For an application of McKeown's

thesis to an American setting, see Judith Walzer Leavitt, *The Healthiest City: Milwaukee and the Politics of Health Reform* (Princeton: Princeton University Press, 1982). Increased access to health care has come primarily from two sources: (1) private and government-assisted construction of health care facilities; and (2) private, individually purchased or employer-provided health insurance and government-provided health insurance (Medicaid) for those poor who qualify.

8. Institute of Medicine, Committee to Study the Prevention of Low Birthweight, *Preventing Low Birthweight* (Washington, D.C.: National Academy Press, 1985), p. 1. For a survey of the major medical advances aiding infant survival, see Thomas E. Cone, Jr., *History of American Pediatrics,* (Boston: Little, Brown, 1979), pp. 201–27, 232–40.

9. This ranking is subject to some dispute, depending on which figures are used and which countries are counted in the comparison. To rank the United States twenty-second, I employ the most recent mortality figures available from the Population Reference Bureau, Inc., and count all countries and protectorates with complete death registration rather than only those defined as "more developed" by the United Nations. Doing so, the United States ranks behind the following: Japan (5.2), Finland (5.2), Iceland (5.4), Sweden (5.9), Switzerland (6.8), Taiwan (6.9), Hong Kong (7.7), Netherlands (7.7), Canada (7.9), Luxembourg (7.9), France (8.0), Denmark (8.4), Norway (8.5), W. Germany (8.6), Ireland (8.7), Spain (9.0), E. Germany (9.2), Singapore (9.4), United Kingdom (9.5), Belgium (9.7), and Australia (9.8). Moreover, only three developed countries—Italy (10.1), New Zealand (10.8), and the USSR (25.0)—rank below the United States. *World Population Data Sheet, 1988* (Washington, D.C.: Population Reference Bureau, 1988).

10. In 1986 the infant mortality rate in Central Harlem was 27.6. In 1985 the infant mortality rate (deaths under one year of age per 1,000 live births in a single year) among blacks in the United States was 18.2 compared to 9.3 among whites. Similarly, black neonatal mortality (deaths in the first 28 days per 1,000 live births) was 12.1 compared to 6.1 for whites. "Baby Death Rate Rising in New York After a Dip," *New York Times,* November 3, 1988, sect. B, p. 3; National Center for Health Statistics, *Health, United States, 1987* (Washington, D.C.: Government Printing Office, 1988), p. 45.

11. For a recent review of the evidence and issues, see James C. Cramer, "Social Factors and Infant Mortality: Identifying High-Risk Groups and Proximate Causes," *Demography* 24 (1987): 299–322.

12. "Prenatal Care Is Declining, Agency Finds," *New York Times,* January 8, 1984, section E, p. 5.

13. For three good summaries of the arguments of both sides see C. Arden Miller, "Infant Mortality in the U.S.," *Scientific American* 253 (July 1985): 31–37; Stephen Budiansky, "A Measure of Failure," *The Atlantic* 257 (January 1986): 32–35; George C. Graham, "Poverty, Hunger, Malnutrition, Prematurity and Infant Mortality in the United States," *Pediatrics* 75 (1985): 117–25.

14. See, for instance, William M. Schmidt, "The Development of Health Services for Mothers and Children in the United States," *American Journal of Public Health* 63 (1973): 419–27.

15. Specifically, maternal and infant health and assistance programs fall under Titles IV and V of the Social Security Act (1935). Title IV provides federal assistance to states to aid families with dependent children. Title V authorizes funds to help states establish and maintain maternal, infant, and child health services and programs as well as special services for crippled and mentally retarded children. Both titles have been amended a number of times since they were included in the 1935 legislation. Perhaps most important were the Mental and Child Health Planning Amendments of 1963 and the Child Health Act of 1967. Also of critical importance was the 1965 amendment of the Social Security Act establishing Medicare and Medicaid. Similarly, the development of private health

insurance and the government-assisted construction of pediatric and neonatal care facilities are largely post–World War II phenomena.

16. Most recent histories of public health in America do touch upon infant welfare. Moreover, a few historians have rediscovered the Sheppard-Towner Act, maternal reform, and the Children's Bureau, while others have examined various aspects of the turn-of-the-century debates over infant feeding and the contemporaneous emergence of pediatrics as a medical specialty. Nevertheless, no substantial and focused analysis of American infant mortality and public health reform has yet appeared. See, for instance, Barbara Gutmann Rosenkrantz, *Public Health and the State: Changing Views in Massachusetts, 1842–1936* (Cambridge: Harvard University Press, 1972), pp. 148–61; John Duffy, *A History of Public Health in New York City, 1866–1966* (New York: Russell Sage, 1974), pp. 208–37; Stuart Galishoff, *Safeguarding the Public Health: Newark, 1895–1918* (Westport, Conn.: Greenwood, 1975), pp. 107–19; Leavitt, *The Healthiest City*, pp. 156–89; Sheila Rothman, "Women's Clinics or Doctors' Offices: The Sheppard-Towner Act and the Promotion of Preventive Health Care," in *Social History and Social Policy*, ed. David J. Rothman and Stanton Wheeler (New York: Academic Press, 1981), pp. 175–201; Molly Ladd-Taylor, ed., *Raising a Baby the Government Way: Mothers' Letters to the Children's Bureau, 1915–1932* (New Brunswick, N.J.: Rutgers University Press, 1986); idem, "'Grannies' and 'Spinsters': Midwife Education Under the Sheppard-Towner Act," *Journal of Social History* 22 (Winter 1988): 255–75; Harvey Levenstein, "'Best for Babies' or 'Preventable Infanticide'? The Controversy over Artificial Feeding of Infants in America, 1880–1920," *The Journal of American History* 70 (1983): 75–94; Cone, *History of American Pediatrics*; Kathleen W. Smith, "Sentiment and Science: The Late Nineteenth-Century Pediatrician as Mother's Advisor," *Journal of Social History* 17 (1983): 97–114; and Sydney Halpern, *American Pediatrics: The Social Dynamics of Professionalism, 1880–1980* (Berkeley: University of California Press, 1988).

Somewhat more attention has been given to infant welfare in other countries. George D. Sussman discusses French infant welfare, albeit somewhat indirectly, in his *Selling Mother's Milk: The Wet-Nursing Business in France, 1715–1914* (Urbana: University of Illinois Press, 1982). Anthony S. Wohl devotes a chapter to English infant welfare in his *Endangered Lives: Public Health in Victorian Britain* (Cambridge: Harvard University Press, 1983). And Deborah Dwork provides an in-depth analysis in her *War Is Good for Babies and Other Children: A History of the Infant and Child Welfare Movement in England, 1898–1918* (London: Tavistock, 1987).

Moreover several monographs have been written analyzing public health policy and programs in regard to a host of specific diseases and health problems, including hookworm, pellagra, scurvy, poliomyelitis, tuberculosis, venereal disease, influenza, and cancer. And yet others have been written on public health campaigns to combat various environmental problems, ranging from insanitation to narcotics to pesticides. See: John Ettling, *Germ of Laziness: Rockefeller Philanthropy and Public Health in the New South* (Cambridge: Harvard University Press, 1981); Elizabeth W. Etheridge, *The Butterfly Caste: A Social History of Pellagra in the South* (Westport, Conn.: Greenwood, 1972); Kenneth J. Carpenter, *History of Scurvy and Vitamin C* (New York: Cambridge University Press, 1986); John R. Paul, *A History of Poliomyelitis* (New Haven, Conn.: Yale University Press, 1971); René and Jean Dubos, *The White Plague: Tuberculosis, Man, and Society* (New Brunswick, N.J.: Rutgers University Press, 1987); Michael E. Teller, *The Tuberculosis Movement: A Public Health Crusade in the Progressive Era* (Westport, Conn.: Greenwood, 1988); Mark Caldwell, *The Last Crusade: The War on Consumption, 1862–1954* (New York: Atheneum, 1988); Allan Brandt, *No Magic Bullet: A Social History of Venereal Disease in the United States Since 1880* (New York: Oxford University Press, 1985); Alfred W. Crosby, Jr., *Epidemic and Peace, 1918* (Westport, Conn.: Greenwood, 1976);

James T. Patterson, *The Dread Disease: Cancer and Modern American Culture* (Cambridge: Harvard University Press, 1987); Martin V. Melosi, *Garbage in the Cities: Refuse, Reform, and the Environment, 1880–1980* (College Station: Texas A & M University Press, 1982); Louis P. Cain, *Sanitation Strategy for a Lakefront Metropolis: The Case of Chicago* (Dekalb: Northern Illinois University Press, 1978); David F. Musto, *The American Disease: Origins of Narcotic Control* (New Haven, Conn.: Yale University Press, 1973); James Whorton, *Before Silent Spring: Pesticides and Public Health in Pre-DDT America* (Princeton: Princeton University Press, 1975).

17. The current tendency to make a sharp distinction between race and ethnicity was not one common to the late nineteenth and early twentieth centuries. Indeed, the line between race and ethnicity was quite blurred.

18. The difference between the U.S. approach to combating infant mortality and that adopted by the welfare and socialist states of Europe is less one of definition than of degree of support. As feminist analysts have correctly observed, a pronatalist approach to infant welfare (that is, one which is predicated on a nuclear family ideal and places primary responsibility for infant welfare on the individual mother) is fairly universal. Hence, the differences between the states reside in how comprehensive are their maternal support programs. See, for instance, Alena Hertlinger, *Reproduction, Medicine, and the Socialist State* (New York: St. Martins, 1987).

19. For a sample of the scholarly literature on reform and reform movements see: Robert Asch, *Social Movements in America* (Chicago: University of Chicago Press, 1972); Joseph Ambrose Banks, *The Sociology of Social Movements* (London: Macmillan, 1972); William Bruce Cameron, *Modern Social Movements: A Sociological Outline* (New York: Random House, 1986); Joseph R. Gusfield, ed., *Protest, Reform, Revolt* (New York: Wiley, 1970); Rudolph Heberle, *Social Movements* (New York: Appleton-Century-Crofts, 1951); Armand Moss, *Social Problems as Social Movements* (Philadelphia: Lippincott, 1975); Robert Walker, *Reform in America: The Continuing Frontier* (Lexington: University of Kentucky Press, 1985); and John Wilson, *Introduction to Social Movements* (New York: Basic Books, 1973).

20. Walker, *Reform in America,* p. 7.

21. Although the definition is essentially mine, it owes considerable debt to the large and constantly growing body of theoretical literature on history, culture, and discourse. Most notably, however, it owes a debt to the writings of David Hollinger, specifically his "Historians and the Discourse of Intellectuals," in *New Directions in American Intellectual History,* ed. John Higham and Paul K. Conkin (Baltimore: Johns Hopkins University Press, 1979), pp. 42–63; and to the collected essays in his work, *In the American Province: Studies in the History and Historiography of Ideas* (1985; Baltimore: Johns Hopkins University Press, 1989).

22. For an informative survey of the theories of discourse currently being employed by historians, see John E. Toews, "Intellectual History after the Linguistic Turn: The Autonomy of Meaning and the Irreducibility of Experience," *American Historical Review* 92 (1987): 879–907.

23. Moreover, as with medical evidence, I attempt to demonstrate that statistical evidence is at once both indeterminate and possessed of cumulative power. No single set of statistical data had the ability to still debate and produce consensus but combined and building on each other they did manage to push the discourse on infant mortality in certain directions.

24. I recognize and applaud the recent efforts of some medical and public health historians to reorient historical analysis away from practitioners and reformers and toward patients and reform targets. Judith Walzer Leavitt, for instance, has produced a study of childbirth from the perspective of women rather than from that of obstetricians and

obstetric reformers. Francis B. Smith and Anthony S. Wohl have written excellent and informative histories of public health in Victorian England which focus on the general populace rather than on reformers. Yet as Molly Ladd-Taylor has noted, doing so for infant welfare is exceptionally difficult because virtually all the surviving comments from late nineteenth- and early twentieth-century mothers are from those in the middle and upper classes. What we know about poor and working-class mothers comes primarily from the writings of charity workers and social scientists, or from those working-class women who have "risen" and wish to recall or make a political statement. Indeed, the only source for mothers' responses to infant welfare work may be the letters written to the Children's Bureau. While I employ these letters, they are of limited usefulness since virtually all were written after 1915. Judith Walzer Leavitt, *Brought to Bed: Childbearing in America, 1750–1950* (New York: Oxford University Press, 1986); Francis B. Smith, *The People's Health, 1830–1910* (London: Holmes and Meier, 1979); Wohl, *Endangered Lives;* Ladd-Taylor, *Raising a Baby the Government Way,* pp. 3–4.

25. For three thoughtful analyses of the positions, range, and implications of this debate, see Gerald Grob, "The Social History of Medicine and Disease in America: Problems and Possibilities," *Journal of Social History* 10 (1977): 391–409; L. J. Jordanova, "The Social Sciences and History of Science and Medicine," in *Information Sources in the History of Science and Medicine,* ed. Pietro Corsi and Paul Weindling (Boston: Butterworth, 1983), pp. 81–96; and Daniel M. Fox, "History and Health Policy: An Autobiographical Note on the Decline of Historicism," *Journal of Social History* 18 (1985): 349–64. See also Leonard G. Wilson, "Medical History without Medicine," *Journal of the History of Medicine and Allied Sciences* 35 (1980): 7; Morris J. Vogel, "Introduction," in *The Therapeutic Revolution: Essays in the Social History of American Medicine,* ed. Morris J. Vogel and Charles E. Rosenberg (Philadelphia: University of Pennsylvania Press, 1979), p. x; Paul Starr, *The Social Transformation of American Medicine* (New York: Basic Books, 1982), pp. 3–4.

26. W[illiam] F[arr], "History of the Medical Profession, and Its Influence on Public Health in England," *The Medical Annual, or, British Medical Almanack,* suppl. (1839), p. 113. Quoted in John Eyler, *Victorian Social Medicine: The Ideas and Methods of William Farr* (Baltimore: Johns Hopkins University Press, 1979), p. 3.

1. Cities as Infant Abattoirs:
Anglo-American Sanitary Reform and the Discovery of Urban Infant Mortality

1. *New York Times,* July 19, 1876, p. 4. Despite its use of the phrase "little children" the *Times* was referring to infants under one year of age. That it failed to be more exact illustrates the extent to which even in the latter half of the nineteenth century the language of age remained nebulous. The term *infant,* for example, though usually used to refer to a baby that was still nursing, was not limited to that. Carrying a connotation of dependency, it could be and often was used to refer to young children as old as five or six years. It is imperative to keep this in mind when confronted in the following pages with the various comments made by nineteenth-century public health reformers in regard to "infantile mortality." For a discussion on the fluidity of the language of age in the nineteenth century, see Joseph F. Kett, *Rites of Passage: Adolescence in America 1790 to the Present* (New York: Basic Books, 1977), pp. 11–14. See also Howard P. Chudacoff, *How Old Are You? Age in American Culture* (Princeton: Princeton University Press, forthcoming).

2. Irene B. Taeuber and Conrad Taeuber, *People of the United States in the Twentieth Century* (Washington, D.C.: U.S. Bureau of the Census, 1971), pp. 113–18; Ira Rosenwaike, *Population History of New York City* (Syracuse, N.Y.: Syracuse University Press,

1971), p. 16; Massachusetts Bureau of Statistics of Labor, *The Census of Massachusetts, 1885* (Boston: Wright and Potter, 1887), 1: xl; Howard P. Chudacoff, *The Evolution of American Urban Society* (Englewood Cliffs, N.J.: Prentice-Hall, 1975), p. 56.

3. On the making of nineteenth-century urban slums, see David Ward, "The Emergence of Central Immigrant Ghettos in American Cities, 1840–1920," in *Cities in American History*, ed. Kenneth T. Jackson and Stanley K. Shulz (New York: Knopf, 1972), pp. 164–76; for classic descriptions of the conditions prevailing in those slums, see Robert Ernst, *Immigrant Life in New York City, 1825–1863* (Port Washington, N.Y.: Ira J. Freedman, 1965); Oscar Handlin, *Boston's Immigrants: A Study of Acculturation*, rev. ed. (Cambridge: Harvard University Press, 1979), pp. 101–14; idem, *The Uprooted* (Boston: Little, Brown, 1951), pp. 155–56.

4. On the positive views of Americans toward city growth, see Thomas Bender, *Toward an Urban Vision: Ideas and Institutions in Nineteenth-Century America* (1975; Baltimore: Johns Hopkins University Press, 1982); on the negative views, see Morton and Lucia White, *The Intellectual Against the City: From Thomas Jefferson to Frank Lloyd Wright* (New York: Oxford University Press, 1962).

5. There were, of course, exceptions. New Orleans, a major commercial port and immigrant gateway, early experienced many of the same problems plaguing the northeastern cities and was, as a consequence, an early leader in the public health movement. Still, the ongoing prevalence of yellow fever in the city made New Orleans health officials somewhat more concerned with quarantine than with sanitary reform. Indeed, it was not until after 1880 that sanitary reform actually took root in New Orleans. See John Duffy, ed., *The Rudolph Matas History of Medicine in Louisiana* (Baton Rouge: Louisiana State University Press, 1962), pp. 160–97, 459–96. On the tardiness of other southern cities to embrace sanitary reform, see John Ellis, "Business and Public Health in the Urban South During the Nineteenth Century," *Bulletin of the History of Medicine* 44 (1970): 197–212, 346–71.

6. John Duffy, *A History of Public Health in New York City, 1625–1866* (New York: Russell Sage, 1968), p. 163; Barbara Gutmann Rosenkrantz, *Public Health and the State: Changing Views in Massachusetts, 1842–1936* (Cambridge: Harvard University Press, 1974), pp. 11–12.

7. In addition to helping found the American Statistical Association in 1839 and being the prime mover behind Massachusetts' pioneering 1842 vital registration act, Shattuck wrote the abstract of the 1845 Boston Census and the 1850 Report of the Sanitary Commission of Massachusetts. See Lemuel Shattuck, *Report to the Committee of the City Council Appointed to Obtain the Census of Boston for the Year 1845* (Boston, 1848); idem and others, *Report of the Sanitary Commission of Massachusetts, 1850* (facsimile ed.; Cambridge: Harvard University Press, 1948). For accounts of Shattuck's life and influence on the emergence of public health, see James H. Cassedy, *American Medicine and Statistical Thinking, 1800–1860* (Cambridge: Harvard University Press, 1984), pp. 194–98, passim; Rosenkrantz, *Public Health and the State*, pp. 14–23, passim. For an account of the emergence of statistics in antebellum America and their application to health matters, see Cassedy, *American Medicine and Statistical Thinking*. For an account of similar developments in England, see Michael J. Cullen, *The Statistical Movement in Early Victorian Britain: The Foundations of Empirical Social Research* (New York: Barnes and Noble, 1975).

8. Lemuel Shattuck, "The Vital Statistics of Boston, 1810–1841," *American Journal of Medical Sciences*, n.s. 1 (April 1841), 369–400; reprinted in *Bills of Mortality, 1810–1849, City of Boston* (Boston: Registry Department, 1893), pp. xxii, xxv, xxvi.

9. An eminent physician and committed social reformer, Griscom had helped found the New York Academy of Medicine, the New York Medical and Surgical Society, the New

York Home of Refuge and the Society for the Prevention of Pauperism. On Griscom and the history of his report, see Gert H. Brieger, "Sanitary Reform in New York City," *Bulletin of the History of Medicine* 40 (1966): 407–29; and Charles E. Rosenberg and Carrol Smith Rosenberg, "Pietism and the Origins of the American Public Health Movement: A Note on John H. Griscom and Robert H. Hartley," *Journal of the History of Medicine and Allied Sciences* 23 (1968): 18–19.

10. John H. Griscom, *The Sanitary Condition of the Laboring Population of New York* (New York: Harper and Bros., 1845).

11. For a summary of the English discourse and the conditions which inspired it, see M. W. Flinn, "Introduction," in Edwin Chadwick, *Report of the Sanitary Condition of the Labouring Population of Great Britain* [1842], ed. M. W. Flinn (Edinburgh: Edinburgh University Press, 1965), pp. 1–73. Also informative is George Rosen, *A History of Public Health* (New York: MD Publications, 1958), pp. 192–233.

12. Cullen, *The Statistical Movement*, pp. 135–47. For an early example of this argument, see Southwood Smith, *The Common Nature of Epidemics* (Philadelphia: Lippincott, 1866), p. 60.

13. Still the classic study of the English Public Health Movement is William Mowll Frazer, *A History of English Public Health, 1834–1939* (London: Balliere, Tindall, and Cox, 1950). Narrower but also superb are John W. Eyler, *Victorian Social Medicine: The Ideas and Methods of William Farr* (Baltimore: Johns Hopkins University Press, 1979); and Anthony S. Wohl, *Endangered Lives: Public Health in Victorian Britain* (Cambridge: Harvard University Press, 1983). Also a mine of information from one who was a major participant in the movement, is Sir John Simon, *English Sanitary Institutions* (London: Cassell, 1890).

14. Eyler, *Victorian Social Medicine*, pp. 125–30; Chadwick, *Report of the Sanitary Condition*, pp. 219–54.

15. Quoted in Samuel E. Finer, *The Life and Times of Sir Edwin Chadwick* (London: Methuen, 1952), p. 298.

16. My summary of Farr's zymotic theory is based on his comments in the fifth and sixth GRO reports. However, my ability to interpret and summarize those comments was immensely aided by the excellent discussion of Farr's etiological thinking in Eyler, *Victorian Social Medicine*, pp. 97–107.

17. See, for instance, "Diseases of Towns and the Open Air," *Boston Medical and Surgical Journal* 24 (1841), 26–29.

18. "First Report of the Committee on Public Hygiene," *Transactions of the American Medical Association* 2 (1849), 431–42.

19. On the early governmental centralization of English public health, see Jeanne L. Brand, *Doctors and the State: The British Medical Profession and Government Action in Public Health, 1870–1912* (Baltimore: Johns Hopkins Press, 1965), pp. 1–6.

20. For a discussion of the place of radical continental ideas in the English sanitary reform discourse, see John M. Eyler, "Mortality Statistics and Victorian Health Policy: Program and Criticism," *Bulletin of the History of Medicine* 50 (1976): 138–41.

21. On the pietistic roots of early public health reform, see Rosenberg and Rosenberg, "Pietism and the Origins of the American Public Health Movement." On the influence of moral philosophy, see Gerald Grob, *Edward Jarvis and the Medical World of the Nineteenth Century* (Nashville: University of Tennessee Press, 1978), pp. 15–16, 66–67. On that of Romantic self-perfectionism, see Rosenkrantz, *Public Health and the State*, pp. 10, 30–36.

22. New York City Board of Health, *Reports of Hospital Physicians* (New York, 1832), pp. 14–15, quoted in Charles E. Rosenberg, *The Cholera Years: The United States in 1832, 1849, and 1866* (Chicago: University of Chicago Press, 1962), p. 62.

23. Shattuck, "Vital Statistics of Boston," p. xxv. For a discussion of the tendency of nineteenth-century Americans to blame immigrants and immigration for the creation of slums and other urban problems, see Robert H. Bremner, *From the Depths: The Discovery of Poverty in the United States* (New York: New York University Press, 1956), pp. 7–11; and Rosenberg, *The Cholera Years,* pp. 61–64, 136–42, 181–83, passim.

24. Francis B. Smith, *The People's Health, 1830–1910* (New York: Holmes and Meier, 1979), p. 68.

25. "Infantile Mortality in New York," *New York Journal of Medicine and Surgery* 4 (1841), 454–55; Shattuck, "Vital Statistics of Boston," pp. xx–xxvi; Griscom, *The Sanitary Condition of the Laboring Population of New York,* pp. 4, 21.

26. "Mortality of Children in Great Britain," *Boston Medical and Surgical Journal* 54 (1856): 48.

27. D. Meredith Reese, "Report on Infant Mortality in Large Cities, the Sources of Its Increase and the Means of Its Diminution," *Transactions of the American Medical Association* 10 (1857): 102.

28. Smith, *People's Health,* p. 68; Southwood Smith quoted in Wilson G. Smillie, *Public Health: Its Promise for the Future* (New York: Macmillan, 1955), p. 243.

29. Shattuck, "Vital Statistics of Boston," p. xxiv; Griscom, *The Sanitary Condition of the Laboring Population of New York,* pp. 4, 21.

30. William Cadogan, *An Essay on the Nursing and Management of Children from Birth to Three Years of Age* (London, 1748), p. 7.

31. Dewees' *A Treatise on the Physical and Medical Treatment of Children* (Philadelphia: Carey and Lea, 1925) is generally considered the first major American pediatric text.

32. On the Romantic thrust of all antebellum American reform, see John L. Thomas, "Romantic Reform in America, 1815–1865," *American Quarterly* 17 (1965): 656–81; on the Romantic thrust of antebellum health reform, see Ronald G. Walters, *American Reformers, 1815–1860* (New York: Hill and Wang, 1978), pp. 145–72.

33. Alcott was one of antebellum America's best known "health writers." Probably the most popular and widely read of Alcott's many health manuals was *The House I Live In,* first published in 1834 and subsequently revised and reissued seventeen times over the course of the next twenty-three years. Also extremely popular was *The Laws of Health: or Sequel to the House I Live In,* first published in 1857.

34. William A. Alcott, "Mortality among Children," *Boston Medical and Surgical Journal* 54 (1855): 80–81.

35. Boston City Registrar, *Registration Report for 1855* (Boston, 1856), pp. 24–25.

36. "The Health Physician's Fourth Annual Report for the City of Buffalo, 1857," *Buffalo Medical Journal* 13 (1857–58): 700; "Herod in Our Homes," *New York Times,* August 31, 1859, p. 4.

37. Reese, "Report on Infant Mortality," p. 93.

38. Charles E. Rosenberg, "The Therapeutic Revolution: Medicine, Meaning, and Social Change in Nineteenth-Century America," in *The Therapeutic Revolution: Essays in the Social History of Medicine,* ed. Morris Vogel and Charles E. Rosenberg (Philadelphia: University of Pennsylvania Press, 1979), p. 5.

39. Ibid.

40. What follows is a condensation of popular and academic medical views held during the third quarter of the nineteenth century. It is based on no single source, but rather on a wide reading in academic medical texts, popular health manuals, and public health reports. For those interested in pursuing in greater depth the issues raised here, a good place to begin would be with Austin Flint's *A Treatise on the Principles and Practice of Medicine* (1869) and Job Lewis Smith's *A Treatise on the Disease of Infancy and Childhood* (1869),

which were, respectively, the most widely used and influential of the period's general medical and pediatric texts.

41. Cadogan, *An Essay,* p. 3.

42. William Buchan, *Domestic Medicine; Or the Family Physician,* 3d American ed. (Boston, 1778), p. ii.

43. William P. Dewees, *A Treatise on the Physical and Medical Treatment of Children,* 2d ed. (Philadelphia: Carey and Lea, 1826), p. xi.

44. Indeed, a pragmatic orientation—that is, a tendency to opt for what seemed possible given the prevailing social and political climate and the existing state of medical knowledge—remained a prime characteristic of American public health's approach to infant mortality through the twentieth century.

45. Boston City Registrar, *Registration Report for 1864* (Boston, 1865), p. 43.

46. Lemuel Shattuck, *Report . . . Census of Boston for the Year 1845,* p. 146.

47. Reese, "Report on Infant Mortality," p. 100.

48. The National Quarantine and Sanitary Convention, *Proceedings and Debates of the Third National Quarantine and Sanitary Convention* (New York, 1859), p. 526.

49. Citizen's Association of New York, *Sanitary Condition of the City: Report of the Council of Hygiene and Public Health of the Citizen's Association of New York,* 2d ed. (1866; New York: Arno Press, 1970), p. 64.

50. Jerome Walker, "Air for Babies," *Sanitarian* 2 (1874): 154–55.

51. Cadogan, *An Essay,* p. 55.

52. James P. Lynde, "Infantile Mortality: The Causes and Prevention," *Boston Medical and Surgical Journal* 105 (1882): 51.

53. Citizen's Association, *Sanitary Condition of the City,* p. xii.

54. Eyler, *Victorian Social Medicine,* p. 68; John H. Griscom, *Sanitary Legislation, Past and Future* (New York: New York Sanitary Association, 1861), p. 10.

55. Shattuck, for instance, contended that because it is biased by age composition, the crude death rate of a particular population is a "fallacious test of its sanitary condition." Shattuck, *Report of the Sanitary Commission,* p. 141.

56. Edwin Chadwick, "Address on Public Health," *Transactions of the National Association for the Promotion of Social Science* (1860): 580.

57. William Farr, "Mortality of Children in the Principal States of Europe," *Journal of the Statistical Society of London* 29 (1866): 15–18.

58. Edward Jarvis, "Infant Mortality," *Fourth Annual Report of the Massachusetts State Board of Health, 1873* (Boston, 1874), pp. 193–94.

59. New York City Department of Registry, *Annual Report for the Year Ending December 31, 1879* (New York, 1880), p. 212.

60. If not the first to use the statistic, the first to popularize it was the pioneering English demographer John Graunt. Using parish death records, Graunt in 1662 estimated the proportion dying at each age by calculating the percentage of age-specific deaths to all deaths. See John Graunt, *Natural and Political Observations Made upon the Bills of Mortality,* ed. Walter F. Wilcox (Baltimore: Johns Hopkins Press, 1939), pp. 4–5, 18. Other early English demographers, such as Sir William Petty and Gregory King, also adopted the statistic. Indeed, the common wisdom of the eighteenth century—that half of all humanity perished before reaching adulthood—was based on the use of this ratio. For a discussion of early perceptions on the extent of infant mortality, see Henry Seibert, "The Progress of Ideas Relating to the Causation and Control of Infant Mortality," *Bulletin of the History of Medicine* 8 (1940): 549–50.

61. For an analysis of fertility differentials by ethnicity in postbellum urban America, see Tamara K. Hereven and Maris A. Vinovskis, "Marital Fertility, Ethnicity, and Occupation in Urban Families: An Analysis of South Boston and the South End in 1880," in

Studies in American Historical Demography, ed. Maris A. Vinovskis (New York: Academic Press, 1979), pp. 481–506.

62. See, for instance, Appolino's comments on this in Boston City Registrar, *Registration Report for 1865* (Boston, 1866), p. 46.

63. One of the problems that arose in computing the figures for Table 1 was what to do with recorded infant deaths where parentage was unlisted. To eliminate them would have, I feared, greatly reduced the mortality rate of foreign-parented infants, since it seems logical that newly arrived and unacclimated immigrants would be the most likely to provide incomplete death data. This supposition also seems to be supported by the fact that 95 percent of the "parent unknowns" died in Boston, where the immigrant community was by far the largest. Consequently, I decided to add the unknown proportionately to the number of dead infants who had one or both parents foreign.

64. In 1772, for instance, Hugh Smith, using the ratio of infant and child deaths to all deaths, flatly declared that 65 percent of all children born in London died before the age of five years. Hugh Smith, *Letters to Married Women on Nursing and the Management of Their Children,* 1st American ed. (Philadelphia, 1792), p. vi.

65. On the correlation between immigration and urban mortality trends, see Richard A. Meckel, "Immigration, Mortality, and Population Growth in Boston, 1840–1880," *Journal of Interdisciplinary History* 15 (1985): 393–417; and Robert Higgs, "Cycles and Trends of Mortality in Eighteen Large American Cities, 1871–1900," *Explorations in Economic History* 16 (1979): 381–408.

66. On the 1870s origins of the late-nineteenth- and early-twentieth-century child welfare movement, see Richard A. Meckel, "Protecting the Innocents: Age Segregation and the Early Child Welfare Movement," *Social Service Review* 59 (1985): 455–75.

67. On nineteenth-century French efforts to protect infant life, see George D. Sussman, *Selling Mother's Milk: The Wet-Nursing Business in France, 1715–1914* (Urbana: University of Illinois Press, 1982), esp. pp. 121–29. On English efforts, see George K. Behlmer, "Deadly Motherhood: Infanticide and Medical Opinion in Mid-Victorian England," *Journal of the History of Medicine and Allied Sciences* 34 (1979): 403–27.

68. "Infanticide," *Boston Medical and Surgical Journal* 70 (1864): 66–67; *New York Times,* January 25, 1868, p. 2; ibid., February 2, 1868, p. 8.

69. *New York Times,* March 15, 1868, p. 2. One of the reasons that Madame Parselle's trial attracted so much attention was that it followed closely upon a similar and widely publicized trial of an English "baby farmer." Behlmer, "Deadly Motherhood," p. 426.

70. On the establishment of foundling hospitals and infant asylums, see Duffy, *Public Health in New York City, 1625–1866,* pp. 209–14; and Peter Romonovsky, "Saving the Lives of the City's Foundlings: The Joint Committee and New York City Child Care Methods, 1860–1907," *New York Historical Quarterly* 61 (1977): 49–68.

71. Abraham Jacobi, "On Foundlings and Foundling Institutions," *Medical Record* (1873): 481. The horrendous survival rate of committed infants was chiefly due to two causes: (1) the tendency of infant asylums to serve as incubators of disease and to facilitate its transmission; and (2) the generally poor physical condition of the infants committed.

72. Public health officials were not alone in realizing the provocative power and political usefulness of infant and child mortality rates. That realization was also shared by many of their allies in urban reform, especially Republican newspapers. The *New York Times,* for instance, never tired of citing infant and child mortality levels as proof of the corrupt callousness of Tammany Hall. See *New York Times,* June 29, 1873, p. 4; July 23, 1873, p. 8; July 12, 1875, p. 4; July 28, 1875, p. 4.

73. Jerome Walker, "Causes and Prevention of Infant Mortality," *Brooklyn Medical Journal* 4 (1890): 515.

74. Siebert, "The Progress of Ideas," pp. 546–52.

75. Shattuck, *Report of the Sanitary Commission,* p. 141.

76. Smith, *A Treatise,* pp. 23–27.

77. Henry Hartshorne, "Infant Mortality in Cities," *American Public Health Association: Papers and Reports* 2 (1874–75): 211.

78. H. B. Baker, "Infant Mortality in Michigan," ibid., pp. 139–40.

79. Joseph F. Kett, *Rites of Passage,* pp. 11–14; and Howard P. Chudacoff, *How Old Are You?*

80. Secretary of the Commonwealth of Massachusetts, *Registry and Returns of Births, Marriages, and Deaths in the Commonwealth for the Year Ending December 31, 1843* (Boston, 1844), p. 42.

81. Rose A. Cheney, "Seasonal Aspects of Infant and Childhood Mortality: Philadelphia, 1865–1920," *Journal of Interdisciplinary History* 14 (1984): 572.

82. Indeed, Rose Cheney has shown that mortality among urban children two to five years of age actually decreased during the summer. Ibid., p. 565.

83. See, for instance, *New York Times,* July 19, 1876, p. 4; July 9, 1879, p. 4.

84. William Clendenin, "The General Causes of Disease," *American Public Health Association: Papers and Reports* 1 (1873): 47.

85. Raymond Mohl, *The New City: Urban America in the Industrial Age, 1860–1920* (Arlington Heights, Ill.: Harlan Davidson, 1985), p. 88.

86. Duffy, *Public Health in New York City, 1625–1866,* pp. 221–25.

87. Roy Lubove, *The Progressives and the Slums: Tenement House Reform in New York City, 1890–1917* (Pittsburgh: University of Pittsburgh Press, 1962), pp. 8–11. For a recent and perceptive analysis of the reasons behind the failure of American cities to adopt effective public housing reforms during the late nineteenth and early twentieth centuries, see Howard P. Chudacoff, "Absence of Public Housing Policy in U.S. Cities, 1870–1935," paper presented at a symposium on Anglo-American public housing policy. University of Edinburgh, January 10, 1987.

88. On English housing reform, see Anthony S. Wohl, *The Eternal Slum: Housing and Social Policy in Victorian London* (London: Edward Arnold, 1977). On that in France and Germany, see Nicholas Bullock and James Read, *The Movement for Housing Reform in Germany and France* (Cambridge: Cambridge University Press, 1985); and Ann-Louise Shapiro, *Housing the Poor of Paris, 1850–1902* (Madison: University of Wisconsin Press, 1985).

89. Boston City Registrar, *Registration Report for 1870* (Boston, 1871), p. 38.

90. Quoted in Walker, "Causes and Prevention of Infant Mortality," p. 519.

91. It seems immaterial whether such was actually the case or whether, as some demographers suggest, it was the product of improved registration of infant deaths. Public health reformers responded to what they perceived the infant mortality rate to be, not to what it may have actually been.

92. New York City Department of Registry, *Registration Report, 1879,* p. 213.

93. Boston City Registrar, *Registration Report for 1879* (Boston, 1880), p. 4.

94. John Duffy, *A History of Public Health in New York City, 1866–1966* (New York: Russell Sage, 1974), pp. 71–72.

95. "Relief of the Sick Children of New York," *Sanitarian* 4 (1876): 327.

96. New York State Board of Health, *Annual Report for the Year Ending December 31, 1890* (Albany, 1891), pp. 11–14.

2. Improper Aliment:
American Pediatrics and Infant Feeding

1. L. Emmett Holt, "The Diarrheal Diseases, Acute and Chronic," in *Cyclopaedia of the Diseases of Children, Medical and Surgical*, 15 vols., ed. John M. Keating (Philadelphia: Lippincott, 1889–1899), 3: 63–64.

2. Edward Jarvis, "Infant Mortality," *Fourth Annual Report of the Massachusetts State Board of Health, 1873* (Boston, 1874), pp. 197–201.

3. Abraham Jacobi, *Infant Feeding and Infant Foods: The Anniversary Address Delivered before the New York State Medical Society, February 11, 1882* (Philadelphia, 1882).

4. In his 1869 general medical text, Austin Flint speculated that despite popular opinion, cholera infantum was not peculiar to the United States and noted that English physicians had long described a similar disease though they had called it, variously, watery gripes, weaning brash, and choleric fever. However, Flint did believe that the disease was more prevalent in the United States and suggested that this was primarily the result of the heat of its summers. Austin Flint, *A Treatise on the Principles and Practices of Medicine* (Philadelphia: Lea, 1869), p. 417.

Given the inferior quality of nineteenth-century nosological data, it is virtually impossible to determine with any accuracy whether or not American urban infants died more frequently from cholera infantum than did infants in the rest of the industrial West. If they did, however, it may well have been because of the heat of our summers: not because heat was a direct cause of the disease, but rather because there is a direct correlation between temperature and bacterial contamination of milk. This may have been accentuated by the fact that Americans tended to consume more raw milk than their English and continental counterparts. In 1900, for instance, the per capita annual consumption of milk by Philadelphians was 23 gallons whereas that of Londoners in 1892 was 11.5. Moreover, among the continental urban poor it was common practice to boil milk given to infants. And among the English urban poor, especially after 1860, the use of condensed milk for infant feeding was much more common than in the United States, where "loose" or "bulk" raw milk was the staple of artificially fed urban poor infants. For further discussion, see J. M. Eager, "Morbidity and Mortality as Influenced by Milk," in *Milk and Its Relation to Public Health*, rev. and enlarged, ed. Milton J. Roseneau (Washington, D.C.: U.S. Marine Hospital and Public Health Service, 1909), p. 235; M.W. Beaver, "Population, Infant Mortality, and Milk," *Population Studies* 27 (1973): 243–54.

5. John Duffy, *Epidemics in Colonial America* (Baton Rouge: Louisiana State University Press, 1953), pp. 214–22.

6. Benjamin Rush, *An Inquiry into the Case and Cure of the Cholera Infantum* (Philadelphia, 1777), cited in Thomas E. Cone, Jr., *History of American Pediatrics* (Boston: Little, Brown, 1979), p. 44.

7. For a nineteenth-century account of the symptoms and course of cholera infantum, see M. Trousseau, "A Few Words on Cholera Infantum," *Boston Medical and Surgical Journal* 60 (1857): 74–76.

8. John Gordon et al., "Acute Diarrheal Disease in Less Developed Countries and Epidemiological Basis for Control," *Bulletin of the World Health Organization* 31 (1964): 1–17; William Spivik, "Diarrhea," in *Pediatrics*, 3rd ed., ed. Mohsen Ziai (Boston: Little, Brown, 1984), pp. 286–92; Abraham M. Rudolph, ed., *Pediatrics*, 17th ed. (Norwalk, Conn.: Appleton-Century-Crofts, 1982), pp. 552, 615–16, 924.

9. Cone, *History of American Pediatrics*, pp. 205–8.

10. William P. Dewees, *Treatise on the Physical and Medical Treatment of Children*, 2d ed. (Philadelphia: Carey and Lea, 1826), pp. 353–56.

11. Cone, *History of American Pediatrics*, p. 81.

12. David Francis Condie, *A Practical Treatise on the Diseases of Children* (Philadelphia: Lea and Blanchard, 1844), p. 221.

13. "Infant Mortality," *Boston Medical and Surgical Journal* 58 (1858): 344–46.

14. J. Lewis Smith, *A Treatise on the Diseases of Infancy and Childhood* (Philadelphia: Lea, 1869), p. 26.

15. Idem, "Causes of the Great Mortality of Young Children in Cities During the Summer Season, and the Hygienic Measures Required for Prevention," in *The Sanitary Care and Treatment of Children and Their Diseases: Being a Series of Five Essays by Drs. Elizabeth Gault-Addison, Samuel Busey, A. Jacobi, J. Forsyth Meigs, and J. Lewis Smith* (Boston: Houghton Mifflin, 1881), p. 253.

16. Idem, *A Treatise*, p. 359.

17. Ibid., p. 360.

18. C.H.F. Routh, *Infant Feeding and Its Influence on Life: Or the Causes and Prevention of Infant Mortality* (London: John Churchill, 1860).

19. Eustace Smith, *On the Wasting Diseases of Infants and Children*, 2d American ed. (Philadelphia: Lea, 1871), p. 29.

20. Arthur Abt and Fielding H. Garrison, *The History of Pediatrics* (Philadelphia: Saunders, 1965), pp. 119–22.

21. Samuel X. Radbill, "A History of Children's Hospitals," *American Journal of the Diseases of Children* 90 (1955): 415–16.

22. A. Jacobi, "Claims of Pediatric Medicine," *Transactions of the American Medical Association* 31 (1880): 713. Interestingly, Jacob himself did not limit his practice to infants and children, but also treated adults and delivered babies. So too did Smith. Indeed, of the forty-three "pediatrists" who founded the American Pediatric Society in 1887, only two had practices exclusively devoted to children. Harold Kniest Faber and Rustin McIntosh, *History of the American Pediatric Society, 1887–1965* (New York: McGraw-Hill, 1966), pp. 7–8.

23. Cone, *History of American Pediatrics*, pp. 127–28; Faber and McIntosh, *American Pediatric Society*, p. 7. New and excellent, but unfortunately published after this chapter was written, is Sydney Halpern, *American Pediatrics: The Social Dynamics of Professionalism, 1880–1980* (Berkeley: University of California Press, 1988).

24. Still the classic study of the process of specialization in American medicine is George Rosen, *The Specialization of Medicine with Particular Reference to Ophthalmology* (New York: Froben, 1944). On the emergence of a culture of professionalism among the late nineteenth-century middle class, see Burton J. Bledstein, *The Culture of Professionalism: The Middle Class and the Development of Higher Education in America* (New York: W. W. Norton, 1976), esp. pp. 80–128.

25. On the development of age-specific educational and welfare policies, see Michael S. Shapiro, *Child's Garden: The Kindergarten Movement from Froebel to Dewey* (University Park: Pennsylvania State University Press, 1983), pp. 85–105; and Richard A. Meckel, "Protecting the Innocents: Age Segregation and the Early Child Welfare Movement," *Social Service Review* 59 (1985): 455–75.

26. Theodore von Escherereich, "The Foundation and Aims of Modern Pediatrics," *American Medicine* 9 (1905): 58.

27. L. Emmett Holt, *The Diseases of Infancy and Childhood: For the Use of Students and Practitioners of Medicine* (New York: D. Appleton, 1897), p. 31.

28. Abraham Jacobi, "Introductory," in Keating, *Cyclopaedia of the Diseases of Children*, 1: 2.

29. William Cadogan, *An Essay Upon the Nursing and Management of Children: From Birth to Three Years of Age* (London, 1748), p. 3.

30. Dewees, *A Treatise*, p. 64.

31. Abt and Garrison, *Pediatrics,* p. 122.

32. Thomas Morgan Rotch, "General Principles Underlying All Good Methods of Infant Feeding," *Boston Medical and Surgical Journal* 129 (1893): 506.

33. Luther Emmett Holt, *The Diseases of Infancy and Childhood: For Use of Students and Practitioners of Medicine,* 6th ed. (New York: D. Appleton, 1914), p. 122.

34. Harvey Levenstein, "'Best for Babies' or 'Preventable Infanticide'? The Controversy over Artificial Feeding of Infants in America, 1880–1920," *The Journal of American History* 70 (1983): 76.

35. Francis B. Smith, *The People's Health, 1830–1910* (New York: Holmes and Meier, 1979), pp. 88–89.

36. Hugh Smith, *Letters to Women on Nursing and the Management of the Children,* 1st American ed. (Philadelphia 1792), pp. 59–61; William Buchan, *Domestic Medicine: Or the Family Physician,* 3rd American ed. (Boston 1778), p. 18.

37. Andrew Combe, "Food for Infants at Birth," *The Mother's Assistant and Young Lady's Friend* (July, 1842): 175–76; Dewees, *A Treatise,* p. ix.

38. William A. Cornell, "Management of Infants," *The Mother's Assistant and Young Lady's Friend* (June, 1858): 121. On the role that maternal association periodicals played in disseminating information on infant and child management, see Richard A. Meckel, "Educating a Ministry of Mothers: Evangelical Maternal Associations, 1815–1860," *Journal of the Early Republic* 2 (1983): 403–23.

39. Routh, *Infant Feeding,* pp. 1–11, 40, 11.

40. Ibid., p. 115.

41. Abraham Jacobi, *Infant Diet: A Paper Read Before the Public Health Association of New York, May 8, 1873* (New York: G. P. Putnam's Sons, 1873). Jacobi's paper was revised and enlarged by Mary Putnam Jacobi and published the following year as Abraham Jacobi, *Infant Diet: Revised, Enlarged and Adopted for Popular Use by Mary Putnam Jacobi* (New York: G. P. Putnam, 1874).

42. Ibid., pp. 10–12.

43. Catherine Beecher, "Statistics of Female Health," in *The Oven Birds: American Women on Womanhood, 1820–1920,* ed. Gail Parker (Garden City, N.Y.: Anchor/Doubleday, 1972), p. 165.

44. On late nineteenth-century American physicians' views of female health, see Barbara Ehrenreich and Deirdre English, eds., *For Her Own Good: One Hundred Fifty Years of Experts' Advice to Women* (Garden City, N.Y.: Anchor/Doubleday, 1978), pp. 100–140.

45. Jacobi, *Infant Feeding: Revised,* p. 17.

46. Rotch, "The General Principles," p. 505.

47. See, for instance, Harmon Knox Root, *The People's Medical Lighthouse,* 8th ed. (New York: H. K. Root, 1854), p. 337.

48. Levenstein, "'Best for Babies,'" p. 76.

49. George T. Gream, *Remarks on the Diet of Children and On the Distinctions Between the Digestive Powers of the Infant and the Adult* (London: Longmans, 1847), p. 66.

50. Typical of that concern was this comment by a turn-of-the-century physician: "Even when fresh cow's milk is used, the differences in chemical composition between it and mother's milk so often set up functional disturbances of the stomach that digestion and absorption are rendered impossible." Nathan Oppenheim, *The Medical Diseases of Children* (New York: Macmillan, 1900), p. 214.

51. Cone, *History of American Pediatrics,* p. 134.

52. Elmer V. McCollum, *A History of Nutrition: The Sequence of Ideas in Nutrition Investigations* (New York: Houghton Mifflin, 1957), p. 92; Reay Tannahill, *Food in History* (New York: Stein and Day, 1973), pp. 345–46.

53. My discussion of artificial foods is much indebted to Levenstein, "'Best for

Babies' "; and Rima D. Apple, " 'How Shall I Feed My Baby?' Infant Feeding in the United States, 1870–1940" (Ph.D. diss., University of Wisconsin, 1981), pp. 1–40. Apple's dissertation, revised, has recently been published as *Mothers and Medicine: A Social History of Infant Feeding, 1890–1950* (Madison: University of Wisconsin Press, 1987).

54. As early as 1865, the *Boston Medical and Surgical Journal* published a report by *Lancet* endorsing Liebig's "soup for infants." See, "Baron Liebig's Soup for Children," *Boston Medical and Surgical Journal* 72 (1865): 141–42.

55. Quoted in Levenstein, " 'Best for Babies,' " p. 78.

56. Probably contributing to the popularity of proprietary foods was the growing concern of urbanites over the safety and quality of commercial milk supplies. See below, chapter 3.

57. Smith, *The People's Health*, pp. 92–93; Levenstein, " 'Best for Babies,' " pp. 78–79.

58. Prompting particular concern was the 1890s realization among physicians that they had for sometime been seeing cases of infantile scurvy or "Barrow's disease" as it was called. Since it seemed to be most pronounced among the middle class, physicians were quick to blame the increasing use of proprietary foods. For a discussion of the discovery of infantile scurvy and the resultant medical outcry over proprietary foods, see Kenneth J. Carpenter, *History of Scurvy and Vitamin C* (New York: Cambridge University Press, 1986), pp. 161–64. For a turn-of-the century attempt to link scurvy to types of feeding, see J.P.C. Griffith, C. G. Jennings, and J. L. Morse, "The American Pediatric Society's Investigation of Infantile Scurvy in North America," *Archives of Pediatrics* 15 (1898): 481–508.

59. Whether a proprietary food was nutritionally deficient depended on how it was processed and whether or not it was mixed with cow's milk. The nutritional quality of condensed milk also depended on how it was processed. Moreover, although probably not as dangerous as charged, condensed milk did contain a high level of sucrose which was difficult for infants to digest (indeed impossible for malnourished infants) and which created a dependency on sweet-tasting foods.

60. Rotch, "General Principles," p. 506.

61. Gream, *Remarks on the Diet*, p. 65.

62. Cone, *History of American Pediatrics*, p. 83.

63. Ibid., p. 134; Levenstein, " 'Best for Babies,' " p. 81.

64. Fritz Talbot, "Pediatric Profiles: Thomas Morgan Rotch," *Journal of Pediatrics* 49 (1956): 109–12.

65. Thomas Morgan Rotch, "The Artificial Feeding of Infants," *Archives of Pediatrics* 4 (1887): 459.

66. Apple, "How Shall I Feed My Baby?" p. 44.

67. Rotch, "The Artificial Feeding of Infants," pp. 458–80.

68. Ibid. Fitting the formula to the baby was essentially a process of trial and error. The percentage of each constituent element was changed ever so slightly until a mixture was found that the baby seemed to thrive upon.

69. Jacoby quoted in Cone, *History of American Pediatrics*, p. 138.

70. Quoted in Levenstein, " 'Best for Babies,' " p. 82.

71. A. H. Wentworth, "The Importance of Milk Analysis in Infant Feeding," *Boston Medical and Surgical Journal* 146 (1902): 683–86; and 147 (1903): 5–10.

72. Apple, "How Shall I Feed My Baby?" pp. 64–65.

73. Cone, *History of American Pediatrics*, p. 156; Minnie Ahrens, "Infant Welfare or Milk Stations," *Transactions of the American Association for Study and Prevention of Infant Mortality, 1911* (Baltimore: AASPIM, 1912), p. 288.

74. Levenstein, " 'Best for Babies,' " p. 84.

75. Cone, *History of American Pediatrics*, pp. 162–63.

3. Pure Milk for Babes:
Improving the Urban Milk Supply

1. Henry Hartshorne, "Infant Mortality in the Cities," *Public Health* 2 (1874): 214.

2. J. H. Mason Knox, "The Claims of the Baby in the Discussion of the Milk Question," *Charities and the Commons* 16 (1906): 493.

3. Norman Shaftel, "A History of the Purification of Milk in New York; or, 'How Now Brown Cow,'" in *Sickness and Health in America: Readings in the History of Medicine and Public Health*, ed. Judith Walzer Leavitt and Ronald J. Numbers (Madison: University of Wisconsin Press, 1978), pp. 275–80; John Duffy, *A History of Public Health in New York City, 1625–1866* (New York: Russell Sage, 1968), pp. 427–28; Robert M. Hartley, *An Historical, Scientific, and Practical Essay on Milk as an Article of Human Sustenance* (New York: J. Leavitt, 1842), pp. 305–6.

4. Hartley, *Essay on Milk*, pp. 310, 331–32.

5. Mitchell Okun, *Fair Play in the Market Place: The First Battle for Pure Food and Drugs* (Dekalb: Northern Illinois University Press, 1986), pp. 9–10.

6. See, for instance, John Mullaly, *The Milk Trade in New York and Vicinity* (New York: Fowler and Wells, 1853); and Hartley's study reissued as *The Cow and the Dairy* (New York, 1850). Newspapers also took up the issue again. See the *New York Tribune*, June 6, 1849; January 18, 1853; and the *New York Times*, March 9, 1854; August 18, 1854; September 7, 1857.

7. *Leslie's Illustrated*, May 8, 15, 22, July 17, August 7, October 9, 1858; March 5, July 9, September 3, 1859; April 6, 1861; March 22, July 5, 1862.

8. Okun, *Fair Play*, pp. 18–19. Actually, New York was not the site of the first anti-swill-milk legislation. Three years earlier, following a year-long debate among physicians and sanitarians, Massachusetts passed a law proscribing the sale and production of swill milk. Nevertheless, the New York law and the debate surrounding it served as the primary catalyst and model for those laws subsequently passed by other state legislatures. For a description of the Massachusetts law and other laws, see Arthur H. Nichols, "A Report on the Adulteration of Milk," *Fourth Annual Report of the State Board of Health, 1872* (Boston, 1873), pp. 300–301.

For a good illustration of the extent to which swill milk was still being sold and still eliciting concern among public health officials in the late nineteenth century, see the swill-milk series published in *Science* in 1887. Near the beginning of that year the editors sent a letter to most of the prominent public health advocates in the United States and Canada requesting their views on whether milk produced by cows fed on distillery swill was harmful to infant life. Over forty recipients of the letter responded and *Science* abstracted and published their comments in a serialized report that spread over several issues.

For a detailed account of a battle over swill milk that took place somewhat later and in a smaller midwestern city, see Judith Walzer Leavitt, *The Healthiest City; Milwaukee and the Politics of Health Reform* (Princeton: Princeton University Press, 1982), pp. 156–67.

9. Willard W. Cochrane, *The Development of American Agriculture: An Historical Analysis* (Minneapolis: University of Minnesota Press, 1979), p. 74; Eric E. Lampard, *The Rise of the Dairy Industry in Wisconsin: A Study of Agricultural Change, 1820–1920* (Madison, Wis.: the State Historical Society, 1963), pp. 59–63.

10. Percy W. Bidwell and John Falconer, *History of Agriculture in the Northern United States, 1620–1860* (Washington, D.C.: The Carnegie Institution, 1925), pp. 421–34; Mullaly, *The Milk Trade*, pp. 25–30; Fred Bateman, "The 'Marketable Surplus' in Northern Dairy Farming: New Evidence by Size of Farm in 1860," *Agricultural History* 52 (1978): 345–52.

11. By and of themselves dirt and manure are not inherently harmful. However, many

cows themselves were sick with diarrheal diseases, and thus the manure and mud that caked their flanks and udders were frequently contaminated with pathogens that in turn contaminated milk.

12. Leavitt, The Healthiest City, pp. 157–58.

13. While there seems little doubt that the skimming of cream and the addition of water were fairly common practices, some uncertainty exists as to the frequency of other adulterations. Okun suggests that little proof exists to support reformers' claims that market milk was a veritable witches' brew of sophisticants. The one exception, he admits, may have been the addition of bicarbonate of soda, which was an effective and inexpensive method for neutralizing the acidity—and therefore the telltale taste—of spoiled milk. Okun, Fair Play, pp. 116–19.

14. Horatio Newton Parker, City Milk Supply (New York: McGraw-Hill, 1917), pp. 229–30.

15. Quoted in Thomas E. Cone, Jr., History of American Pediatrics (Boston: Little, Brown, 1979), p. 142.

16. Again events in England helped awaken American interest in reforming an existing social condition. In 1850, Arthur Hill Hassell, a member of the Royal College of Surgeons, presented a paper reporting the results of his investigation into adulteration in the London coffee trade. Combining a scientific method of inquiry with sensational charges, Hassell's paper attracted a great deal of attention; and as a consequence, Hassell was approached by Thomas Wakely, the editor of Lancet, with the proposition that he conduct an in-depth investigation into food adulteration which would be sponsored by and published in the medical journal. Between 1851 and 1854 Hassell published in Lancet a series of shocking essays on food adulteration (which in 1855 he collected and published in book form as Food and Adulteration). The Hassell-Lancet investigations provoked widespread public indignation and led Parliament to sponsor its own investigations in 1855 and 1856 and subsequently to pass the Adulteration of Food Act of 1860. Both the investigations and the passing of the food law were widely reported in the American press. On Hassell and the parliamentary investigations, see Anthony S. Wohl, Endangered Lives: Public Health in Victorian England (Cambridge: Harvard University Press, 1983), p. 54; Okun, Fair Play, pp. 15–18.

17. Richard J. Hooker, Food and Drink in America: A History (Indianapolis: Bobbs-Merrill, 1981), pp. 212–13; Carl L. Alsberg, "Progress in Federal Food Control," in A Half Century of Public Health: Jubilee Historical Volume of the American Public Health Association, ed. Mazyck P. Ravenel (New York: American Public Health Association, 1921), p. 211.

18. "What We Eat," Harper's Weekly, January 25, 1879, p. 74.

19. Journal of The American Medical Association 1 (1883): 319.

20. John Duffy, A History of Public Health in New York City, 1866–1966, (New York: Russell Sage, 1974), p. 71.

21. On public health's adoption of the guise of scientific objectivity, see Barbara Gutmann Rosenkrantz, Public Health and the State: Changing Views in Massachusetts, 1842–1936 (Cambridge: Harvard University Press, 1974), pp. 74–96.

22. Okun, Fair Play, pp. 74–75.

23. Austin Flint, A Treatise on the Principles and Practices of Medicine (Philadelphia: Lea, 1869), p. 417. Flint's textbook went through several editions and revisions between 1869 and 1886, but included the comment on sophisticated milk in all of them.

24. J. Chesterton Morris, "The Milk Supply of Our Large Cities: The Extent of Adulteration and Its Consequences," The American Public Health Association: Reports and Papers 10 (1885): 251.

25. Okun, Fair Play, p. 197n; Rosenkrantz, Public Health and the State, p. 83n.

26. Those cities were Boston, Massachusetts; Providence, Rhode Island; Syracuse, Buffalo, Rochester, and New York, New York; Newark and Montclair, New Jersey; Pittsburgh and Philadelphia, Pennsylvania; Washington, D.C.; Detroit, Michigan; Chicago, Illinois; Milwaukee, Wisconsin; Topeka, Kansas; St. Louis, Missouri; Minneapolis, Minnesota; Nashville, Tennessee; Louisville, Kentucky; New Orleans, Louisiana; Denver, Colorado; and Los Angeles and San Francisco, California.

27. Prior to the 1890s, when more effective devices were developed, milk inspectors in the field had to rely on the lactometer. The lactometer was a device that supposedly could establish whether milk had been watered or not by measuring the specific gravity of the liquid, thereby determining the percentage of milk fats it contained. (Raw whole milk consists of approximately 87 percent water and 13 percent "solids," consisting of butterfat, casein or albumin (protein), milk sugar, and minerals. On average it has a specific gravity of 1.032; that is, a certain volume of milk weighs approximately 103.2 percent of what the same volume of water does.) However, since removing butterfat (which weighs 90 percent of what water does) raises the specific gravity of milk while adding water lowers it, the two processes carefully done in conjunction could provide a batch of skimmed and watered milk with the same specific gravity as unadulterated whole milk. Johan D. Frederiksen, *The Story of Milk* (New York: Macmillan, 1919), p. 18.

28. Parker, *City Milk Supply*, p. 373.

29. James A. Tobey, *Public Health Law: A Manual for Sanitarians* (Baltimore: Williams and Wilkins, 1926), p. 99; Joseph M. Kaestle, "The Chemistry of Milk," in *Milk and Its Relation to Public Health*, rev. and enlarged, ed. Milton J. Roseneau (Washington, D.C.: United States Marine Hospital and Public Health Service, 1909), p. 380.

30. Leavitt, *The Healthiest City*, pp. 173–74. Indeed, dominance of the milk market by large dealers soon followed, with the result that after 1910 there was rising concern over the "milk monopoly" and escalating milk prices. See, for instance, "The Cost of Milk," *Survey* 30 (1913): 386; "What Does Milk Cost?" *Independent* 74 (1913): 1208; and "Market Milk: How Farmers Are Driven Out of Business," *Current Opinion* 59 (1915): 355–56.

31. Milton J. Roseneau, "The Number of Bacteria in Milk and the Value of Bacteria Counts," in Roseneau, ed., *Milk and Its Relation to Public Health*, p. 435.

32. William H. Park, "The Great Bacterial Contamination of the Milk in Cities. Can It Be Lessened by the Action of Health Authorities?" *Journal of Hygiene* 1 (1901): 402.

33. George Rosen, *A History of Public Health* (New York: MD Publications, 1958), p. 287; Wilson G. Smillie, *Public Health: Its Promise for the Future* (New York: Macmillan, 1955), p. 360.

34. See J. K. Crellin, "The Dawn of the Germ Theory: Particles, Infection, and Biology," in *Medicine and Science in the 1860s: Proceedings of the Sixth British Congress on the History of Medicine*, ed. F.N.L. Poynter (London: Welcome Institute of the History of Medicine, 1968), pp. 57–76.

35. *Report of the Metropolitan Board of Health, 1867* (New York, 1868), p. 32.

36. Koch developed the gelatin tube method in 1875 and the solid plate method in 1883. For a brief but good description of his work and its implications, see Charles Singer and E. Ashworth Underwood, *A Short History of Medicine*, 2d ed. (New York: Oxford University Press, 1962), pp. 336–38.

37. Frederick P. Gorham, "The History of Bacteriology and Its Contribution to Public Health Work," in *A Half Century of Public Health*, pp. 77–79; Rosenkrantz, *Public Health and the State*, pp. 98–102.

38. Edward Hart, "The Influence of Milk in Spreading Zymotic Diseases," *Transactions of the International Medical Congress* 4 (1881): 491–544.

39. John W. Trask, "Milk as a Cause of Epidemics of Typhoid Fever, Scarlet Fever, and

Diphtheria," in Roseneau, ed., *Milk and Its Relation to Public Health*, pp. 25–92.

40. Although concern with protecting infants from the milk of cows with tuberculosis was central to milk reform, for the crucial decade between 1900 and 1910, considerable debate took place over whether humans could actually be infected with bovine tuberculosis. The debate began in 1901 when Koch, incorrectly interpreting the meaning of Theobold Smith's 1896 discovery of the different morphologies of human and bovine tuberculosis bacilli, publicly declared that the diseases each caused were distinct and therefore that humans were not susceptible to bovine tuberculosis. Because of Koch's reputation, his theory carried considerable weight, despite the fact that prevailing medical and public health opinion and most existing evidence seemed to contradict it. Indeed, it took epidemiologists a decade and a half to discredit it fully. For a discussion of the bovine tuberculosis debate, see Michael E. Teller, *The Tuberculosis Movement: A Public Health Crusade in the Progressive Era* (Westport, Conn.: Greenwood, 1988); and Mark Caldwell, *The Last Crusade: The War on Consumption, 1862–1954* (New York: Atheneum, 1988).

41. Trask, "Milk as a Cause of Epidemics," pp. 39–41.

42. "Typhoid Fever Spread: The Stamford Epidemic," *New York Times*, April 29, 1895, p. 4; "Epidemics Due to Careless Sanitary Methods," ibid., July 1, 1895, p. 4; "Bacteria and the Dairy," *Popular Science Monthly* 58 (1901): 559; D. S. Hanson, "Milk Contamination and How Best to Prevent It," *Scientific American* 52 (1901): 21339–40; and S. T. Rorer, "Lessons on Milk," *Ladies' Home Journal* 19 (1902): 26.

43. In particular, the typhoid bacillus and the common and nonpathogenic *B. coli* bacillus could not be morphologically distinguished nor differentiated from each other by the size and appearance of the colonies. See Singer and Underwood, *A Short History*, pp. 309–10.

44. Ernest C. Meyer, *Infant Mortality in New York City: A Study of the Results Accomplished by Infant Life-Saving Agencies, 1880–1920* (New York: The Rockefeller Foundation International Health Board, 1921), p. 19.

45. William D. Booker, *A Bacteriological and Anatomical Study of the Summer Diarrhea of Infants* (Baltimore: Johns Hopkins Press, 1896); Simon Flexner and L. Emmett Holt, eds. *Bacteriological and Clinical Studies of the Diarrheal Diseases of Infancy* (New York: Rockefeller Institute for Medical Research, 1904); Linnaeus E. La Fetra and John Howland, "A Clinical Study of Sixty-Two Cases of Intestinal Infection by the Bacillus Dysenteriae (Shiga) in Infants," *Medical News* 84 (1904): 481–86.

46. Booker, *A Bacteriological and Anatomical Study*, p. 91.

47. Charles E. North, "Milk and Its Relation to Public Health," in *A Half Century of Public Health*, p. 243; Herbert W. Conn, *The Fermentations of Milk* (Washington, D.C.: Government Printing Office, 1892).

48. Charles Chapin quoted in North, "Milk and Its Relation to Public Health," pp. 265–66.

49. William T. Sedgwick and John L. Batchelder, "A Bacteriological Examination of the Boston Milk Supply," *Boston Medical and Surgical Journal* 126 (1892): 25–28; Maud J. Frye, "Notes on the Estimation of the Number of Bacteria in Milk," *Medical Record* 2 (1896): 442; Park, "The Great Bacterial Contamination of the Milk in Cities," pp. 309–406; George W. Goler, "The Influence of the Municipal Milk Supply on the Deaths of Children," *New York Journal of Medicine* 6 (1903): 989–91.

50. Park, "The Great Bacterial Contamination of the Milk in Cities," p. 402.

51. James Curtis, "Infant Hygiene," in *A Treatise on Hygiene and Public Health*, 2 vols., ed. Alfred H. Buck (New York: W. Wood, 1879), 2: 293. Buck was also the American editor of Hugo von Ziemssen's twenty-volume *Cyclopaedia of the Practice of Medicine* (New York: W. Wood, 1874–81), of which his treatise constituted the last two volumes.

52. Roseneau, "The Number of Bacteria in Milk," pp. 429–30.

53. North, "Milk and Its Relation to Public Health," p. 283.

54. Massachusetts Association of Boards of Health, Journal 2 (1892): 30. Quoted in Manfred J. Waserman, "Henry Coit and the Certified Milk Movement in the Development of Modern Pediatrics," Bulletin of the History of Medicine 46 (1972): 359.

55. Milton J. Roseneau, "Pasteurization," in Roseneau, ed., Milk and Its Relation to Public Health p. 642.

56. Abraham Jacobi, "On the Improvement of the Condition of the Poor and Sick Children, in The Sanitary Care and Treatment of Children and Their Diseases: Being a Series of Five Essays by Drs. Elizabeth Gault-Addison, Samuel C. Busey, A. Jacobi, J. Forsyth Meigs, and J. Lewis Smith (Boston: Houghton Mifflin, 1881), p. 175. The following year Jacobi chaired a special committee of the New York State Medical Society that recommended the establishment of depots where poor children could be supplied with food. Medical Record 21 (1882): 14–15.

57. Lina Gutherz Straus, Disease in Milk: The Remedy, Pasteurization, The Life Work of Nathan Straus, 2d ed. (New York: E. P. Dutton, 1917), pp. 75–77.

58. Ibid., p. 79; Joseph W. Schereshewsky, "The Present Status of Infant Welfare Work in the United States," Transactions of the American Association for Study and Prevention of Infant Mortality, 1911 (Baltimore: AASPIM, 1912), 40–43.

59. George W. Goler, "Municipal Milk Work in Rochester," Charities and the Commons 16 (1906): 484–87.

60. Duffy, Public Health in New York City, 1866–1966, p. 258; Mrs. W. H. Barton, "The Work of Infant Milk Stations in Relation to Infant Mortality," Transactions of the American Association for Study and Prevention of Infant Mortality, 1911, pp. 299–300.

61. Rosenkrantz, Public Health and the State, pp. 108–110. Bartley, a steadfast and articulate critic of milk purification, repeatedly railed against it "as best an apology for dirty milk." Goler, who originally favored purifying milk, came to agree and advocated in its place the improvement of methods on the average dairy. See Elias Bartley, "Some Causes of Infant Mortality in Nurseries and Asylums," American Public Health Association: Reports and Papers 27 (1901): 306–13; and Goler, "Municipal Milk Work," p. 486.

62. The process and temperatures described here are that of "batch" pasteurization of regular milk. Liquids with higher sugar contents (e.g., chocolate milk) demand higher temperatures. Also commonly used is "continuous" pasteurization, in which milk is run continuously through heated pipes and raised to 161°F (71.7°C) for 15 seconds.

63. Ernest Kelly and Clarence E. Clement, Market Milk (New York: John Wiley and Sons, 1923), p. 281.

64. Abraham Jacobi, quoted in North, "Milk and Its Relation to Public Health," p. 271.

65. Cone, History of American Pediatrics, p. 141.

66. Arthur V. Meigs, Feeding in Early Infancy (Philadelphia: Saunders, 1896), p. 75.

67. Rowland G. Freeman, "Should All Milk Used for Infant Feeding Be Heated for the Purpose of Killing Germs?" Transactions of the American Pediatric Society 10 (1898): p. 35.

68. Cone, History of American Pediatrics, p. 246.

69. Although the following section on milk certification is based on a number of different sources, I am most indebted to Waserman, "Henry Coit," pp. 359–90; and Clarence Bronson Lane, Medical Milk Commissions and the Production of Certified Milk in the United States (Washington, D.C.: Government Printing Office, 1908).

70. Henry L. Coit, "The Origin, General Plan, and Scope of Medical Milk Commissions," Proceedings of the American Association of Medical Milk Commissions (1907), pp. 11–12; Waserman, "Henry Coit," pp. 362–63.

71. Waserman, "Henry Coit," pp. 365–68.

72. North, "Milk and Its Relation to Public Health," p. 268.

73. Roseneau, "Pasteurization," p. 642.

74. Henry L. Coit, *A Plan to Secure Cow's Milk Designed for Clinical Purposes* (Newark, N.J.: L. J. Hardham, 1893).

75. Quoted in Waserman, "Henry Coit," p. 383.

76. Leslie Lunsden, "The Milk Supply in Relation to the Epidemiology of Typhoid Fever," in Roseneau, ed., *Milk and Its Relation to Public Health*, p. 164.

77. The higher grades of milk were now being sold in sealed bottles. Henry Hemholz, "The Pasteurization, Sterilizing, and Boiling of Milk," *Transactions of the American Association for Study and Prevention of Infant Mortality, 1912* (Baltimore: AASPIM, 1913), p. 208.

78. Nathan Straus quoted in Lena Straus, *Disease in Milk*, p. 31.

79. Throughout his long career, Jacobi insisted that medical problems were essentially social problems and therefore could not be rectified with narrow medical solutions, a view that he probably developed early. As a young medical student in Germany, he was part of the circle of medical democrats who surrounded Rudolf Virchow in the heady revolutionary days of the late 1840s. Indeed, Jacobi ended up in the United States because he was forced to flee Germany following the failure of the liberal-nationalist revolution of 1848.

80. Abraham Jacobi, "The Role of Pure Cow's Milk in Infant Feeding," *Charities and the Commons* 16 (1906): 505.

81. *National Encyclopedia of American Biography* (1956), s.v. "Knox, J.[ames] H.[all] Mason, Jr."

82. Knox, "The Claims of the Baby in the Discussion of the Milk Problem," pp. 492–95.

83. North, "Milk and Its Relation to Public Health," p. 272; Roseneau, "Pasteurization," pp. 647–51; Cone, *History of American Pediatrics*, pp. 123–24; J. P.C. Griffiths, C. G. Jennings, J. L. Morse, "The American Pediatric Society's Collective Investigation of Infantile Scurvy in North America," *Archives of Pediatrics* 15 (1898): 481–508.

84. H. W. Conn and W. M. Esten, "The Effect of Different Temperatures in Determining the Species of Bacteria Which Grow in Milk," Storrs Agricultural Experiment Station, *Annual Report, 1904*, pp. 27–88; U.S. Marine Hospital and Public Health Service, *Thermal Death Points of Pathogenic Micro-organisms in Milk*, by Milton J. Roseneau (Washington, D.C.: Government Printing Office, 1906). A synopsis can be found in Roseneau, ed., *Milk and Its Relation to Public Health*, pp. 683–86.

85. Rowland G. Freeman, "The Reduction of Infant Mortality in the City of New York and the Agencies Which Have Been Instrumental in Bringing It About," *Medical News* 83 (1903): 433–34; William H. Park and L. Emmett Holt, "Report upon the Results with Different Kinds of Pure and Impure Milk in Infant Feeding in Tenement Houses and Institutions of New York City: A Clinical and Bacteriological Study," *Archives of Pediatrics* 20 (1903): 881–1909.

86. Roseneau, "Pasteurization," p. 665.

87. Parker, *City Milk Supply*, p. 269.

88. Ibid., p. 313; Kelly and Clement, *Market Milk*, p. 288.

89. One reason for this may be that the regulations gradually abolished the horribly unsanitary practice of selling milk in loose form.

90. Rose A. Cheney, "Seasonal Aspects of Infant and Child Mortality: Philadelphia, 1865–1920," *Journal of Interdisciplinary History* 14 (1984): 565.

91. Meyer, *Infant Mortality in New York City*, pp. 11, 17–21.

4. A Question of Motherhood

1. Patricia Mooney Melvin, "Milk to Motherhood: The New York Milk Committee and the Beginning of the Well-Child Programs," *Mid-America* 65 (October, 1983): 120; Charles R. Henderson, "Infant Morbidity and Mortality with Special Reference to

French Methods," in *The Prevention of Infant Mortality: Being the Papers and Discussion of a Conference Held in New Haven, Conn., November 11, 12, 1909* (Philadelphia: The American Academy of Medicine, 1910), pp. 81–94; Edward Bunnell Phelps, "The World-wide Effort to Diminish Infant Mortality—Its Present Status and Its Possibilities," *Transactions of the Fifteenth International Congress On Hygiene and Demography, 1912*, 6 vols. (Washington, D.C.: Government Printing Office, 1913), 6: 137; George F. McCleary, "The Infants' Milk Depot: Its History and Function," *Journal of Hygiene* 4 (1904): 329–68.

2. Wilbur C. Phillips, "The Mother and the Baby," *Survey* 22 (1909): 624.

3. Idem, "A Plan for Reducing Infant Mortality in New York City," *Medical Record* 73 (1908): 890–94; Melvin, "Milk to Motherhood," p. 121.

4. "To Reduce Infant Mortality," *Charities and the Commons* 20 (1908): 285–86.

5. Charles Chapin, "Municipal Sanitation," *American Journal of Public Hygiene* 18 (1908): 467.

6. L. Emmett Holt, "The Medical Prevention of Infant Mortality," *Transactions of the American Association for Study and Prevention of Infant Mortality, 1910* (Baltimore: AASPIM, 1911), p. 204.

7. Edward Bunnell Phelps, quoted in Ira S. Wile "Health and the Nations," *Survey* 29 (1912): 151.

8. "Report of the Executive Secretary," *Transactions of the American Association for Study and Prevention of Infant Mortality, 1912* (Baltimore: AASPIM, 1913), p. 19.

9. *Congress on Hygiene and Demography, 1912*, 6: 52–55; Josephine Baker, "Reduction of Infant Mortality in New York City," *American Journal of the Diseases of Children* 5 (1913): 159. For an illustration of the new classification system, see U.S. Department of Commerce and Labor, Bureau of the Census, *Mortality Statistics, 1900–1904* (Washington, D.C.: Government Printing Office, 1906), pp. cc–cci.

10. Rose A. Cheney, "Seasonal Aspects of Infant and Childhood Mortality: Philadelphia, 1865–1920," *Journal of Interdisciplinary History* 14 (1984): 573; Baker, "Reduction of Infant Mortality," p. 155.

11. Arthur Newsholme, *Fifty Years in Public Health: A Personal Narrative with Comments* (London: George Allen and Unwin, 1935), p. 347–48.

12. Phillips, "A Plan for Reducing Infant Mortality," p. 892; Jane Lewis, *The Politics of Motherhood: Child and Maternal Welfare in England, 1900–1939* (London: Croom Helm, 1980), p. 65.

13. O. H. Peters "Observations upon the Natural History of Epidemic Diarrhoea," *Journal of Hygiene* 10 (1910): 609–11.

14. J. F. Soothill, "Immunological Aspects of Infant Feeding," in *Pediatric Immunology*, ed. J. F. Soothill, A. R. Hayward, and C. B. S. Wood (Oxford: Blackwell, 1983), p. 114.

15. Peters, "Epidemic Diarrhoea," pp. 621–27, 656; C. W. Hutt, "A Study of Summer Diarrhoea in Warrington, 1911," *Journal of Hygiene* 13 (1913–14): 422–32.

16. In pointing to fecal contamination, early twentieth-century researchers were probably correct. Acute gastritis is highly infectious, and sick infants especially pass large numbers of pathogens in their feces. Contaminating bed sheets, diapers, clothes, and the hands of family members, pathogens are easily transmitted to food. Peters, "Epidemic Diarrhoea," pp. 624–27; Arthur Newsholme, *Fifty Years in Public Health*, pp. 326, 347–60; idem, "A Contribution to the Study of Epidemic Diarrhoea," *Public Health* 12 (1899): 139–213; idem, "Domestic Infection in Relation to Epidemic Diarrhoea," *Journal of Hygiene* 6 (1906): 139–48.

17. Newsholme, *Fifty Years in Public Health*, p. 323.

18. Newsholme's chief opponent in the domestic versus farm contamination debate was Sheridan Delepine, professor of Pathology and director of the Public Health Laboratory at Owens College in Manchester. In studying several outbreaks of epidemic diarrhea, De-

lepine was able to trace those epidemics to milk contaminated on the farm with cow manure containing *E. coli* bacilli. He reported his findings in S. Delepine, "The Bearing of Outbreaks of Food Poisoning upon the Etiology of Epidemic Diarrhoea," *Journal of Hygiene* 3 (1903): 68–91.

19. Newsholme, "Domestic Infection," p. 144; idem, *Fifty Years in Public Health,* p. 348.

20. Abraham Jacobi, quoted in William H. Davis, "Statistical Comparison of the Mortality of Breast-fed and Bottle-fed Infants," *Congress on Hygiene and Demography, 1912,* 6: 185.

21. The debate over maternal employment was most heated in England, and the chief English critic of such employment was George Reid, the medical officer of health of Staffordshire. Beginning in the early 1890s Reid conducted and published a series of studies purporting that when all other factors were the same, employment of mothers revealed itself to be detrimental to infant survival. For a summary of Reid's arguments, see his "Infant Mortality in Relation to Factory Labor," *Congress on Hygiene and Demography, 1912,* 3: 943–46. For a discussion of the overall debate, see Carol Dyhouse, "Working-class Mothers and Infant Mortality in England, 1895–1914," *Journal of Social History* 12 (1978): 251–57.

22. As early as 1859, England's John Simon declared to the Privy Council:

The extensive factory employment of female labour is a sure source of very large infantile mortality, both diarrhoeal and convulsive; that where mothers are engaged in factories, infants who should be at the breast are commonly ill-fed or starved, and have their cries of hunger and distress quieted by those fatal opiates which are in such request at the centre of our manufacturing industry.

John Simon, quoted in Anthony S. Wohl, *Endangered Lives: Public Health in Victorian Britain* (Cambridge: Harvard University Press, 1983), p. 26.

23. U.S. Department of Labor, Children's Bureau, *Maternity Benefit Systems in Certain Foreign Countries,* by Henry J. Harris (Washington, D.C.: Government Printing Office, 1919), pp. 21, 31, 38, 49, 67, 121, 153; idem, *Infant Welfare Work in Europe,* by Nettie McGill (Washington, D.C.: Government Printing Office, 1921), pp. 16, 82; U.S., Congress, Senate, *Report on the Condition of Women and Child-Wage Earners in the United States,* 61st Cong., 2d sess., S. Doc. 645, vol. 13: *Infant Mortality and Its Relation to the Employment of Mothers, Part 1, A Study of Massachusetts,* by Edward Bunnell Phelps (Washington, D.C.: Government Printing Office, 1912), pp. 48–49, 72–74.

24. George Newman, *Infant Mortality: A Social Problem* (London: Methuen, 1906), pp. 217–25.

25. Ibid., p. vi.

26. Ibid., p. 221.

27. Ibid., p. 257. The idea was not original to Newman, however. B. Seebohm Rowntree, in his classic study of poverty in York, had earlier declared, "the high general [infant mortality] rate is chiefly due to ignorance of the feeding and management of infants rather than causes arising out of the poverty of the people." B. Seebohm Rowntree, *Poverty: A Study of Town Life,* (London: Macmillan, 1901), p. 207.

28. George F. McCleary, *The Early History of the Infant Welfare Movement* (London: H. K. Lewis, 1933), p. 35.

29. For a recent discussion of the ways in which various national maternal and infant health programs are similar in ideology but different in degree of support, see Alena Hertlinger, *Reproduction, Medicine, and the Socialist State* (New York: St. Martins, 1987).

30. McCleary, *Early History,* pp. 14–15.

31. Newsholme, *Fifty Years in Public Health*, p. 321; Daniel J. Kevles, *In the Name of Eugenics: Genetics and the Uses of Human Heredity* (New York: Knopf, 1985), p. 72.

32. George D. Sussman, *Selling Mothers' Milk: The Wet-Nursing Business in France, 1715–1914* (Urbana: University of Illinois Press, 1982), p. 7.

33. John Spargo, *The Common Sense of the Milk Problem* (New York: Macmillan, 1908), pp. 2–3. See also Irving Fisher, "On the Duty of a Nation to Its Potential Citizens," *Transactions of the American Association for Study and Prevention of Infant Mortality, 1910,* p. 40; M. Jusserand, "Some Checks on Infant Mortality," ibid., pp. 33–34; Mc-Cleary, *Early History,* p. 12.

34. Newsholme, *Fifty Years in Public Health*, p. 330. See also H. Lewellyn Heath, *The Infant, the Parent, and the State* (London: P. S. King and Son, 1907), pp. 45–46. Similarly, McCleary stated categorically that "it was largely from the fear of depopulation that public interest in infant welfare began." See George F. McCleary, *The Maternity and Child Welfare Movement* (London: P. S. King and Son, 1935), p. 8.

35. Francis B. Smith, *The People's Health, 1830–1900* (New York: Holmes and Meier, 1979), p. 118; Lewis, *The Politics of Motherhood,* pp. 15, 27.

36. New York Milk Committee, *Fifth Annual Report, 1911* (New York, 1912), p. 4.

37. On the early child welfare movement, see Richard A. Meckel, "Protecting the Innocents: Age Segregation and the Early Child Welfare Movement," *Social Service Review* 59 (1985): 455–75. On Progressive child welfare, see Susan Tiffin, *In Whose Best Interest? Child Welfare Reform in the Progressive Era* (Westport, Conn.: Greenwood, 1982).

38. Robert H. Wiebe, *The Search for Order, 1877–1920* (New York: Hill and Wang, 1967), p. 169.

39. Edward T. Devine, *Misery and Its Causes* (New York: Macmillan, 1910), p. 244.

40. See, for example, Felix Adler, "The Attitude Toward the Child as an Index of Civilization," *Annals of the American Academy of Political and Social Science* 29 (1907): 135–40; and Edward T. Devine, "The New View of the Child," *Proceedings of the Fourth Annual Meeting of the National Labor Committee, 1907* (Philadelphia: The American Academy of Political and Social Science, 1908), pp. 4–10.

41. Public and official concern with demographic conditions rarely remains constant, even when those conditions do. Rather it surges, ebbs, and surges, as conditions are highlighted, forgotten, and highlighted again. For an analysis of this process in a currently "rediscovered" social problem, see Barbara J. Nelson, *Making an Issue of Child Abuse: Political Agenda Setting for Social Problems* (Chicago: University of Chicago Press, 1984).

42. "The German Exposition on Infant Mortality," *Charities and the Commons* 17 (1906): 111–12.

43. The recorded increase in English infant mortality during the last quarter of the century may have been due significantly to improved death registration following reform of the registration law in 1876. Early twentieth-century infant welfare activists were aware of this possibility but tended to discount it. For a discussion of their reasons, see McCleary, *The Maternity and Child Welfare Movement,* pp. 8–12.

44. McCleary, *Early History,* p. 112.

45. U.S. Department of Interior, Census Office, *Report on Vital and Social Statistics in the United States at the Eleventh Census: 1890,* by John S. Billings (Washington, D.C.: Government Printing Office, 1896), pp. 7–9.

46. By 1933 the death registration area included 100 percent of the population. On the history and development of the area, see U.S. Department of Health, Education and Welfare, National Office of Vital Statistics, *Vital Statistics of the United States, 1950,* 2 vols. (Washington, D.C.: Government Printing Office, 1954), 1: 12–14.

47. U.S. Department of Interior, Census Office, *Twelfth Census of the United States:*

1900 (Washington, D.C.: Government Printing Office, 1902), 3: 286–564.

48. On the creation of the census bureau and its mandate to compile and publish data on mortality, see A. Ross Eckler, *The Bureau of the Census* (New York: Praeger, 1972), pp. 9–10.

49. Phelps, "The World-wide Effort," pp. 138, 142, 154–56.

50. McCleary, *Early History,* pp. 99–103, 133.

51. "Infant Mortality in American Cities: A Symposium," *Annals of the American Academy of Political and Social Science* 31 (1908): 484–94; Melvin, "Milk to Mother-hood," pp. 116–120.

52. Edward Thompson Caswell, *Reform in Medical Education: The Aim of the Acade-my* (Philadelphia: The American Academy of Medicine, 1889). Shortly after the 1909 conference the academy changed the name of its journal from the *Bulletin of the American Academy of Medicine* to the *Journal of Sociologic Medicine.* Despite its influence and socially progressive orientation, until recently the AAM had all but escaped the attention of medical historians. For the only scholarly treatment of the organization, see Steven J. Peitzman, "Forgotten Reformers: The American Academy of Medicine," *Bulletin of the History of Medicine* 58 (Winter 1984): 516–28.

53. Ernest K. Thomas, *A Brief Sketch of the Life of Helen C. Putnam* (Providence: privately printed, 1948), pp. 1–7. Putnam's election to the presidency of the AAM has special historical significance, for it took place at a time when, according to Mary Roth Walsh and other medical historians, women physicians were being increasingly excluded from the organizational power structure of American medicine. See Mary Roth Walsh, *"Doctors Wanted: No Women Need Apply": Sexual Barriers in the Medical Profession, 1835–1975* (New Haven: Yale University Press, 1977), pp. 213–14.

54. *The Prevention of Infant Mortality,* p. 3.

55. Newsholme, *Fifty Years in Public Health,* pp. 144–50, 347–60; Thomas, *Life of Helen Putnam,* pp. 6–8.

56. *Prevention of Infant Mortality,* p. 3.

57. *National Encyclopedia of American Biography* (1956), s.v. "Knox, J.[ames] H.[all] Mason, Jr.."

58. On Folks, see Walter I. Trattner, *Homer Folks: Pioneer in Social Welfare* (New York: Columbia University Press, 1968).

59. Charles-Edward Amory Winslow, *The Evolution and Significance of the Modern Public Health Campaign* (New Haven: Yale University Press, 1923), pp. 57–59.

60. *The Prevention of Infant Mortality,* p. 313.

61. Harold M. Cavins, *National Health Agencies: A Survey with Especial Reference to Voluntary Agencies* (Washington, D.C.: Public Affairs Press, 1945), pp. 11–12. Still the most complete work on the organization and evolution of the AMA is James G. Burrow, *AMA: Voice of American Medicine* (Baltimore: Johns Hopkins Press, 1963). It should, however, be supplemented by his *Organized Medicine and the Progressive Era: The Move Toward Monopoly* (Baltimore: Johns Hopkins University Press, 1977); and by Oliver Garceau, *The Political Life of the American Medical Association* (Cambridge: Harvard University Press, 1941).

62. Richard H. Shryock, *National Tuberculosis Association, 1904–1954: A Study of the Voluntary Health Movement in the United States* (New York: National Tuberculosis Association, 1957), p. 182n.

63. *Prevention of Infant Mortality,* p. 333. A number of AASPIM's founders (for instance, William H. Welch and Homer Folks) had also been founders of NASPT.

64. Charles R. Henderson, "Address of the President for 1911," *Transactions of the American Association for Study and Prevention of Infant Mortality, 1910,* pp. 17–18.

65. J. H. Mason Knox, "Address of the President," ibid., p. 30.

66. Edward Bunnell Phelps, "A Statistical Study of Infant Mortality's Call for Action," ibid., pp. 165–70.

67. Created in 1915, the birth registration area grew to encompass all the states by 1933. On its origin and development, see *Vital Statistics of the United States, 1950*, 1: 12–14; and Sam Shapiro, "Development of Birth Registration and Birth Statistics in the United States," *Population Studies* 4 (June 1950): 86–111.

68. Julia C. Lathrop, "The Federal Children's Bureau," *Transactions of the American Association for Study and Prevention of Infant Mortality, 1912* (Baltimore: AASPIM, 1913), p. 47.

69. At AASPIM's 1910 meeting it was decided to focus on enforcing existing registration laws rather than lobby for new ones since all major American municipalities and fifteen states had fully adequate birth registration statutes. As in other areas of public health, the problem was less the lack of rules and regulations than the unwillingness of state legislatures and city councils to appropriate funds for the enforcement of those rules and regulations.

70. U.S. Department of Labor, Children's Bureau, *Birth Registration: An Aid in the Lives and Rights of Children* (Washington, D.C.: Government Printing Office, 1913), p. 9.

71. William H. Welch, "Address," *Transactions of the American Association for Study and Prevention of Infant Mortality, 1910*, p. 52.

72. Knox, "Address of President," p. 30. In 1910, for instance, 55,504 people (of whom 1,918 were infants) died from lumbular tuberculosis. In the same year, 111,687 infants died in the first year of life and another 26,722 died in the second year. U.S. Department of Commerce and Labor, Bureau of the Census, *Mortality Statistics, 1900–1904* (Washington, D.C.: Government Printing Office, 1906), p. 82.

73. "Report of the Executive Secretary," *Transactions of the American Association for Study and Prevention of Infant Mortality, 1912*, pp. 15–17.

74. "Report of the Executive Secretary," *Transactions of the American Association for Study and Prevention of Infant Mortality, 1914* (Baltimore: AASPIM, 1915), p. 27.

75. "Reports of the Affiliated Associations," *Transactions of the American Association for Study and Prevention of Infant Mortality, 1910, 1912, 1914*.

76. "Report of the Executive Secretary," *Transactions of the American Association for Study and Prevention of Infant Mortality, 1910*, p. 21.

77. George Goler, "But a Thousand a Year—the Cost and the Results in Rochester of Feeding Clean Milk as Food for the Hand-Fed Baby," *Charities* 14 (1905): 967–73; S. Josephine Baker, *Fighting for Life* (New York: Macmillan, 1939), pp. 82–87.

78. "Report of the Executive Secretary," *Transactions of the American Association for Study and Prevention of Infant Mortality, 1910*, p. 21.

79. Grace Abbott, "The Federal Government in Relation to Maternity and Infancy," *Annals of the American Academy of Political and Social Science* 151 (September, 1930): 94.

80. On the campaign to establish a national health department, see Manfred Waserman, "The Quest for a National Health Department in the Progressive Era," *Bulletin of the History of Medicine* 49 (1975): 353–80. On the creation of the United States Children's Bureau, see Nancy Pottishman Weiss, "Save the Children": A History of the Children's Bureau, 1903–1918 (Ph.D. diss., University of California, Los Angeles, 1974).

81. R. L. Duffus, *Lillian Wald: Neighbor and Crusader* (New York: Macmillan, 1939), pp. 93–104; Weiss, "Save the Children," pp. 49–50.

82. Waserman, "The Quest for a National Health Department," 357–68.

83. "Resolution in Support of the Establishment of a National Department of Health," *Transactions of the American Association for Study and Prevention of Infant Mortality, 1910*, p. 14.

84. Mark H. Haller, *Eugenics: Hereditarian Attitudes and American Thought* (New Brunswick, N.J.: Rutgers University Press, 1963), p. 173.

85. The scholarly literature on eugenics is considerable and growing. For bibliographic summaries of it, see Lyndsay Farrall, "The History of Eugenics: A Bibliographical Review," *Annals of Science* 36 (1979): 111–17; and Kevles' "Essay on Sources," in his *In the Name of Eugenics*, pp. 383–405. In addition to Kevles' monograph, two other useful book-length studies are Haller, *Eugenics*; and Kenneth M. Ludmerer, *Genetics and American Society* (Baltimore: Johns Hopkins Press, 1972). Also insightful and informative is Charles E. Rosenberg, "Charles B. Davenport and the Irony of American Eugenics," in *No Other Gods: On Science and American Social Thought*, ed. Charles E. Rosenberg (Baltimore: Johns Hopkins University Press, 1976), pp. 89–97.

86. Henderson, "Address of the President for 1911," pp. 18–19.

87. Eugenicists were split over the question of whether infant welfare activities were beneficial or harmful to national efficiency. Karl Pearson, Galton Professor of Eugenics at University College, England was a leading proponent of the view that they were the latter, arguing that infant mortality was a sign of hereditary weakness and thus was nature's way of weeding out the unfit. Others, however, disagreed. For instance, C. W. Saleeby, who was often quoted by American infant welfare activists, labeled Pearson and his followers "the better-dead-school," and argued that preventable maternal ignorance and environmental factors were probably more important than heredity. See Lewis, *The Politics of Motherhood*, pp. 29–31.

88. L. Emmett Holt, "Infant Mortality, Ancient and Modern: An Historical Sketch," *Transactions of the American Association for Study and Prevention of Infant Mortality, 1913*, p. 25.

89. Charles Darwin, *The Descent of Man, and Selection in Relation to Sex* (London: J. Murray, 1871), p. 501.

90. Ibid.

91. Holt, "Infant Mortality, Ancient and Modern," p. 25.

92. *Transactions of the American Association for Study and Prevention of Infant Mortality, 1911*, p. 114.

93. Newman, *Infant Mortality*, p. 47.

94. William H. Welch, "Address," *Transactions of the American Association for Study and Prevention of Infant Mortality, 1910*, p. 52.

95. Knox, "Address of the President," p. 30.

96. "Report of the Executive Secretary," *Transactions of the American Association for Study and Prevention of Infant Mortality, 1912*, p. 19.

97. Quoted in F. Freeze, "Caroline Rest and School for Mothers," ibid., p. 295.

98. Newsholme, *Fifty Years in Public Health*, p. 326.

99. On the new public health, see George Rosen, *A History of Public Health* (New York: MD Publications, 1958), pp. 393–404; Barbara Gutmann Rosenkrantz, *Public Health and the State: Changing Views in Massachusetts, 1842–1936* (Cambridge: Harvard University Press, 1972), pp. 128–76; James H. Cassedy, *Charles V. Chapin and the Public Health Movement* (Cambridge: Harvard University Press, 1962), pp. 126–42; C.-E. A. Winslow, *The Evolution and Significance of the Modern Public Health Campaign* (1923; reprint ed., Burlington, Vt: *Journal of Public Health Policy*, 1984), pp. 49–65.

100. Quoted in George Newman, *Infant Mortality*, pp. 263–64.

101. Cassedy, *Charles V. Chapin*, pp. 126–27.

102. Rosenkrantz, *Public Health and the State*, p. 128.

103. J. Whitridge Williams, "The Midwife Problem and Medical Education in the United States," *Transactions of the American Association for Study and Prevention of Infant Mortality, 1911*, pp. 165–94. The following year Williams published a shortened

version of his address as "Medical Education and the Midwife Problem," *Journal of the American Medical Association* 58 (1912): 1–7. On the quality of early twentieth-century obstetrics and efforts to reform it, see Richard W. and Dorothy C. Wertz, *Lying-In: A History of Childbirth in America* (New York: Schocken, 1977), pp. 132–77; Jane Pact Brickman, "Mother Love—Mother Death: Maternal and Infant Care: Social Class and the Role of Government" (Ph.D. diss., City University of New York, 1978), pp. 350–430; Judith Walzer Leavitt, "Science Enters the Birthing Room: Obstetrics in America since the Eighteenth Century," *Journal of American History* 70 (1983): 281–304; and Nancy Schrom Dye, "Modern Obstetrics and Working-Class Women: The New York Midwife Dispensary, 1890–1920," *Journal of Social History* 20 (1987): 549–64.

104. Mary Richmond, "Charitable Cooperation," in National Conference of Charities and Corrections, *Proceedings of the Twenty-Eighth Annual Conference* 28 (1901): 301.

105. Mary P. Ryan, *Womanhood in America: From Colonial Times to the Present*, 3d ed. (New York: Franklin Watts, 1983), pp. 138–44; George Rosen, *Preventive Medicine in the United States, 1900–1975: Trends and Interpretations* (New York: Science History Publications, 1975), p. 47; Frank J. Bruno, *Trends in Social Work, 1874–1956* (New York: Columbia University Press, 1957), pp. 138–44.

106. George Newman, quoted in National Conference of Charities and Corrections, "Report of the Sub-Committee on Infant Mortality," *Proceedings of the Thirty-Ninth Annual Conference* 39 (1912): 323.

107. Ida Tarbell, *The Business of Being a Woman* (New York: Macmillan, 1910), p. 198.

108. Sheila Rothman, *Woman's Proper Place: A History of Changing Ideals and Practices, 1870 to the Present* (New York: Basic Books, 1978), pp. 97–106.

109. Lathrop, "The Federal Children's Bureau," p. 50.

110. Katherine Graves Busby, *Home Life in America* (New York: Macmillan, 1910), pp. 118–19.

111. Rothman, *Woman's Proper Place*, pp. 97–132.

112. Robert Bruere, "Discussion," *Transactions of the American Association for Study and Prevention of Infant Mortality, 1910*, p. 64.

113. Sherman C. Kingsley, "Economic Aspects of Infant Mortality," *Transactions of the American Association for Study and Prevention of Infant Mortality, 1915* (Baltimore: AASPIM, 1916), pp. 162–72.

5. Better Mothers, Better Babies, Better Homes

1. U.S. Department of Labor, Children's Bureau, *Baby-Saving Campaigns: A Preliminary Report on What American Cities Are Doing to Prevent Infant Mortality* (Washington, D.C.: Government Printing Office, 1913), pp. 20–21; idem, *A Tabular Statement of Infant-Welfare Work by Public and Private Agencies in the United States*, by Etta R. Goodwin (Washington, D.C.: Government Printing Office, 1916), p. 26.

2. Although the fly's role in the transmission of typhoid in military camps had been suggested by American doctors during the Spanish-American War and corroborated by British medical officers during the Boer War, it was not until a 1907 study by the New York City Water Pollution Committee that flies were directly implicated in the spread of summer diarrhea among infants. Plotting cases of infant diarrhea on a map, the study showed that not only did the number of such cases increase at those times when fly infestation increased, but also that they were most heavily concentrated in areas where flies bred and massed. Within a short time, the need to combat the "fly menace" had become widely accepted among public health authorities and infant welfare activists and had inspired an educational campaign that included lectures, circulars, newspaper and magazine stories, and even a motion picture, *The Fly Pest*, which was shown in hundreds

of movie halls throughout the country. The message of such educational materials was simple and direct. The only way to combat the fly menace was through cleanliness, especially cleanliness in the home. This meant keeping kitchens and nurseries spotless, putting food away, cleaning drains, and covering garbage. In short, only if domestic hygiene improved would flies cease to spread death to the nation's infants. Indeed, after conducting a 1915 experiment involving 480 infants in the southwest Bronx, the NYMC concluded that the fly menace made it even more imperative that infant welfare work center on instructing mothers in hygienic prophylaxis. On this, see Edward Hatch, Jr., "The House Fly as a Carrier of Disease," *Annals of the American Academy of Political and Social Science* 37 (1911): 412–23; and New York Association for Improving the Condition of the Poor, *Flies and Diarrheal Disease* (New York: NYAICP, 1915).

3. Children's Bureau, *Baby-Saving Campaigns*, p. 22.

4. Ira S. Wile, "The Educational Responsibilities of the Milk Depot," in *The Prevention of Infant Mortality* (Philadelphia: The American Academy of Medicine, 1910), pp. 139–53; Patricia Mooney Melvin, "Milk to Motherhood: The New York Milk Committee and the Beginning of Well-Child Programs," *Mid-America* 65 (1983), 125–26; Children's Bureau, *Baby-Saving Campaigns*, pp. 22–24; George F. McCleary, "The Infants' Milk Depot: Its History and Its Function," *Journal of Hygiene* 4 (1904): 329–68; George Rosen, *A History of Public Health* (New York: MD Publications, 1958), pp. 354–56.

5. Responding to the 1915 Children's Bureau survey, Boston public health officials pleaded lack of funds in explanation for their nonsupport of milk stations. However, given that they were one of the best-financed city health departments, that explanation rings hollow.

6. Children's Bureau, *Baby-Saving Campaigns*, p. 24; Melvin, "Milk to Motherhood," pp. 125–26; New York Milk Committee, Committee for the Reduction of Infant Mortality, *Infant Mortality and Milk Stations* (New York: NYMC, 1912).

7. For a short but informative discussion of the development of that guiding principle in the early nineteenth century, see Walter I. Trattner, *From Poor Law to Welfare State: A History of Social Welfare in America*, 2d ed. (New York: The Free Press, 1979), pp. 42–66. For another short but equally informative discussion of the way it guided Progressive era philanthropy, see James T. Patterson, *America's Struggle Against Poverty, 1900–1980* (Cambridge: Harvard University Press, 1981), pp. 20–34. On the Progressive emphasis on saving the family, see Susan Tiffin, *In Whose Best Interest? Child Welfare Reform in the Progressive Era* (Westport, Conn.: Greenwood, 1982), pp. 110–40.

8. Lillian D. Wald, *The House on Henry Street* (New York: Henry Holt, 1915), pp. 55–56.

9. S. Josephine Baker, *Fighting for Life* (New York: Macmillan, 1939), p. 139.

10. Sherman C. Kingsley, "On the Trail of the White Hearse," *Survey* 22 (1909): 687.

11. Wald, *House on Henry Street*, pp. 30–35; Minnie Ahrens, "Infant Welfare or Milk Stations," *Transactions of the American Association for Study and Prevention of Infant Mortality, 1910* (Baltimore: AASPIM, 1911), p. 292.

12. S. W. Newmeyer, "Erroneous Ideas on Infant Mortality and Methods of Reducing It," *Transactions of the American Association for Study and Prevention of Infant Mortality, 1910*, p. 231.

13. Children's Bureau, *Tabular Statement*, pp. 23, 40–95; Rowland G. Freeman, discussion following J. P. Crozer Griffiths, "The Influence of Diet on Infant Mortality," in *The Prevention of Infant Mortality*, p. 51. For a discussion of the role of the charitable clinic and dispensary in early twentieth-century medical education, see Charles E. Rosenberg, "Social Class and Medical Care in Nineteenth-Century America: The Rise and Fall of the Dispensary," *Journal of the History of Medicine and Allied Sciences* 29 (1974): 32–49.

14. Children's Bureau, *Tabular Statement*, pp. 27, 37.

15. Ibid., pp. 40–95; Philip Van Ingen, "Recent Progress in Infant Welfare Work," *Journal of the Diseases of Children* 9 (1914): p. 493.

16. Patterson, *America's Struggle Against Poverty*, p. 24.

17. Allan Davis, *Spearheads for Reform: The Social Settlements and the Progressive Movement, 1890–1914* (New York: Oxford University Press, 1967), pp. 40–59; Sheila M. Rothman, *Woman's Proper Place: A History of Changing Ideals and Practices, 1870 to the Present* (New York: Basic Books, 1978), pp. 114–20; Barbara Ehrenreich and Deirdre English, *For Her Own Good: One Hundred Fifty Years of the Experts' Advice to Women* (Garden City, N.Y.: Anchor/Doubleday, 1979), p. 173.

18. William H. Guilfoy, "Infant Mortality in New York City," *Transactions of the Fifteenth International Congress on Hygiene and Demography, 1912,* 6 vols. (Washington, D.C.: Government Printing Office, 1913), 6: 194.

19. Mrs. W. H. Barton, "The Work of Infant Milk Stations in Relation to Infant Mortality," *Transactions of the American Association for Study and Prevention of Infant Mortality, 1911* (Baltimore: AASPIM, 1912), p. 301.

20. George Rosen, *Preventive Medicine in the United States, 1900–1975* (New York: Science History Publications, 1975), p. 47.

21. In publishing statistics on infant mortality, both the Census Bureau and the Children's Bureau detailed deaths by parental nativity and race. For late-nineteenth- and early-twentieth-century discussions of the relation between infant mortality and race and ethnicity, see, for instance, Frederick L. Hoffman, "Race Traits and Tendencies of the American Negro," *Publications of the American Statistical Association* 11 (1896): 37–45, passim.; R. C. Cabot and E. K. Ritchie, "The Influence of Race on Infant Mortality in Boston in 1909," *Boston Medical and Surgical Journal* 162 (1910): 199–202; F. H. McCarthy, "A Study of Mortality and Vitality of Infants of Different Racial Groups," *New England Medical Gazette* 52 (1917): 366–71; P. R. Eastman, "The Relation of Parental Nativity to the Infant Mortality of New York," *American Journal of the Diseases of Children* 17 (1919): 195–211; Philip Van Ingen, "The Melting Pot and Babies Lives," *Mother and Child* 4 (1923): 165, 205; J. H. Mason Knox, "Morbidity and Mortality in the Negro Infant," *American Journal of the Diseases of Children* 27 (1924): 398–400; and J. V. DePorte, "Inter-Racial Variations in Infant Mortality," *American Journal of Hygiene* 5 (1925): 454–96.

22. Hoffman, "Race Traits," p. 63; Knox, "Morbidity and Mortality of the Negro Infant," p. 399.

23. Hoffman, "Race Traits," p. 50.

24. Ibid., p. 95.

25. Robert Morse Woodbury, *Infant Mortality and Its Causes* (Baltimore: Williams and Wilkins, 1926), pp. 117–19.

26. Arthur Newsholme, *Fifty Years in Public Health: A Personal Narrative with Comments* (London: George Allen and Unwin, 1935), p. 374.

27. William Bunnell Phelps, "The World-wide Effort to Diminish Infant Mortality—Its Present Status and Possibilities," *Congress on Hygiene and Demography, 1912,* 6: 142–44; U.S. Department of Labor, Children's Bureau, *Infant Welfare Work in Europe,* by Nettie McGill (Washington, D.C.: Government Printing Office, 1921), pp. 110–11.

28. Children's Bureau, *Infant Welfare in Europe,* pp. 82–86.

29. Ibid., pp. 17–21; McCleary, *Early History,* pp. 88, 140–43.

30. "Infant Mortality in American Cities: A Symposium," *Annals of the American Academy of Political and Social Science* 31 (1908), 484–94. The cities polled were New York, Philadelphia, St. Louis, Baltimore, Cincinnati, Milwaukee, Minneapolis, Providence, and Rochester.

31. Children's Bureau, *A Tabular Statement,* pp. 7, 21; Grace Abbott, "The Federal

Government in Relation to Maternity and Infancy," *Annals of the American Academy of Political and Social Science* 151 (September, 1930): 94.

32. Baker, *Fighting for Life*, pp. 44, 54–63, 84–85.

33. Ibid., pp. 84–86.

34. Children's Bureau, *A Tabular Statement*, pp. 37, 40–95.

35. Children's Bureau, *Baby-Saving Campaigns*, p. 34; S. Josephine Baker, "The Reduction of Infant Mortality in New York City," *Congress on Hygiene and Demography, 1912*, 3: 141; idem, *Fighting for Life*, pp. 91–92.

36. Elsa G. Herzfield, "Superstitions and Customs of the Tenement House Mother," *Charities and the Commons* 14 (1905): 985.

37. Baker, *Fighting for Life*, p. 86. For a good discussion of the way in which immigrant mothers responded to social workers and visiting nurses, see Elizabeth Ewen, *Immigrant Women in the Land of Dollars: Life and Culture on the Lower East Side* (New York: Monthly Review Press, 1985). For a similar discussion of the response of English working-class mothers to the infant care advice of health visitors, see Anthony S. Wohl, *Endangered Lives: Public Health in Victorian Britain* (Cambridge: Harvard University Press, 1983), pp. 41–42.

38. Alice Hamilton, *Exploring the Dangerous Trades: The Autobiography of Alice Hamilton, M.D.* (Boston: Little, Brown, 1943), pp. 69–70; Rothman, *Woman's Proper Place*, p. 118.

39. Ewen, *Immigrant Women*, p. 139.

40. New York Association for Improving the Condition of the Poor, *Sixty-Fifth Annual Report* (New York, 1909), pp. 62–63.

41. Ernest C. Meyer, *Infant Mortality in New York City* (New York: The Rockefeller Foundation International Health Board, 1921), p. 116.

42. Quoted in Joseph S. Neff, "Recent Public Health Work in the U. S. Especially in Relation to Infant Mortality," *American Journal of Public Health* 5 (1915): 973.

43. Melvin, "Milk to Motherhood," pp. 127–28; Barton, "The Work of Infant Milk Stations in Relation to Infant Mortality," pp. 299–300; Baker, *Fighting for Life*, pp. 127–28.

44. Baker, "The Reduction of Infant Mortality," p. 146.

45. Ibid.; Melvin, "Milk to Motherhood," p. 127; *Report of the Babies Welfare Association, 1912–1915* (New York: Russell Sage Foundation, 1915), p. 1.

46. Joseph S. Neff, "A City's Duty in the Prevention of Infant Mortality," *Transactions of the American Association for Study and Prevention of Infant Mortality, 1910*, pp. 156–58.

47. George Thomas Palmer, "The Shortcomings of Municipal Public Health Administration," *American City* 5 (1911): 65.

48. "Report of the Special Public Health Commission," quoted in Children's Bureau, *Baby-Saving Campaigns*, p. 11.

49. Selskar M. Gunn, "Modern Board of Health Methods in Small Cities," *Journal of the American Public Health Association*, n.s. 1 (1911), 376.

50. Those states were Maine, New Hampshire, Vermont, Massachusetts, Rhode Island, Connecticut, New York, New Jersey, Pennsylvania, Ohio, Indiana, Illinois, Michigan, and Wisconsin.

51. Children's Bureau, *Tabular Statement*, pp. 23–25, 36. By the South, I mean here the states of Delaware, Maryland, Virginia, West Virginia, North Carolina, South Carolina, Georgia, Florida, Kentucky, Tennessee, Alabama, Mississippi, Arkansas, Louisiana, Oklahoma, and Texas, plus the District of Columbia.

52. That this was so only began to be appreciated toward the end of the second decade

of the century. See, for instance, John C. Gebbart, "Filling the Gaps in Childlife," *Survey* 43 (1919): 313.

53. Hoffman, "Race Traits," p. 45.

54. The four cities were Savannah, New Orleans, Charleston, and Richmond. Ibid., pp. 42–48.

55. The birth registration area was established in 1915 and included Minnesota, Michigan, Pennsylvania, New York, Connecticut, Rhode Island, Massachusetts, New Hampshire, Vermont, and Maine, plus the District of Columbia. By 1920 it also included Maryland, Virginia, North Carolina, South Carolina, Kentucky, Ohio, Indiana, Wisconsin, Nebraska, Kansas, Washington, Oregon, and California. In 1920 black infant mortality in the registration area was 135.6 compared to 82.1 for whites and 89.6 for nonwhites. U.S. Department of Commerce, Bureau of the Census, *Birth Statistics, 1920* (Washington, D.C.: Government Printing Office, 1922), pp. 6–7, 36–37.

56. Mrs. H. A. to Children's Bureau, July 2, 1918, in Molly Ladd-Taylor, ed., *Raising a Baby the Government Way: Mothers' Letters to the Children's Bureau, 1915–1932* (New Brunswick, N. J.: Rutgers University Press, 1986), p. 163.

57. Children's Bureau, *Tabular Statement*, pp. 8–17; Franz Schneider, "The Seventh Baby Campaign," *American City* 17 (1917): 129.

58. Ibid., pp. 52, 62; Samual Hopkins Adams, "Tomfoolery with Public Health: The Present Pittsburgh Situation," *Survey* 25 (1910): 455; Children's Bureau, *Baby-Saving Campaigns*, pp. 34–35; Ernst C. Meyer, *Infant Mortality in New York City*, pp. 77–79.

59. Baker, *Fighting for Life*, pp. 132–33; idem, "Little Mothers' Leagues," *Transactions of the American Association for Study and Prevention of Infant Mortality, 1911*, pp. 308–309.

60. Children's Bureau, *Tabular Statement*, pp. 29–30.

61. Baker, "The Reduction of Infant Mortality," p. 154; *Report of the Babies Welfare Association*, p. 1; J. H. Larson, "New York's Balance Sheet of Infant Life Saving," *American City* 12 (1915): 193–94.

62. Baker, "The Reduction of Infant Mortality," p. 158.

63. Homer Folks, "The Foundling," *Congress on Hygiene and Demography, 1912*, 3: 88. That institutionalization had harmful effects on children was fairly widely accepted in the social service community by the first decade of the century and was one of the basic themes articulated and agreed upon at the first White House Conference on the Care of Dependent Children held in 1909.

64. Henry D. Chapin, "The Speedwell Plan of Child Saving in Theory and Practice," *Survey* 41 (1917): 88–91; Baker, *Fighting for Life*, p. 121.

65. U.S. Department of Labor, Children's Bureau, *Child Welfare Exhibits: Types and Preparation* (Washington, D.C.: Government Printing Office, 1915), pp. 7–13; Samuel McC. Hamill, "Discussion of the Baby-Saving Show Held in Philadelphia in May, 1912," *Congress on Hygiene and Demography, 1912*, 3: 90–102.

66. Baker, *Fighting for Life*, p. 122.

67. "Chicago's Baby Week," *Survey* 32 (1914): 296; "Baby Week," ibid., p. 355.

68. "Campaigning for Better Babies," *Survey* 34 (1915): 382.

69. U.S. Department of Labor, Children's Bureau, *Baby-Week Campaigns*, rev. ed. (Washington, D.C.: Government Printing Office, 1917), p. 3.

70. Ibid., pp. 35–62, and passim.

71. Ehrenreich and English, *One Hundred Fifty Years*, p. 144; Helen Campbell, quoted in Daniel Beekman, *The Mechanical Baby: A Popular History of the Theory and Practice of Child Raising* (New York: New American Library, 1977), p. 113.

72. Two caveats are required here. The first is that there is currently some debate as to whether the invention of so-called labor-saving devices actually served to lessen the

amount of work required of the middle-class wife and mother. For an argument that it did not, see Susan Strasser, *Never Done: A History of American Housework* (New York: Pantheon, 1982). The second caveat is that only a minority of American households had access to labor-saving devices. The home of the urban working-class woman was hardly filled with labor-saving devices nor characterized by a consumer rather than a producer orientation. Nor was the home of the rural or farm woman.

73. For a good general discussion of the decline of American fertility, see Carl N. Degler, *At Odds: Women and the Family in America from the Revolution to the Present* (New York: Oxford University Press, 1980), pp. 178–88.

74. Nancy Woloch, *Women and the American Experience* (New York: Knopf, 1984), p. 295.

75. For an example of the *Good Housekeeping* articles, see J. P. C. Griffiths, "Mistakes of Young Mothers," *Good Housekeeping* 48 (1909): 82–86. In addition to publishing similar articles, the *Ladies Home Journal* ran a regular advice feature by E. L. Coolidge called the "Young Mothers Home Club" and another by the home economist Christine Frederick. On kindergarten clubs, see Rothman, *Woman's Proper Place*, pp. 98–104. For an example of the discussion on motherhood and the educated woman, see M. M. Tuttle, "Maternity and the Intellectual Woman," *Colliers* 44 (1910): 18–19. For an example of a child welfare advocate's concern over improperly trained mothers, see Florence Kelley, "Unskilled Mothers," *Century* 73 (1907): 640–42.

76. Helen Watterson Moody, "The True Meaning of Motherhood, *Ladies Home Journal* 16 (1899): 12.

77. Mary Holland Kinkaid, in discussion following Lillian Wald, "The District Nurses' Contribution to the Reduction of Infant Mortality," in *The Prevention of Infant Mortality*, p. 221–22. Schneider, "The Seventh Baby Campaign," pp. 129–30.

78. Schneider, "The Seventh Baby Campaign," pp. 129–32.

79. J. J. Biddison, "Better Babies," *Woman's Home Companion* 40 (March 1913): 26–27; Anne S. Richardson, "Finest Babies in Colorado: First Better Babies Show," *Woman's Home Companion* 40 (April 1913): 26; "Human Cattle Shows," *Literary Digest* 55 (1913): 127–28; "Perfect Babies," *Independent* 74 (1913): 1069–70.

80. Thomas E. Cone, Jr., *History of American Pediatrics* (Boston: Little, Brown, 1979), p. 127.

81. Aside from Holt's, another popular advice manual written by a respected pediatrician was J. P. Crozer Griffith's *The Care of Baby* (Philadelphia: Saunders, 1895). The list of manuals written by less well-known physicians and lay writers is a long one, but a sampling would be: Frances Sage Bradley, *The Care of Baby* (New York: Russell Sage Foundation, 1913); Daniel Rollins Bell, *The Baby* (Boston: Whitcomb and Burrows, 1908); Roger Herbert Dennett, *The Healthy Baby* (New York: Macmillan, 1912); Thomas N. Gray, *Common Sense and the Baby* (New York: Berwick, 1907); Leonard K. Hirshberg, *What You Ought to Know About Your Baby* (New York: Butterick, 1910); Setrak G. Eghian, *The Mother's Nursery Guide* (New York: Putnam's, 1907); Mrs. Burton Chance, *Self-Training for Mothers* (Philadelphia: Lippincott, 1914).

82. Mrs. H. S. to the Children's Bureau, December 4, 1917, in Ladd-Taylor, *Raising a Baby the Government Way*, p. 103.

83. Rima Apple, "'How Shall I Feed My Baby?' Infant Feeding in the United States, 1870–1940" (Ph.D. diss., University of Wisconsin, 1981), pp. 278–80.

84. Beekman, *The Mechanical Baby*, pp. 109–33.

85. Alice Hamilton, "Excessive Child-Bearing as a Factor in Infant Mortality," in *The Prevention of Infant Mortality*, pp. 74–80.

86. Havelock Ellis, *The Task of Social Hygiene* (Boston: Houghton Mifflin, 1912), p. 128; Florence Kiper, "The New Motherhood," *Forum* 52 (1914): 207.

87. This is obviously a rough estimate and is based on the infant mortality rates by fathers' earnings computed by the Children's Bureau in its studies of Brockton, Manchester, New Bedford, and Saginaw. I define the poor as those earning $649 or less a year, the working class as those earning $650 to $1,049, and the middle class as those earning over $1,050. For a table detailing the infant mortality rate by fathers' earnings for all the cities, see U.S. Department of Labor, Children's Bureau, *Infant Mortality: Results of a Field Study in Brockton, Mass., Based on Births in One Year*, by Mary V. Dempsey (Washington, D.C.: Government Printing Office, 1919), p. 32.

88. Nancy Schrom Dye and Daniel Blake Smith, "Mother Love and Infant Death, 1750–1920," *Journal of American History* 73 (1986): 347. I would also suggest that the relationship between parental fear of and response to infant death and the level of infant mortality extant at a particular time needs much more analysis than it has been given by demographic and social historians. Totally inadequate is the generalization that the higher the rate the more fatalistic the response. About the only certainty is that a high rate of infant mortality does require a response. What determines that response, though, remains in question.

89. Ladd-Taylor, *Raising a Baby the Government Way*, pp. 2–3, n. 5.

90. Ibid., pp. 78–79, Mrs. N. B. to Children's Bureau, July 20, 1926.

91. U.S. Department of Commerce, Bureau of the Census, *Mortality Statistics, 1910* (Washington, D.C.: Government Printing Office, 1913), p. 59; idem, *Mortality Statistics, 1920* (Washington, D.C.: Government Printing Office, 1922), p. 52.

92. Rose A. Cheney, "Seasonal Aspects of Infant and Childhood Mortality: Philadelphia, 1865–1920," *Journal of Interdisciplinary History* 15 (1984): 565–72.

93. Children's Bureau, *Tabular Statement*, pp. 40–95.

94. Although there is considerable uncertainty as to when the first baby was kissed in an election campaign, *Survey* reported in 1917 that the practice was new to the political arena. Describing the reelection campaign of New York Mayor John P. Mitchell, *Survey* noted that the mayor had made an issue of his administration's efforts to conserve child life and that he was touring the city embracing and kissing all infants proffered. "Votes for Babies," *Survey* 39 (1917–18): 118–19.

6. Before the Baby Comes:
Neonatal Mortality and the Promotion of Prenatal Care

1. Philip Van Ingen, "Recent Progress in Infant Welfare Work," *American Journal of the Diseases of Children* 9 (1914): 481.

2. S. Josephine Baker, "The Reduction of Infant Mortality in New York City," *Transactions of the Fifteenth International Congress on Hygiene and Demography, 1912*, 6 vols. (Washington, D.C.: Government Printing Office, 1913), 3: 146.

3. "Report of the Executive Secretary," *Transactions of the American Association for Study and Prevention of Infant Mortality, 1912* (Baltimore: AASPIM, 1913), p. 19.

4. Ann Oakley, *The Captured Womb: A History of the Medical Care of Pregnant Women* (Oxford: Basil Blackwell, 1984), pp. 11–12; Henri Seibert, "The Progress of Ideas Regarding the Causation and Control of Infant Mortality," *Bulletin of the History of Medicine* 8 (1940): 546–48.

5. Alexander Hamilton, *Treatise on Midwifery* (London, 1781), pp. 159–62; William Dewees, *Treatise on the Physical and Medical Treatment of Children*, 9th ed. (Philadelphia: Lea and Blanchard, 1847), p. 25; Andrew Combe, *Treatise on the Physiological and Moral Management of Infancy* (Philadelphia: Carey and Hart, 1840), p. 28.

6. Edward Jarvis, "Infant Mortality," *Fourth Annual Report of the Massachusetts State Board of Health, 1873* (Boston, 1874), p. 198.

7. *Encyclopaedia Britannica* (1842), 17: 684, quoted in Oakley, *Captured Womb,* p. 11.

8. Walter Radcliffe, *Milestones in Midwifery* (Bristol: J. Wright, 1967), p. 97.

9. Richard W. Wertz and Dorothy C. Wertz, *Lying-In: A History of Childbirth in America* (New York: Schocken Books, 1979), pp. 90–92.

10. Lawrence D. Longo and Christina M. Thompsen, "Prenatal Care and Its Evolution in America," *Proceedings of the Second Motherhood Symposium* (Madison, Wis: Women's Research Center, 1982), p. 33.

11. J. W. Ballantyne, "A Plea for a Pro-Maternity Hospital," *British Medical Journal* 6 (1901): 813–14.

12. J. W. Ballantyne, *Manual of Ante-Natal Pathology and Hygiene,* vol. 1: *The Foetus* (Edinburgh: William Green and Sons, 1902), p. 465.

13. For an example of the former description, see Radcliffe, *Milestones in Midwifery,* p. 91. For an example of the latter, see Oakley, *Captured Womb,* especially Chapters 1–2.

14. J. W. Ballantyne, quoted in Jane Lewis, *The Politics of Motherhood: Child and Maternal Welfare in England, 1900–1939* (London: Croom Helm, 1980), p. 19.

15. Williams's textbook, *Obstetrics: A Text-Book for the Use of Students and Practitioners* (New York: D. Appleton, 1903), which has gone through numerous editions and revisions since it was first published, is still a standard and highly regarded obstetric text.

16. Ibid., 3d and enlarged edition (1912), p. 207.

17. Ibid., p. 210.

18. Henry Hartshorne, "Infant Mortality in Cities," *Reports and Papers of the American Public Health Association* 2 (1874–75): 212.

19. I am concerned here only with gestation and the development of prenatal obstetric care, but a similar argument can be made in regard to obstetric intervention in the birthing process.

20. Hartshorne, "Infant Mortality in Cities," p. 215.

21. For a discussion of that transformation, see Wertz, *Lying-In,* pp. 132–77; Judith Walzer Leavitt, "Science Enters the Birthing Room: Obstetrics in America Since the Eighteenth Century," *Journal of American History* 60 (1983): 281–304; and Nancy Schrom Dye, "Modern Obstetrics and Working-class Women: The New York Midwifery Dispensary, 1890–1920," *Journal of Social History* 20 (1987): 549–64.

22. Longo and Thompson, "Prenatal Care," pp. 34–35; Dye, "Modern Obstetrics," pp. 551–53; Van Ingen, "Recent Progress," p. 481; John M. Glenn, Lillian Brandt, F. Emerson Andrews, *Russell Sage Foundation, 1907–1946,* 2 vols. (New York: Russell Sage Foundation, 1947), 1: 106.

23. "Resolutions of the Section on Nursing and Social Work," *Transactions of the Association for Study and Prevention of Infant Mortality, 1911* (Baltimore: AASPIM, 1912), p. 282; U.S. Department of Labor, Children's Bureau, *Baby-Saving Campaigns* (Washington, D.C.: Government Printing Office, 1913), pp. 38–39; New York Milk Committee, *Ten Years' Work, 1907–1916* (New York: NYMC, 1916), pp. 14–15; Van Ingen, "Recent Progress," p. 482.

24. Van Ingen, "Recent Progress," p. 483; Margaret N. McClure, "The Prenatal Work of the Visiting Nurse Association of St. Louis," *Transactions of the American Association for Study and Prevention of Infant Mortality, 1912,* pp. 292–94; "Reports of the Affiliated Societies," ibid., pp. 332–48; F. Freeze, "Caroline Rest and School for Mothers," ibid., pp. 295–307.

25. Children' Bureau, *Baby-Saving Campaigns,* pp. 40–41; idem, *Prenatal Care,* by Mrs. Max B. West (Washington, D.C.: Government Printing Office, 1913).

26. Newman, for instance, continued to argue this line through the 1920s.

27. Mrs. Max B. West, "The Development of Prenatal Care in the United States,"

Transactions of the American Association for Study and Prevention of Infant Mortality, *1914* (Baltimore: AASPIM, 1915), p. 70.

28. In 1910 the registration area included twenty-one states, the District of Columbia, and forty-three cities outside the registration states. The population of the registration area was 53,843,896, or 58.3 percent of the total U.S. population.

29. U.S. Department of Commerce, Bureau of the Census, *Mortality Statistics, 1910* (Washington, D.C.: Government Printing Office, 1913), p. 533.

30. Ibid.; U.S. Department of Commerce, Bureau of the Census, *Mortality Statistics, 1912* (Washington, D.C.: Government Printing Office, 1913), p. 335.

31. Children's Bureau, *Baby-Saving Campaigns,* p. 38.

32. Van Ingen, "Recent Progress," p. 481.

33. Indeed, it was not until the 1940s that the medical treatment of neonates achieved any sort of prominence as an effective strategy for reducing mortality within the first month of life. Thomas E. Cone, Jr., *History of the Care and Feeding of the Premature Infant* (Boston: Little, Brown, 1985), pp. 61–62. Moreover, since the mid-1960s and the proliferation of neonatal intensive care units, such treatment has probably been the major factor in the continued reduction of infant mortality.

34. Children's Bureau, *Prenatal Care,* pp. 1–4.

35. J. Whitridge Williams, "The Limitations and Possibilities of Prenatal Care," *Transactions of the American Association for Study and Prevention of Infant Mortality, 1914,* pp. 32–48.

36. Cone, *History of the Care and Feeding of the Premature Infant,* pp. 4–5.

37. Lewis, *Politics of Motherhood,* p. 119.

38. Abraham Flexner, *Medical Education in the United States and Canada: A Report to the Carnegie Foundation for the Advancement of Teaching* (New York: The Carnegie Foundation, 1910), p. 117.

39. J. Whitridge Williams, "Medical Education and the Midwife Problem in the United States," *Journal of the American Medical Association* 58 (1912): 4. Also quoted in Wertz, *Lying-In,* p. 145.

40. On early twentieth-century obstetric reform, see Wertz, *Lying-In,* pp. 145–48; Leavitt, "'Science' Enters the Birthing Room," pp. 290–99; and idem, *Brought to Bed,* Chapters 5–7; Lawrence D. Longo, "Obstetrics and Gynecology," in *The Education of American Physicians: Historical Essays,* ed. Ronald L. Numbers (Berkeley, University of California Press, 1980), pp. 216–25; and Joyce Antler and Daniel M. Fox, "The Movement Toward Safe Maternity: Physician Accountability in New York City, 1915–1940," *Bulletin of the History of Medicine* 50 (1976): 569–95.

41. Of the 58,089 neonatal deaths that occurred in the registration area in 1910, injuries at birth accounted for 3,689, while prematurity accounted for 19,498, congenital debility for 10,273, and malformation for 5,901. Bureau of the Census, *Mortality Report for 1910,* p. 533.

42. For discussion of female midwifery in early America and its gradual decline in the nineteenth century see Wertz, *Lying-In,* pp. 1–131; Jane B. Donegan, *Women & Men Midwives: Medicine, Mortality, and Mysogeny in Early America* (Westport, Conn.: Greenwood, 1978); and Judy Barrett Litoff, *American Midwives: 1860 to the Present* (Westport, Conn.: Greenwood, 1978), pp. 3–47.

43. Elizabeth Crowell, "The Midwives of New York," *Charities and the Commons* 17 (1907): 670–71; "The Midwives of Chicago," *Journal of the American Medical Association* 50 (1908): 1346.

44. Elizabeth Ewen, *Immigrant Women in the Land of Dollars: Life and Culture on the Lower East Side, 1890–1925* (New York: Monthly Review Press, 1985), pp. 131–33; Crowell, "Midwives of New York," p. 668; Litoff, *American Midwives,* pp. 28–29.

45. Carolyn Connant Van Blarcon, "Midwives in America," *American Journal of Public Health* 4 (1914): 197–207.

46. For a comprehensive survey of the arguments advanced by both sides in that debate, see Litoff, *American Midwives,* pp. 64–121. Also extremely informative is Francis E. Kobrin, "The American Midwife Controversy: A Crisis in Professionalization," *Bulletin of the History of Medicine* 40 (1966): 350–63.

47. J. Whitridge Williams, "The Midwife Problem and Medical Education in the United States," *Transactions of the American Association for Study and Prevention of Infant Mortality, 1911,* pp. 165–94. The following year he published a shortened version of the talk as "Medical Education and the Midwife Problem in the United States," *Journal of the American Medical Association* 58 (1912): 1–7. This shortened version has been reprinted in Judy Barrett Litoff, ed., *The American Midwife Debate: A Sourcebook of Its Modern Origins* (Westport, Conn.: Greenwood, 1986), pp. 86–101. Virtually all those involved in the debate over midwifery considered Williams' paper a seminal one. Indeed, it was still being quoted ten years after it was first published.

48. Williams, "The Midwife Problem," p. 188.

49. Charles Edward Ziegler, "The Elimination of the Midwife," *Transactions of the American Association for Study and Prevention of Infant Mortality, 1912,* p. 232.

50. Joseph B. DeLee, "Progress Toward Ideal Obstetrics," *Transactions of the American Association for Study and Prevention of Infant Mortality, 1915* (Baltimore: AASPIM, 1916), p. 116.

51. "The Case of the Midwife," *Boston Medical and Surgical Journal* 164 (1911): 276.

52. S. Josephine Baker, *Fighting for Life* (New York: Macmillan, 1939), pp. 111–15; idem, "Schools for Midwives," *Transactions of the American Association for Study and Prevention of Infant Mortality, 1912,* pp. 232–42; Litoff, *American Midwives,* pp. 91–95; Philip Van Ingen, Discussion following George D. Kosmak, "Does the Average Midwife Meet the Requirements of a Patient in Confinement?" *Transactions of the American Association for Study and Prevention of Infant Mortality, 1911,* p. 256; Abraham Jacobi, "The Best Means of Combating Infant Mortality," *Journal of the American Medical Association* 58 (1912): 1735–44.

53. Josephine Baker, discussion following West, "The Development of Prenatal Care," p. 112.

54. The four states were Massachusetts, New York, Vermont, and Connecticut.

55. West, "The Development of Prenatal Care," p. 75.

56. Baker, discussion following West, "The Development of Prenatal Care," p. 113.

57. Homer Folks, "Address to the Mass Meeting," *Transactions of the American Association for Study and Prevention of Infant Mortality, 1914,* pp. 273–74.

7. The Steps Not Taken:
The Rediscovery of Poverty and the Rejection of Maternity Insurance

1. Robert Morse Woodbury, *Infant Mortality and Its Causes* (Baltimore: Williams and Wilkins, 1926), pp. 23–24.

2. The studies were published in the following order: Johnstown (1915), Montclair (1915), Manchester (1917), Waterbury (1918), Brockton (1919), Saginaw (1919), New Bedford (1920), Akron (1920), Baltimore (1921), and Gary (1923).

3. Computed by dividing the number of infant deaths during a year into the number of births during the same year, the standard infant mortality statistic only approximates the percentage of infants born in a year who die, since a significant number of the deaths used in the computation will be of infants born during the previous year.

4. Bureau investigators defended their decision to limit in this way the population of infants studied by arguing the critical importance of information gathered from parental

interviews and by noting that the survival of those infants who moved away was significantly influenced by conditions other than those obtaining within the community under investigation.

5. Although the precise investigatory procedures employed in each study varied slightly, they were for the most part similar. For a detailed accounting of those procedures, see Woodbury, *Infant Mortality and Its Causes*, pp. 23–37.

6. Although the Children's Bureau studies followed the lead of the Bureau of the Census mortality reports and listed deaths from congenital malformations as separate from the other three pathological conditions of early infancy, in actually discussing the causes of mortality, they tended to include them: and with good reason. Seventy-eight percent of all registration area infant deaths ascribed to congenital malformation in 1912 occurred during the first month of life. As a consequence, I include them also. Bureau of the Census, *Mortality Statistics, 1912*, p. 335.

7. Exclusive of Montclair, New Jersey, and Gary, Indiana, and describing only the eight other cities studied. Calculated from data presented in Woodbury, *Infant Mortality and Its Causes*, pp. 38–39.

8. Based on a total of 2,555 infant deaths among 22,967 live births in the cities studied exclusive of Gary, Indiana, and Montclair, New Jersey. According to the published figures of the Bureau of the Census, the undifferentiated infant mortality rate for the registration area (exclusive of Rhode Island) was 99.55 in 1915, 99.95 in 1916, 105.83 in 1918, 88.74 in 1919, and 80.92 in 1920.

9. Nancy Pottishman Weiss, "Save the Children: A History of the Children's Bureau, 1903–1918" (Ph.D. diss., University of California, Los Angeles, 1974), p. 58.

10. In Brockton, for instance, where the Board of Health was extremely active, sewerage and garbage disposal were quite good, the milk supply was closely regulated and inspected, and considerable infant welfare work was carried out under the direction of the Brockton Milk and Baby Hygiene Association, the infant mortality rate was 96.7 compared to an average of 127.0 for the four other cities to that point studied. U.S. Department of Labor, Children's Bureau, *Infant Mortality: Results of a Field Study in Brockton, Mass.*, by Mary V. Dempsey (Washington, D.C.: Government Printing Office, 1919), pp. 15, 48–55.

11. Ibid., pp. 44–47.

12. U.S. Department of Labor, Children's Bureau, *Infant Mortality: Results of a Field Study in Johnstown, PA*, by Emma Duke (Washington, D.C.: Government Printing Office, 1915), p. 53.

13. Ibid., p. 42.

14. Idem, *Infant Mortality: Results of a Field Study in Montclair, N.J.* (Washington, D.C.: Government Printing Office, 1915), p. 19.

15. Idem, *Infant Mortality: Results of a Field Study in Manchester, N.H.*, by Beatrice Sheets Duncan and Emma Duke (Washington, D.C.: Government Printing Office, 1917), pp. 47–52.

16. Ibid., p. 47.

17. U.S. Department of Labor, Children's Bureau, *Infant Mortality: Results of a Field Study in Waterbury, Conn.*, by Estelle B. Hunter (Washington, D.C.: Government Printing office, 1918), p. 66.

18. The figures exclude data from Gary, Indiana, which was the last city studied, and data from Montclair, which as a suburban community had little female employment. For infants whose mothers were gainfully employed away from home during pregnancy, the overall mortality rate was 176.1 and neonatal mortality rate 67.2. For those whose mothers were not gainfully employed during pregnancy, the respective rates were 98.0 and 43.2. Woodbury, *Infant Mortality and Its Causes*, pp. 49, 147.

19. Ibid., p. 145.

20. Ibid., p. 146.

21. Charles H. Verrill, "Infant Mortality and Its Relation to the Employment of Mothers in Fall River, Mass.," *Transactions of the Fifteenth International Congress on Hygiene and Demography,* 6 vols. (Washington, D.C.: Government Printing Office, 1913), 3, part 1: 337. That Verrill shaped many of the conclusions of the congressional study may explain why they differed so radically from the public positions of the study's official author, Edward Bunnell Phelps.

22. Louis I. Dublin, "Infant Mortality in Fall River, Massachusetts: A Survey of the Mortality Among 833 Infants Born in June, July, and August, 1913," *Publications of the American Statistical Association* 14 (1914–15): 518.

23. U.S. Department of Labor, Children's Bureau, *Maternity Benefit Systems in Certain Foreign Countries,* by Henry J. Harris (Washington, D.C.: Government Printing Office, 1919), p. 9.

24. The first such law was enacted by Switzerland in 1877 and prohibited employment for eight weeks, at least six of which had to be after confinement. L. Emmett Holt, "Infant Mortality, Ancient and Modern," *Transactions of the American Association for Study and Prevention of Infant Mortality, 1913* (Baltimore: AASPIM, 1914), p. 41.

25. Even in Italy, however, it is clear that the maternity benefit system was designed to offset income disruption caused by the proscriptive employment laws since the only women eligible for coverage were those prohibited by the 1907 Factory Act from working during the weeks around confinement.

26. Jeanne L. Brand, *Doctors and the State: The British Medical Profession and Government Action in Public Health, 1870–1912* (Baltimore: Johns Hopkins Press, 1965), p. 211; Ronald L. Numbers, *Almost Persuaded: American Physicians and Compulsory Health Insurance* (Baltimore: Johns Hopkins University Press, 1978), p. 10.

27. Children's Bureau, *Maternity Benefit Systems,* p. 50.

28. Paul Starr, *The Social Transformation of American Medicine* (New York: Basic Books, 1982), p. 237.

29. David Lloyd George, *The People's Insurance,* 3d ed. (London: Hodder and Stoughton, 1912), p. 183; Children's Bureau, *Maternity Benefit Systems,* pp. 67–77, 114.

30. George F. McCleary, *The Maternity and Child Welfare Movement* (London: P. S. King and Son, 1935), pp. 17–23.

31. Starr, *The Social Transformation of American Medicine,* pp. 236–44; Numbers, *Almost Persuaded,* pp. 14–26.

32. American Association for Labor Legislation, *Health Insurance: Standards and Tentative Draft of an Act* (New York: AALL, 1915), pp. 6–15.

33. Isaac M. Rubinow, *Social Insurance* (New York: Henry Holt, 1913), p. 273.

34. Rubinow declared that he was convinced by such evidence that "if wage-work of mothers was undesirable it is one hundredfold more undesirable during the few months immediately preceding and succeeding the act of childbirth." Ibid., p. 443. The estimate of less than .9 percent of total women's wages is that calculated by Edward B. Phelps in "The New Statute for the Protection of Child-Bearing Factory-Workers and Means of Making It Effective," *Second Report of the New York State Factory Investigating Commission* (Albany, 1913).

35. AALL, *Standards and Tentative Draft of an Act,* p. 10.

36. George Rosen, *A History of Public Health* (New York: MD Publications, 1958), p. 453; Numbers, *Almost Persuaded,* pp. 81, 91.

37. Although no single reason explains the mounting opposition of the medical profession, Ronald Numbers has persuasively argued that of critical importance was that between 1916 and 1920 American physicians' incomes dramatically increased and as a

consequence individual doctors no longer found attractive an insurance scheme that would ensure them patients but tightly control fees. Numbers, *Almost Persuaded*, pp. 110–14.

38. Ibid., pp. 256–57.

39. While sickness insurance received the support of many local and state labor leaders, it provoked impassioned opposition from Samuel Gompers, national head of the influential American Federation of Labor. Ibid., pp. 249–51; Patterson, *America's Struggle Against Poverty*, pp. 33–34.

40. On the influence of the different social and political organization in the two countries, see J. Rogers Hollingsworth, *A Political Economy of Medicine: Great Britain and the United States* (Baltimore: Johns Hopkins University Press, 1986), p. 188, passim.

41. From a tract published by the California League for the Conservation of Public Health, an independent organization of physicians opposing the adoption of sickness insurance in that state. Quoted in Numbers, *Almost Persuaded*, p. 80.

42. Numbers, *Almost Persuaded*, pp. 56, 89–94; Rosen, *History of Public Health*, p. 455.

43. Starr, *The Social Transformation of American Medicine*, p. 247; Numbers, *Almost Persuaded*, p. 57.

44. Julius Levy, "The Reduction of Infant Mortality by Economic Adjustment and by Health Education," in National Conference on Social Work, *Proceedings of the Forty-sixth Annual Conference* 46 (1920): 202–3.

45. "Report of the Special Commission to Investigate Maternity Benefits," *Massachusetts House Documents, No. 1835* (December 1920), quoted in Barbara Gutmann Rosenkrantz, *Public Health and the State: Changing Views in Massachusetts, 1842–1936* (Cambridge: Harvard University Press, 1974), p. 153.

46. S. Adolphus Knoph, "The Smaller Family," *Survey* 37 (1916): 161.

47. Lee K. Frankel, "Maternity Insurance," *Transactions of the American Association for Study and Prevention of Infant Mortality, 1915* (Baltimore: AASPIM, 1916), pp. 193–95.

48. Numbers, *Almost Persuaded*, p. 37.

49. For comment on the persistence of opposition within the social service community to cash payments to mothers, see Walter I. Trattner, *Homer Folks: Pioneer in Social Welfare* (New York: Columbia University Press, 1968), p. 114. For a good discussion of mothers' pensions, see Mark H. Leff, "Consensus for Reform: The Mothers'-Pension Movement in the Progressive Era," *Social Service Review* 47 (1973): 397–417.

50. See, for instance, Anna Rochester, "Infant Mortality as an Economic Problem," in *Proceedings of the Forty-Sixth Annual Conference*, pp. 197–202. After carefully laying out evidence supporting the conclusion that many "babies are sacrificed to the family's inability to purchase for the mother the rest and care and trained advice and supervision necessary for her own safety and the vigor of her children," Rochester, who was the author of the Children's Bureau's Baltimore study, backpeddled when asked whether the bureau was in favor of maternal wage compensation and other cash subsidies, noting that it had never specifically recommended that such compensation and subsidies be paid when fathers were present and able to work.

51. Julia Lathrop, quoted in Molly Ladd-Taylor, ed., *Raising a Baby the Government Way: Mothers' Letters to the Children's Bureau, 1915–1932* (New Brunswick, N.J.: Rutgers University Press, 1986), p. 21.

52. Bureau analysts seemed particularly fond of pointing out that, despite relatively similar socioeconomic conditions in the two countries, infant mortality in Australia, which relied on cash benefit payments to new mothers, was considerably higher than it was in New Zealand, which did not give cash benefits but did have a nationwide system of instructional and supervisory maternity and infancy centers. See for instance, Children's

Bureau, *Maternity Benefit Systems,* pp. 17–20, 149–52; Children's Bureau, *Children's Year,* pp. 14–15; Woodbury, *Infant Mortality and Its Causes,* pp. 178–79.

53. In particular Lathrop and her bureau had a bitter enemy in Samuel Winslow, the powerful chairman of the House Committee on Interstate and Foreign Commerce. An ardent antifeminist and antisocialist, Winslow considered Lathrop and her bureau a dire threat to fundamental American institutions and worked tirelessly in opposition.

54. U.S. Department of Labor, Children's Bureau, *Children's Year: A Brief Summary of Work Done and Suggestions for Follow-Up Work* (Washington, D.C.:Government Printing Office, 1920), p. 15.

55. Julia Lathrop, "Letter of Transmittal," in U.S. Department of Labor, Children's Bureau, *New Zealand Society for the Health of Women and Children: An Example of Methods of Baby-Saving Work in Small Towns and Rural Districts* (Washington, D.C.: Government Printing Office, 1914), p. 3. For an analysis of New Zealand's influence on American Progressive reform, see Peter J. Coleman, *Progressivism and the World of Reform: New Zealand and the Origins of the American Welfare State* (Lawrence: University of Kansas Press, 1987).

56. Children's Bureau, *New Zealand Society for the Health of Women and Children,* pp. 9–14; Woodbury, *Infant Mortality and Its Causes,* pp. 153–79.

57. It was also an issue in England. Yet the English response was not to deny such payments but to make them the legal property of the mother, thereby offering some assurance that they would be used for that which they were intended.

58. The tendency during the last two decades among historians and other analysts of the evolution of American health care policy to focus on the Progressive era rejection of sickness insurance as the critical turning point has received much-needed counter balance in the recent writings of Daniel M. Fox. See especially his *Health Policies, Health Politics: The British and American Experience, 1911–1965* (Princeton: Princeton University Press, 1986).

59. Starr, *The Transformation of American Medicine,* p. 287, passim.

60. The reasons behind the waning of the reformist impulse in medicine are complex. Some scholars have argued that it followed from changes in medical education and an abdication of leadership by medical academics. Others have suggested it resulted from a rank-and-file takeover of the profession. And yet others have suggested that it was primarily due to the increasing economic well-being of American physicians. For a review of the arguments, see Numbers, *Almost Persuaded,* pp. 110–14.

61. For a discussion of medicine's continuing commitment to social reform, see Lloyd C. Taylor, Jr., *The Medical Profession and Social Reform* (New York: St. Martin's, 1974), pp. 103–62.

62. For a good illustration of the extent to which the political power of the AMA currently dwarfs that of progressive medical organizations, see Shari I. David, *With Dignity: The Search for Medicare and Medicaid* (Westport, Conn.: Greenwood, 1985), pp. 11–12, 42, 56–57, 103–4, and passim.

63. On the history of the AMA see James G. Burrow, *AMA: Voice of American Medicine* (Baltimore: Johns Hopkins Press, 1963); idem, *Organized Medicine in the Progressive Era: The Move Toward Monopoly* (Baltimore: Johns Hopkins University Press, 1977); and Morris Fishbein, *History of the American Medical Association, 1847–1947* (Philadelphia: Saunders, 1947).

64. Roy Lubove, *The Struggle for Social Security, 1900–1935* (Cambridge: Harvard University Press, 1968), pp. 89–90.

8. Defeat in Victory, Victory in Defeat:
The Sheppard-Towner Act

1. S. Josephine Baker, *Fighting for Life* (New York: Macmillan, 1939), p. 165.

2. U.S. Department of Labor, Children's Bureau, *Children's Year: A Brief Summary of Work Done and Suggestions for Follow-up Work* (Washington, D.C.: Government Printing Office, 1920), pp. 5, 13–15.

3. It is a mark of the continuing fluidity of age conceptions that the child aged one to two was caught in something of a borderland between infancy and early childhood.

4. Robert M. Tank, "Young Children, Families and Society in America During the 1920s: The Evolution of Health, Education and Child Care Programs for Preschool Children (Ph.D. diss., University of Michigan, 1980), pp. 164–82; John Duffy, "School Building and the Health of the American School Child in the Nineteenth Century," in *Healing and History: Essays for George Rosen,* ed. Charles E. Rosenberg (New York: Science History Publications, 1979), pp. 161–78.

5. Philip Van Ingen, *The Story of the American Child Health Association* (New York: American Child Health Association, 1936), p. 9; Mrs. William Palmer Lucas and J. H. Mason Knox, Jr., "The Work of the Children's Bureau of the American Red Cross in France," *Transactions of the American Association for Study and Prevention of Infant Mortality, 1918* (Baltimore: AASPIM, 1919), pp. 33–44.

6. S. Josephine Baker, "Lessons from the Draft," *Transactions of the American Association for Study and Prevention of Infant Mortality, 1918,* pp. 181–88; Albert G. Love and Charles B. Davenport, "Defects Found in Drafted Men," *Scientific Monthly* 10 (1920): 5–25; Van Ingen, *The Story of the American Child Health Association,* p. 10. In 1923 the American Child Hygiene Association combined with the Child Health Organization and became the American Child Health Association. It kept that name until it disbanded in 1935.

7. For an analysis of attitudes toward death in child-bed before the twentieth century, see Richard W. and Dorothy C. Wertz, *Lying-In: A History of Childbirth in America* (New York: Schoeken, 1979), pp. 1–28; and Judith Walzer Leavitt, "Under the Shadow of Maternity: Women's Responses to Death and Debility Fears in Nineteenth-Century Childbirth," *Feminist Studies* 12 (1986): 129–54.

8. U.S. Department of Labor, Children's Bureau, *Maternal Mortality from All Conditions Connected with Childbirth in the United States and Certain Other Countries,* by Grace L. Meigs (Washington, D.C.: Government Printing Office, 1917), p. 9.

9. Ibid., pp. 14–20, 22–23.

10. Ibid., p. 24.

11. According to the Census Bureau records, puerperal septicemia accounted for 5,211 and eclampsia for 3,409 of the 12,528 puerperal deaths that occurred in the birth registration area in 1917.

12. Children's Bureau, *Maternal Mortality,* p. 10.

13. Indeed, Williams enjoyed a great deal of respect and influence with the bureau. Not only were his opinions constantly quoted in bureau publications, but he also played a leading part in a number of bureau sponsored conferences. Moreover, that respect and influence was to a great extent justified, for in most ways Williams was at the socially progressive edge of the medical profession. While committed to reforming obstetrics from within and uneasy with the idea of "socialized medicine," he was also convinced that government must take responsibility for providing medical services both to indigent women and to those who lived in geographic areas where private practitioners and hospitals were few and far between. See, for instance, J. Whitridge Williams, "Standard Requirements for Obstetrical Care," in U.S. Department of Labor, Children's Bureau,

Standards of Child Welfare (Washington, D.C.: Government Printing Office, 1919), pp. 145–48.

14. In addition to the respect that the bureau had for Williams and other medical progressives, its emphasis on the medical causes of maternal mortality can also be explained, in part, by the orientation of some influential staff members. Meigs, for instance, was a trained physician and thus inclined to look first to medical solutions.

15. Children's Bureau, *Maternal Mortality*, p. 24.

16. Ibid., p. 25.

17. U.S. Department of Labor, Children's Bureau, *Minimum Standards for Child Welfare* (Washington, D.C.: Government Printing Office, 1919), p. 6.

18. Idem, *Maternity and Infant Care in a Rural County in Kansas,* by Elizabeth Moore (Washington, D.C.: Government Printing Office, 1917); idem, *Maternity Care and the Welfare of Young Children in a Homesteading County in Montana,* by Viola I. Paradise (Washington, D.C.: Government Printing Office, 1919); idem, *Maternity and Infant Care in Two Rural Counties in Wisconsin,* by Florence Brown Sherbon and Elizabeth Moore (Washington, D.C.: Government Printing Office, 1919). Particularly influential in getting the bureau and other infant and maternal welfare organizations to expand the focus of their concern to include rural America was Dr. Frances Sage Bradley. Appointed in 1915 by Lathrop as a special agent to investigate rural infant health, Bradley worked tirelessly to explode the myth that country babies and their mothers enjoyed good health because they lived closer to nature. See for instance: U.S. Department of Labor, Children's Bureau, *Rural Children in Selected Counties of North Carolina,* by Frances Sage Bradley and Margaretta A. Williamson (Washington, D.C.: Government Printing Office, 1918); and her "Save the Country Baby," *Survey* 51 (1923): 321–30.

19. Children's Bureau, *Maternal Mortality*, p. 26.

20. Walter I. Trattner, *From Poor Law to Welfare State: A History of Social Welfare in America,* 2d ed. (New York: Free Press, 1979), p. 182; Joseph B. Chepaitis, "The First Federal Social Welfare Measure: The Sheppard-Towner Maternity and Infancy Act, 1918–1932" (Ph.D. diss., Georgetown University, 1968), p. 17.

21. U.S. Department of Labor, Children's Bureau, *The Promotion of the Welfare and Hygiene of Maternity and Infancy, 1927* (Washington, D.C.: Government Printing Office, 1928), p. 6.

22. U.S. Congress, House Committee on Labor, *A Bill to Encourage Instruction in the Hygiene of Maternity and Infancy and to Extend Proper Care for Maternity and Infancy, Hearings Before the Committee on Labor on H. R. 12634,* 65th Cong., 3rd sess., 1919, pp. 5–28.

23. J. Stanley Lemons, *The Woman Citizen: Social Feminism in the 1920s* (Urbana: University of Illinois Press, 1973), p. 154.

24. Chepaitis, "The First Federal Social Welfare Measure," pp. 33–34; Lemons, *Woman Citizen,* pp. 155–56.

25. Lemons, *Woman Citizen,* p. 160; U.S. Congress, House Committee on Interstate and Foreign Commerce, *A Bill for the Public Protection of Maternity and Infancy, Hearings Before the Committee on Interstate and Foreign Commerce on HR 2366,* 67th Cong., 1st sess., 1921, pp. 100, 115–16 (hereafter cited as, CIFC, *Hearings,* 67th Cong.).

26. CIFC *Hearings,* 67th Cong., pp. 9–13, 266–67; *Congressional Record,* 67th Cong., 1st sess., 1921, 61, pt. 5: 7932–33; Chepaitis, "The First Federal Social Welfare Measure," p. 158; Sheila M. Rothman, "'Women's Clinics or Doctors' Offices': The Sheppard-Towner Act and the Promotion of Preventive Health Care," in *Social History and Social Policy,* ed. David J. Rothman and Stanton Wheeler (New York: Academic Press, 1981), pp. 179–80.

27. CIFC, *Hearings*, 67th Cong., p. 68; Mary Kilbreth quoted in Lemons, *Woman Citizen*, p. 160.

28. *Congressional Record*, 67th Cong., 1st sess., 1921, 61, pt. 9: 8764.

29. Ibid., p. 8765.

30. Ibid., pp. 8759–60. Reed's charges were not only misogynistically slanderous, but also inaccurate. Although, like many social welfare agencies, the bureau was staffed by a large number of young single women, it also had staffers whose "maternal credentials" were beyond question. Mary Mills (Mrs. Max B.) West, for instance, was the widowed mother of five children. Similarly, Dorothy Reed Mendenhall, the bureau's medical officer from 1917 to 1936, was a mother who had lost two children in infancy and who herself suffered from puerperal septicemia as a result of a clumsy and botched delivery by a male physician.

31. *Transactions of the American Child Hygiene Association, 1920*, (Baltimore: ACHA, 1921), pp. 17–18; R. L. Duffus and L. Emmett Holt, Jr., *L. Emmett Holt: Pioneer of a Children's Century* (New York: Appleton-Century, 1940), pp. 214–31; U.S. Department of Labor, Children's Bureau, *Minimum Standards for Child Welfare* (Washington, D.C.: Government Printing Office, 1920), pp. 6–7; Lemons, *Woman Citizen*, p. 165; CIFC, *Hearings*, 67th Cong., p. 58.

32. Quoted in Lemons, *Woman Citizen*, p. 155.

33. Charles A. Selden, "The Most Powerful Lobby in Washington," *Ladies Home Journal* 39 (April 1922): 5, 93–96.

34. Florence Kelley, "My Philadelphia," *Survey* 55 (1926): 50.

35. Lemons, *Woman Citizen*, pp. 165–66, 177–78, n. 2.

36. Herod Is Not Dead," *Good Housekeeping* 71 (December 1920): 4; Anne Martin, "We Couldn't Afford a Doctor," ibid. 70 (April 1920): 19–20; Anne S. Monroe, "Adventuring in Motherhood," ibid. (May 1920): 28–29; Mary S. Boyd, "Let's Stop, Now, the Casualties of Motherhood," ibid. 71 (December 1920): 43.

37. Selden, "The Most Powerful Lobby in Washington," pp. 5, 95.

38. Chepaitis, "The First Federal Social Welfare Measure," pp. 66, 73.

39. The prohibition against federal agents violating the home was a verbatim copy of that contained in the bill establishing the Children's Bureau. It would also be incorporated, again verbatim, into the 1935 Social Security Act.

40. "Appendix A—Text of the Act for the Promotion of the Welfare and Hygiene of Maternity and Infancy," in U.S. Department of Labor, Children's Bureau, *The Promotion of the Welfare and Hygiene of Maternity and Infancy, 1923* (Washington, D.C.: Government Printing Office, 1924), p. 37.

41. U.S. Department of Labor, Children's Bureau, *The Promotion of the Welfare and Hygiene of Maternity and Infancy, 1922*, (Washington, D.C.: Government Printing Office, 1923), pp. 35–37.

42. "Text of the Act," pp. 37–38.

43. Chepaitis, "The First Federal Social Welfare Measure," pp. 161–64; Lemons, *Woman Citizen*, pp. 169–72.

44. U.S. Department of Labor, Children's Bureau, *The Promotion of the Welfare and Hygiene of Maternity and Infancy, 1925* (Washington, D.C.: Government Printing Office, 1926), p. 19.

45. Idem, *The Promotion of the Welfare and Hygiene of Maternity and Infancy, 1926* (Washington, D.C.: Government Printing Office, 1927), pp. 5–10.

46. Ibid., p. 10.

47. U.S. Senate, *Maternity and Infancy Act: Letters and Extracts from Letters Commending the Maternity and Infancy Act*, S. Doc. 120, 69th Cong., 1st sess., 1926, pp. 1, 5–6.

48. Children's Bureau, *The Promotion of the Welfare of and Hygiene of Maternity and*

Infancy, 1926, p. 6. The same or similar statement was contained in all the other annual reports.

49. Ibid., p. 11.

50. Perhaps more than any other single goal, prohibiting child labor was at the center of Progressive child welfare reform. Beginning in the 1880s, Progressives began lobbying for and achieving passage of state laws establishing a minimum age for entry into the labor force and regulating the types of labor children could legally do. Such laws, however, were uneven in their stringency and enforcement. As a consequence, beginning in 1906, reformers made a number of efforts to get federal legislation enacted which would standardize child labor regulations. In 1916 they succeeded with the passage of the Keating-Owen Act. However, in 1918 the U.S. Supreme Court declared the Act unconstitutional, thus compelling child labor reformers to work for a constitutional amendment. In 1924 that amendment (the twentieth) passed both houses of Congress and was sent to the states for ratification, where after some initial success, it encountered widespread opposition. By 1926 it was clear to all that, at least for the time being, the amendment was not going to be ratified. For a specific account of the rise and fall of the amendment, see Richard B. Sherman, "The Rejection of the Child Labor Amendment," *Mid-America* 45 (1963): 3–17.

51. Central to the Republican effort to reduce what they saw as war-inflated government spending was the goal of reducing federal income. With the Revenue Act, which cut income and inheritance taxes as well as abolished many wartime surtaxes, they achieved this goal.

52. On the historical opposition of Catholics (and Jews) to "nonsectarian" welfare activities aimed at dependent children, see Richard A. Meckel, "Protecting the Innocents: Age Segregation and the Early Child Welfare Movement," *Social Service Review* 59 (1985); 455–75.

53. Lemons, *Woman Citizen,* p. 173; Barbara Gutmann Rosenkrantz, *Public Health and the State: Changing Views in Massachusetts, 1842–1936* (Cambridge: Harvard University Press, 1974), p. 156; U.S. Congress, House Committee on Interstate and Foreign Commerce, *On the Extension of Public Protection of Maternity and Infancy, Hearings Before the Committee on Interstate and Foreign Commerce on H.R. 7555,* 69th Cong., 1st sess., 1926, pp. 21–24.

54. "Federal Care of Maternity and Infancy: The Sheppard-Towner Bill," *Journal of the American Medical Association* 76 (1921): 383.

55. Lemons, *Woman Citizen,* p. 164; Rothman, "Women's Clinics or Doctors' Offices," p. 180.

56. Quoted in Numbers, *Almost Persuaded,* pp. 107–8.

57. "Minutes of the Seventy-Third Annual Session of the American Medical Association, Held at St. Louis, May 22–26, 1922," *Journal of the American Medical Association* 78 (1922): 1715.

58. Thomas E. Cone, Jr., *History of American Pediatrics* (Boston: Little, Brown, 1979), p. 203.

59. Charles E. Rosenberg, "Social Class and Medical Care in Nineteenth-Century America: The Rise and Fall of the Dispensary," *Journal of the History of Medicine and Allied Sciences* 29 (1974): 48–51; Rothman, "Women's Clinics or Doctors' Offices," p. 181.

60. Rothman, "Women's Clinics or Doctors' Offices," pp. 187–88.

61. Ibid., pp. 188, 190.

62. Children's Bureau, *The Promotion of the Welfare and Hygiene of Maternity and Infancy, 1926,* pp. 6, 11, passim.

63. These were Senators King (Utah), Reed (Missouri), Wadsworth (New York), Bin-

gham (Connecticut), Broussard (Louisiana), Bayard (Delaware), and Phipps (Colorado). "The Common Welfare," *Survey* 57 (1927): 623.

64. Lemons, *Woman Citizen*, pp. 172–73.

65. Hoover's failure to push for reviving Sheppard-Towner was a bitter disappointment for many in infant and maternal welfare because they considered him one of their own—and with good reason. From the time he was selected to run the World War I Relief Administration Children's Fund, he had been actively involved in infant, child, and maternal welfare. Indeed, in 1921 he had been elected president of the American Child Hygiene Association.

66. In 1928 Representatives John G. Cooper and Walter H. Newton and Senator Wesley L. Jones each introduced bills that would allow for the continuation of funding for Sheppard-Towner programs. None of the bills, however, generated enough congressional support to be enacted into law.

Epilogue. Progress along a Narrow and Bumpy Path: Infant and Maternal Welfare after Sheppard-Towner

1. "Child Parley Split over Bureau Shift," *New York Times*, November 21, 1930, p. 1.

2. Arthur J. Altmeyer, *The Formative Years of the Social Security Act* (Madison: University of Wisconsin Press, 1962), pp. 6–8; Paul Starr, *The Social Transformation of American Medicine* (New York: Basic Books, 1982), pp. 266–70.

3. U.S. Department of Labor, Children's Bureau, *Grants to the States for Maternal and Child Welfare Under the Social Security Act of 1935 and the Social Security Act Amendments of 1939* (Washington, D.C.: Government Printing Office, 1940), pp. 1–5.

4. Idem, *Maternal and Child Health Services Under the Social Security Act: Development of Program, 1936–39* (Washington, D.C.: Government Printing Office, 1941), pp. 1–3.

5. Children's Bureau, *Maternal and Child Health Services Under the Social Security Act*, pp. 12–14.

6. After interviewing those in the Children's Bureau responsible for administering the program, the AMA's Committee on Legislative Activities reported in 1915: "The gentlemen with whom we talked are physicians of years experience in private practice and give evidence of a sympathetic point of view in considering the medical profession in the administration of this activity. They pointed out that the wording of the Social Security Act and the instructions of their superiors is to the effect that the medical profession shall under all circumstances be consulted, their wishes respected and their cooperation sought." At the same time, however, the committee advised that continued vigilance was necessary, noting that: "The wrong plan, however, based on a few unsound principles, could easily prove to be an opening wedge for further inroads on the private practice of medicine which would be difficult to stop." *Journal of the American Medical Association* 106 (1936): 1915.

7. One of the most influential of the many Depression-era sociomedical analyses expressing alarm over rising medical costs was *Medical Care for the American People*, published in 1932. The final majority report of the prestigious Committee on the Costs of Medical Care, set up in 1927, it recommended among other things the founding of cooperative, nonprofit community health centers to provide quality low-cost medical care. For a discussion of the CCMC's recommendations and the AMA's response to them, see Lloyd C. Taylor, Jr., *The Medical Profession and Social Reform, 1885–1945* (New York: St. Martin's, 1974), pp. 121–27.

8. Roy Lubove, "The New Deal and National Health," *Current History* 45 (1963): 77–86.

9. Specifically, the conference called on Congress "to authorize a larger sum to be

appropriated annually to the States for maternal and child health services with provision that the increased payments to the States should be used for the improvement of maternal care and care of newborn infants." U.S. Department of Labor, Children's Bureau, *Proceedings of the Conference on Better Care for Mothers and Babies: Held in Washington, D.C., January 17–18, 1928* (Washington, D.C.: Government Printing Office, 1938), p. 136.

10. U.S. Interdepartmental Committee to Coordinate Health and Welfare Activities, *The Need for a National Health Program* (Washington, D.C.: Government Printing Office, 1938), pp. 5–9. The ICCHWA was created by Roosevelt in 1935 and was comprised of representatives from the Social Security Board and the Departments of Interior, Agriculture, and Labor.

11. In July 1938 the ICCHWA called a National Health Conference at which it was recommended that Title V of the Social Security Act be amended to authorize an increased appropriation for matching grants to states to enable them to provide "facilities for care in two general areas: (a) Medical and nursing care of mothers throughout the period of maternity and of their newborn infants throughout the neonatal period, and (b) health supervision and medical care of children." It was estimated that the cost of providing such care would be $95 million. "Recommendation I: Expansion of Public Health and Child Welfare Services Submitted to the Conference by the Technical Committee on Medical Care," *Proceedings of the National Health Conference, July 18, 19, 20, 1938, Washington, D.C.* (Washington, D.C.: Government Printing Office, 1938), pp. 41–42.

12. U.S. Congress, Senate Subcommittee of the Committee of Education and Labor, *To Establish a National Health Program, Hearings on S. 1620*, 76th Cong., 1st. sess., 1939, pp. 1–2.

13. "Executive Session, House of Delegates, Minutes of the Nineteenth Annual Session of the American Medical Association, Held at St. Louis, May 15–19, 1939," *Journal of the American Medical Association* 112 (1939): 2296–97; Starr, *The Social Transformation of American Medicine*, p. 277. See also Daniel S. Hirshfield, *The Lost Reform: The Campaign for Compulsory Health Insurance in the United States, 1932–1943* (Cambridge: Harvard University Press, 1970), pp. 120–30.

14. On the Beveridge Committee report and the establishment of England's National Health Service, see A. J. Willocks, *The Creation of the National Health Service* (London: Routledge, Kegan Paul, 1967); Brian Watkin, *The National Health Service: The First Phase* (London: George Allen and Unwin, 1978); and Daniel M. Fox, *Health Policies, Health Politics: The British and American Experience, 1911–1965* (Princeton: Princeton University Press, 1986), pp. 104–14, 132–48.

15. On the Wagner-Murray-Dingell bills and on Truman's proposal for a national health program, see Monty M. Poen, *Harry S. Truman Versus the Medical Lobby: The Genesis of Medicare* (Columbia: University of Missouri Press, 1979). On EMIC and the Pepper bill, see Taylor, *The Medical Profession and Social Reform*, pp. 152–59.

16. For an analysis of the effects of the Hospital Survey and Construction Act (known as Hill-Burton after its sponsors, Senators Lister Hill and Harold Burton), see Judith R. and Lester B. Lave, *The Hospital Construction Act: An Evaluation of the Hill-Burton Program, 1948–1973* (Washington, D.C.: American Enterprise Institute, 1974).

17. Starr, *The Social Transformation of American Medicine*, pp. 331–34; Sam Shapiro, Edward R. Schlesinger, and Robert E. L. Nesbitt, Jr., *Infant, Perinatal, Maternal, and Childhood Mortality in the United States* (Cambridge: Harvard University Press, 1968), p. 268.

18. This is not to suggest that there were not serious problems with the orientation and emphasis of such care. Because government assistance emphasized facility construction and because most private health insurance plans paid only for in-patient care, preventive care, in general, and prenatal care, in particular, tended to get slighted. The result was a

medical care system oriented towards correcting problems after they occurred, rather than preventing them.

19. Barbara J. Nelson, *Making an Issue of Child Abuse: Political Agenda Setting for Social Problems* (Chicago: University of Chicago Press, 1984), p. 37.

20. In 1963 responsibility for researching child and maternal health issues was vested in the newly created National Institute of Child Health and Human Development. In 1969 administration of child and maternal health and crippled children's programs was given to the Public Health Service, thus effecting a transfer that opponents of the Children's Bureau had been advocating for close to half a century.

21. Those nations and their 1950 infant mortality rates were: Australia (24.5), Canada (41.5), Denmark (30.7), England and Wales (29.9), Finland (43.5), the Netherlands (26.7), New Zealand (22.7), Norway (28.2), Sweden (21.0), Switzerland (31.2), United States (29.2). Shapiro et al., *Infant, Perinatal, Maternal, and Childhood Mortality*, p. 116.

22. Ibid. In 1950 Canada, Denmark, England and Wales, Finland, and Switzerland had higher infant mortality rates than the United States. In 1960 only Canada did.

23. See, for example, I. M. Moriyama, "Recent Change in Infant Mortality Trend," *Public Health Reports* 75 (1960): 391–405; E. P. Hunt and A. D. Chenoweth, "Recent Trends in Infant Mortality in the United States," *American Journal of Public Health* 51 (1961): 190–207; E. Oppenheimer, "Population Changes in Perinatal Mortality," ibid., 208–16; I.S. Shapiro and I. M. Moriyama, "International Trends in Infant Mortality and Their Implication for the United States," *American Journal of Public Health* 53 (1963): 747–60; U.S. Department of Health, Education, and Welfare, Children's Bureau, *Trends in Infant and Childhood Mortality, 1961*, by E. P. Hunt and S. M. Goldstein (Washington, D.C.: Government Printing Office, 1964).

24. See, for instance, "Infant Mortality," *Scientific American* 203 (July 1960): 81–82; "Too Many Babies Die," *Ladies' Home Journal* 78 (May 1961): 41; "We Can Save More Babies," *Saturday Evening Post* 235 (February 3, 1962): 43–47; "Infant Mortality: No Change; U.S. Death Rate, *Time* 82 (September 6, 1963): 48; Lawrence Engel, "We Could Save 40,000 Babies a Year," *New York Times Magazine*, November 17, 1963, p. 31.

25. John F. Kennedy, "Special Message to the Congress on Health and Hospital Care, February 9, 1961," *Public Papers of the Presidents of the United States, John F. Kennedy, 1961* (Washington, D.C., 1962), p. 86.

26. Wilbur J. Cohen and Charles E. Hawkins, "The Maternal and Mental Retardation Planning Amendments, 1963," *Welfare in Review* (November 1963): 16–21; "New Institute to Study Childhood," *Science Newsletter* 84 (August 10, 1963): 329.

27. For a discussion of the history and effect of NICUs, see Thomas E. Cone, Jr., *A History of the Care and Feeding of the Premature Infant* (Boston: Little, Brown, 1985), pp. 179–82.

28. Shapiro et al., *Infant, Perinatal, Maternal, and Childhood Mortality*, pp. 136–37; Sar A. Levitan and Robert Taggart, *The Promise of Greatness* (Cambridge: Harvard University Press, 1976), p. 82.

29. In New York City from 1961–63, infant mortality in white families where the fathers were service-workers and laborers was 18.7, or 53.3 percent higher than in white families where fathers were managers or professionals. For black families the respective rates were 28.7 and 18.0. Nationally, infant and neonatal mortality among whites in 1959–61 was 22.8 and 17.1. Among nonwhites the respective rates were 42.5 and 26.6. Shapiro et al., *Infant, Perinatal, Maternal, and Childhood Mortality*, pp. 76, 79–82. See also Jean E. Bedger, Abraham Gilperin, and Eveline E. Jacobs, "Socioeconomic Characteristics in Relation to Maternal and Child Health," in *Poverty and Health in the United States* (New York: Medical and Health Research Association, 1962), pp. 829–33.

30. Between 1953 and 1963, hospital costs nearly doubled and the average cost of

confinement increased from $193 to $316. This increase was considerably higher than increases in family income at the lower end of the economic ladder during that decade. Shapiro et al., *Infant, Perinatal, Maternal, and Childhood Mortality*, pp. 266–67.

31. For a detailed if somewhat dated analysis of the different levels of care provided by the private and public systems, see New York Academy of Medicine, *Infant and Maternal Care in New York City: A Study of Hospital Facilities* (New York: Columbia University Press, 1952).

32. Arthur J. Lesser, "Closing the Gaps in the Nation's Health Services for Mothers and Children," *Bulletin of the New York Academy of Medicine* 41 (1965): 1248–54; idem, "Progress in Maternal and Child Health," *Children Today* (March–April, 1972): 8–12.

33. Randall R. Bovbjerg and John Holahan, *Medicaid in the Reagan Era: Federal Policy and State Choices* (Washington, D.C.: The Urban Institute, 1982), p. 15; Starr, *The Social Transformation of American Medicine*, pp. 372–73; Karen Davis, "Achievements and Problems of Medicaid," in *The Medicaid Experience*, ed. Allen D. Spiegel (Germantown, Md.: Aspen Systems Corp., 1979), p. 350; C. Arden Miller, "Infant Mortality in the U.S.," *Scientific American* 253 (July, 1985): 31, 34–35; National Center for Health Statistics, *Vital Statistics of the United States, 1985,* vol. 2, *Mortality,* Part A, sect. 2, p. 1.

34. Sheri I. David, *With Dignity: The Search for Medicare and Medicaid* (Westport, Conn.: Greenwood, 1985), p. 148. The categorical assistance programs were AFDC (Aid to Families with Dependent Children); AB (Aid to the Blind); APTD (Aid to the Permanently and Totally Disabled); AABD (Aid to the Blind and Disabled); and OAA (Old Age Assistance). In 1974 the AB, APTD, AABD, and OAA categories were combined into a single supplemental security income (SSI) category.

35. Until 1986 the "medically needy" were defined as those with incomes no higher than 33 percent above eligibility ceilings who had medical bills of such amount as to reduce their incomes below the eligibility ceiling.

36. Stephen F. Loebs, "Medicaid—A Survey of Indicators and Issues," in *The Medicaid Experience*, pp. 5–7.

37. While nationally in 1980, for instance, 54 percent of those below the poverty line were receiving Medicaid, coverage varied tremendously from state to state. In California 97 percent were covered while in South Dakota only 23 percent were. Moreover, the rules governing eligibility varied from state to state. As late as February 1982, women pregnant with their first child were not eligible for Medicaid coverage in nineteen states. U.S. Department of Health and Human Services, Health Care Financing Administration, Office of Research and Demonstrations, *The Medicare and Medicaid Data Book, 1983* (Baltimore, 1983), pp. 78–79, 125.

38. Although the reasons for this unexpected cost are numerous, the three most often given are: (1) Medicaid has been utilized by many more people than anticipated, in part because the welfare rolls (particularly AFDC) expanded dramatically during the 1970s; (2) American medical costs in general have skyrocketed in the last few decades; (3) Medicaid has assumed the costly responsibility of nursing home care for many elderly and disabled. (Ibid., pp. 349–50.)

39. Unlike the Medicare statute, which mandated that physicians be paid their "usual and customary" fees, Medicaid allowed states to set reimbursement schedules. Hence, during the fiscal crises of the mid and late 1970s, states sought to save money by cutting reimbursement to physicians. In 1975, for instance, Massachusetts slashed Medicaid physicians' fees by 30 percent. Other states consciously declined to raise reimbursement fees in accordance with either general or medical inflation. See Bovbjerg and Holahan, *Medicaid in the Reagan Era*, pp. 49–53.

40. Bovbjerg and Holahan, *Medicaid in the Reagan Era*, pp. xvii–xx, 1–10; "Infant Death Rate: Rise Linked to Health Care Cuts," *U.S. News and World Report* (February

24, 1986): 72; Michael Robin, "A Right to the Tree of Life," *Nation* 238 (June 9, 1984): 699.

41. "Prenatal Care Is Declining Agency Finds," *New York Times*, January 1, 1984, sect. E, p. 5; "Casualties," *Scientific American* 249 (September 1983): 86. See also the Senate testimony of representatives from the Food Research and Action Center in Subcommittee on Rural Development, Oversight and Investigation, Committee on Agriculture, Nutrition, and Forestry, U.S. Senate, *Oversight on Federal Programs* (Washington, D.C.: Government Printing Office, 1983), pp. 167–82; and Food Research and Action Center, *The Widening Gap:The Incidence and Distribution of Infant Mortality and Low Birthweight in the United States, 1978–1982* (Washington, D.C.: Food Research and Action Center, 1984).

42. Stephen Budiansky, "A Measure of Failure," p. 32.

43. Since it has always been and continues to be difficult to establish exact gestational age, weight at birth evolved as an accepted alternative index of maturity. In 1935, the American Academy of Pediatrics recommended that for definitional purposes an infant should be considered premature if it weighs less than 2,500 grams at birth, regardless of what the suspected gestational age is. By the 1950s that criterion was accepted throughout the world. For a discussion of the adoption of weight as the accepted index of prematurity, see Cone, *History of the Care and Feeding of the Premature Infant*, pp. 62–63.

44. For 1973–75, 6.3 percent of all white births and 13.2 percent of black births were of babies weighing less than 2,500 grams. For 1978–80, the respective percentages were 5.8 and 12.6; for 1983–85, 5.6 and 12.5. National Center for Health Statistics, *Health, United States, 1987* (Washington, D.C.: Government Printing Office, 1988), p. 38.

45. In 1960–61 the percentage of newborn infants under 2,500 grams was 8.2 in the United States as compared with 6.6 percent in England and Wales and approximately 5 percent in the Netherlands. Shapiro et al., *Infant, Perinatal, Maternal, and Childhood Mortality*, pp. 126–29. While the U.S. percentage has dropped since then, it remains higher than other developed nations. In 1980, for instance, it was 6.8 compared with 5.1 for Switzerland, 4.0 for Sweden, 3.3 for Norway, 5.3 for New Zealand, 5.2 for Japan, 5.5 for West Germany, 6.1 for Canada, and 6.7 for England and Wales. Institute of Medicine, Division of Health Promotion and Disease Prevention, Committee to Study the Prevention of Low Birthweight, *Preventing Low Birthweight* (Washington, D.C.: National Academy Press, 1985), p. viii.

46. Cone, *History of the Care and Feeding of the Premature Infant*, p. 182.

47. In 1966 the ratio of LBW births to all births in the U.S. climbed to a peak of 8.3, before declining to 6.8 in 1983. The rate of decline for whites, however, was greater than it was for blacks. Between 1971 and 1983 the ratio of white LBW births to all white births fell from 6.6 to 5.7, a decline of 13.6 percent. During the same years the ratio for blacks fell from 13.3 to 12.6, a decline of only 5.3 percent. Both rates of decline paled next to that of neonatal infant morality, which dropped 45.8 percent between 1971 and 1982. Cone, *History of the Care and Feeding of Premature Infants*, p. 170; National Center for Health Statistics, *Vital Statistics of the United States, 1983*, vol. 1, *Natality* (Washington, D.C.: Government Printing Office, 1987), p. 65; *Preventing Low Birthweight*, pp. 1, 253; Maternal and Child Health Studies Project, *Infant and Perinatal Mortality Rates by Age and Race, United States, Each State and County, 1971–1975, 1976–1980* (Vienna, Va.: Information Science Research Institute, 1985), p. iii.

48. In calculating savings, proponents of expanded spending for prenatal care assumed that preventing LBW births would not only reduce intensive neonatal care costs but would also reduce the necessary subsequent medical costs for the significant proportion of LBW babies born with congenital problems. Ibid., p. 170; Miller, "Infant Mortality in the U.S.," p. 37; Budiansky, "A Measure of Failure," p. 35. For a good example of 1984–85 cost

benefit thinking, see "Prenatal Care and Low Birthweight: Effects on Health Care Expenditures," in *Preventing Low Birthweight,* pp. 212–37.

49. Between 1970 and 1983, American health care expenditures grew from $75 billion, or 7.4 percent of the GNP to 357.2 billion, or 10.5 percent of the GNP. National Center for Health Statistics, *Health, United States, 1986,* p. 183.

50. "Women's Health Insurance: Old Problems, New Programs," *Ms.* 15 (March, 1987): 24; interview with Jane DeChristopher, Rhode Island, Department of Health, March 29, 1989.

51. "Expanded Right to Medicaid Shatters Link to Welfare," *New York Times,* March 6, 1988, sect. 1, pp. 1, 32.

52. In Providence, Rhode Island, for example, where 97.2 percent of all women giving birth in 1985 received prenatal care (76.5 percent in the first trimester), the ratio of LBW births to total births was 8.1. This is a relatively low figure given that the city has a high percentage of those sociomedical determinants associated with LBW births: a large minority and immigrant population, a large number of residents on public assistance or living near or below the poverty line, and a high proportion of teenage and out-of-wedlock births.

Index

Abt, Isaac, 60
Adulteration: of food, 66–68; of milk, 63, 66–69
Advice manuals, 122, 149–153, 166
African-Americans: ignored by infant welfare, 142; infant mortality among, 2–3, 132, 142; and low-birthweight infants, 233
Age distinctions, 33
Aid to Families with Dependent Children (AFDC), 230–33
Akron, Ohio, 178
Alabama, 212
Alcott, William, 21
American Academy of Medicine, 108, 198; conference on infant mortality, 108–9
American Academy of Political and Social Science, 108, 134
American Association for Labor Legislation (AALL), 189–93
American Association for Study and Prevention of Infant Mortality (AASPIM), 7, 109–22, 124, 130, 158–59, 165, 171, 174–76, 194, 202, 209; criticism of, 122–23; and eugenics, 116–18; founding of, 109–10; goals and activities of, 110–16; and maternal reform, 119–22; new focus and name, 201–2. *See also* American Child Hygiene Association
American Child Hygiene Association, 114, 202, 209
American Eugenics Society, 116
American Gynecological Society, 207
American Medical Association: emergence of, 198–99; and federal infant welfare measures, 207–8, 212–17, 222, 224–25; and maternity insurance, 190–92, 199; policy on state medicine, 216; report on health of cities, 17, 19, 21, 25

American Pediatric Society, 46, 57, 82, 87
American Public Health Association, 32, 35, 62, 66, 68, 71, 76, 110, 141, 164
American Statistical Association, 41
Antenatal care. *See* Prenatal care
Appolino, Nicholas, 21, 38
Archives Pediatrics, 46
Arizona, 212–13
Arkansas, 212, 228
Asian-Americans, 142
Australia, 202
Austria, 47, 98, 188

Baby farming, 30–31
Baby parades, 148
Baby shows, 146
Baby weeks, 147–48
Baby Welfare Association, 140
Bacteria: E. coli, 42, 74; in milk, 70–74, 81–82, 85–88. *See also* Microbial contamination of milk
Baker, H. B., 33
Baker, S. Josephine, 114, 135–37, 139, 144–45, 150, 159, 175–77, 192, 200, 205–6, 215. *See also* New York City, Bureau of Child Hygiene
Ballantyne, John W., 162–63
Ballard, Edward, 170
Baltimore, 21, 63, 74, 85, 105, 112, 142, 165, 178, 184
Bartley, Elias, 81
Batchelder, John, 75
Bath (England), 19
Beecher, Catherine, 52
Belleville Hospital, 92, 138
Berlin (Germany), 72, 96, 104
Bertillon, Jacque, 94
Better baby contests, 122, 151